T0261644

HARBIN

A Cross-Cultural Biography

Harbin

A Cross-Cultural Biography

MARK GAMSA

UNIVERSITY OF TORONTO PRESS

Toronto Buffalo London

ISBN 978-1-4875-0628-5 (cloth)
ISBN 978-1-4875-3376-2 (EPUB)
ISBN 978-1-4875-3375-5 (PDF)

Library and Archives Canada Cataloguing in Publication

Title: Harbin: A cross-cultural biography / Mark Gamsa.
Names: Gamsa, Mark, 1970– author.
Description: Includes bibliographical references and index.
Identifiers: Canadiana (print) 20200307517 | Canadiana (ebook)
20200307584 | ISBN 9781487506285 (cloth) | ISBN 9781487533762 (EPUB) |
ISBN 9781487533755 (PDF)
Subjects: LCSH: Budberg, Baron Roger. | LCSH: Harbin (China) – History. |
LCSH: Harbin (China) – Ethnic relations. | LCSH: Harbin (China) –
Biography. | LCSH: Physicians – China – Harbin – Biography. | LCSH:
Russia – Relations – China. | LCSH: China – Relations – Russia.
Classification: LCC DS797.42.H373 G36 2020 | DDC 951/.84 – dc23

This book was published with the support of the Israel Science Foundation.

University of Toronto Press acknowledges the financial assistance to its
publishing program of the Canada Council for the Arts and the Ontario
Arts Council, an agency of the Government of Ontario.

Canada Council
for the Arts

Conseil des Arts
du Canada

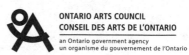

ONTARIO ARTS COUNCIL
CONSEIL DES ARTS DE L'ONTARIO

an Ontario government agency
un organisme du gouvernement de l'Ontario

Funded by the
Government
of Canada

Financé par le
gouvernement
du Canada

Canadä

For my mother

Contents

Illustrations

Armer Europäer, der verdammt ist inmitten dieser fremden Welt zu leben, dem jeder wahre Einblick in diese wunderbar entwickelte Psychologie so völlig verschlossen ist! Daß er gereizt und boshaft wird, darf ihm kaum übelgenommen werden. Wem aber von den Europäern grenzenloser Fleiß im Überwinden grenzenloser Schwierigkeiten, die nicht nur die Sprache mit sich bringt, Eintritt in diese anders denkende und empfindende Welt verschafft hat, der hört auf, seine Stammesgenossen so zu verstehen, wie diese es verlangen. Ich bitte den Leser herzlichst, mich nicht hart zu verurteilen, wenn ich gewiß hier und da ein verändertes Seelenleben an den Tag lege … Mein innigster Wunsch ist, gerecht und wahr zu sein; gerade aber diese Tugenden zeigen im Seelenleben der Menschen viele Verschiedenheiten.

Dr. med. Roger Baron Budberg, *Bilder aus der Zeit der*
Lungenpest-Epidemien in der Mandschurei 1910/11
und 1921. Hamburg: Conrad Behre, 1923, p. 74.

The poor European, condemned to live in the midst of this alien world, to whom any true insight into this wonderfully developed psychology is completely barred! It is hard to blame him for becoming irritated and spiteful. He, however, among the Europeans, to whom unbounded diligence in overcoming unbounded difficulties, which are not only brought by the language, has gained entry into this differently thinking and feeling world, ceases to understand his compatriots as they require. I ask the reader most sincerely not to judge me too severely, if indeed, here and there, I bring to light an altered life of the soul … My deepest wish is to be fair and true; however, precisely these virtues point to many differences in the lives of men's souls.

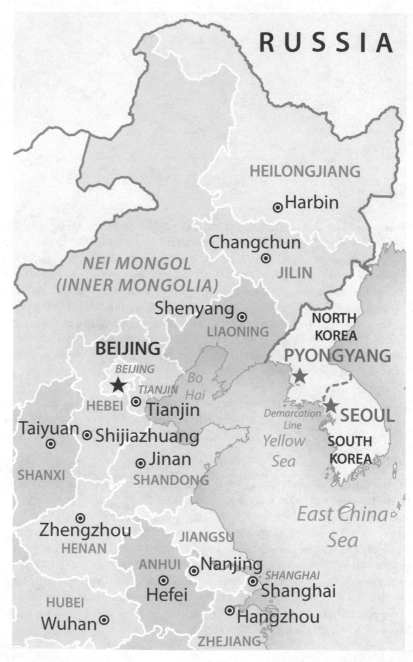

I.1. Northeast China. Adapted from the China Administrative
Map, 2011.

Introduction

The Russians, and the rest of the world, referred to northeastern China as Manchuria. But from the time the Russians started writing "Manchuria," in the mid-nineteenth century, they were unsure how to spell it, wobbling between five or six different transcriptions of this geographical name.[1] By the 1900s, the form *Man'chzhuriia* (standard in modern Russian) was the most common, having been employed, for example, in the corresponding entry in the authoritative encyclopedia *Brockhaus and Efron*.[2] So the use of *Mandzhuriia* by the writer Andrei Bely (1880–1934) in his novel *Petersburg* (written in 1913–14, set in autumn 1905) was meant to convey a message. With its *dzh* sound so exotic to the Russian ear, *Mandzhuriia* symbolized the menacing Orient, which had invaded the streets of the Russian capital, by being attached to the "Manchurian hats" of soldiers returned from the Russo-Japanese War.[3] For the Chinese, Manchuria was usually "the northeast" (Dongbei): a notion that comprised the provinces of Heilongjiang, Jilin, Fengtian (today's Liaoning), and northeastern Inner Mongolia. Japan's conquest of this region in 1932 and its creation of a puppet "Manchurian empire" has done more than anything else to delegitimize references to "Manchuria" in Chinese writing since the 1950s. If used at all as a historical term in China today, *Manzhou* is preceded by the character *wei*, meaning "fake," the standard designation of the Manchukuo state. As for the city of Harbin, which became the epicentre of Russian-Chinese relations in Manchuria (or the northeast) after the completion of the Chinese Eastern Railway (CER) in 1903, we shall see that neither the Chinese nor the Russians knew why it was called what it was.

A Survey of the Scene

Russia and Manchuria did not become close neighbours until 1860. The Treaty of Peking, concluded at the end of the Second Opium War, fixed

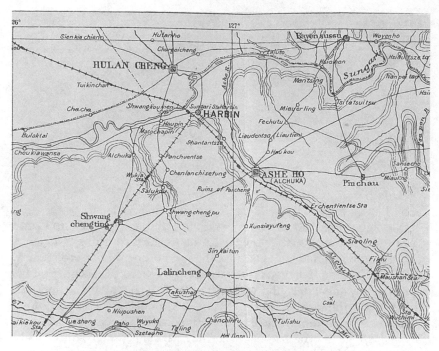

I.2. Detail from *National Geographic* map, "Kirin, Harbin, Vladivostok," 1905.

the eastern border between Russia and the Qing Empire along the Ussuri River. This completed Russia's extensive territorial gains, which the Treaty of Aigun had already brought it two years earlier, by allowing it to annex land north of the Amur River. The liberation of the serfs in Russia, proclaimed in 1861, had a long-term impact on the migration of peasants to Siberia and the Far East, which began in the 1880s. That mass population movement, which peaked around 1910, brought Russian settlers not only to the edges of the country but also beyond them, into China.

After China's defeat in the war against Japan over the domination of Korea in 1894–5, the Treaty of Shimonoseki ceded the island of Taiwan and the Liaodong Peninsula, including Port Arthur (today's Lüshunkou district of Dalian) in southern Manchuria, to Japan. Russia then joined France and Germany in pressuring Japan to return Liaodong to China. But in June 1896, Russia too exploited the weakness of the Qing dynasty by securing the signature of the senior statesman Li Hongzhang (1823–1901) on a secret treaty allowing Russia to complete its great project, the Trans-Siberian Railway, by cutting through Chinese territory.

By 1893, Russia had laid the first stretch of a railway line in its Maritime province. Work on the new Chinese Eastern Railway in Manchuria, intended to link Vladivostok to Chita, began in late August 1897. The following March, after signing another convention with China, Russia took possession of Port Arthur and began building the town of Dal'nii (later Japanese Dairen; present-day Dalian). In the early summer of 1898, the foundations of Harbin were laid. That year and the next were the peak of the scramble for concessions in China, in which Russia participated along with other European powers. In the summer of 1900 the Boxer Uprising against foreigners and Christians in China spilled over into Manchuria; this triggered Russian military occupation of the region. The scheduled evacuation of Russian forces from Manchuria was still not complete when the Japanese fleet attacked Port Arthur in February 1904.[4]

The Russo-Japanese War shook Harbin but also provided a stimulus for its growth from a newly founded town into a large city. The civilian population of Harbin stood at 12,000 in 1901 and 20,000 in 1902. By May 1903, it had reached 44,000.[5] Traffic on the CER opened in June of that year. By 1905, Harbin accommodated over a hundred thousand people.[6] As the city catered to the needs of the Manchurian Front, new commercial possibilities presented themselves and fortunes were made. The profiteering spirit born in the heady atmosphere of a wartime supply centre had not evaporated by 1906, when the defeated Russian army was finally able to leave northeastern China after a long delay caused by a strike on the Trans-Siberian Railway.

Russia's defeat led to the ceding to Japan of the southern branch of the CER: the section from Port Arthur to Changchun was run by the Japanese from then on and renamed the South Manchuria Railway (SMR). Japan's economic control of the region became a springboard for its expansion into northern China. The Chinese villages of Manchuria had been occupied and plundered by the fighting armies, and thousands of lives were lost.[7] After the war, labour migration into Manchuria resumed nonetheless. Migrants fleeing poverty and hunger in rural Shandong sought in Harbin the opportunities that work on the construction of the railway had previously provided. Most of them settled in Fujiadian, initially a Chinese shantytown named after the family Fu, which predated the foreign-dominated city by about a decade and was formally identified in Chinese as Binjiang. Today this quarter of Harbin is called Daowai, "Beyond the Tracks."

Harbin's history was strongly influenced by its function as headquarters of the CER. From Harbin, the railway line stretched almost 1,500 kilometres to the west and (after 1905) 240 kilometres south to Changchun. On both sides of the track, tsarist Russia enjoyed virtual concession powers over land defined as the CER alienation zone, a right-of-way that it had leased for ninety years under the treaty of 1896. In this zone, which included Harbin but not Fujiadian, the Russian inhabitants and their institutions were under Russian jurisdiction. The Diplomatic Bureaux of Jilin and Heilongjiang provinces, which had their main offices in Harbin, handled legal issues involving the Chinese, as well as disputes between Chinese and Russian subjects, by negotiating with Russian officials (until 1905, there was also a bureau in Mukden). Russians and Chinese officials jointly presided over "mixed courts" in Harbin, based on the example of Shanghai.[8] These arrangements continued even after the Qing dynasty fell in 1911.

Over the course of a single night in February 1913, the Russian railway administration conducted a census of the entire population of Harbin (excluding Fujiadian). It counted 68,549 people and interviewed most of them, using interpreters into Russian when necessary. Those interpreters certainly had their work cut out for them, for besides the 43,691 subjects of the Russian empire, who had no trouble understanding the questions, it emerged that the native language of more than 23,000 of Harbin's residents was Chinese. The next-largest community, the Japanese, counted only 757 people. The census established that the young city was home to as many as fifty-three nationalities, speaking no less than forty-five languages.[9] Most of Harbin's Chinese were concentrated in the quarter of town known as Pristan' (the wharf, or quay) in Russian, and as Daoli, "Within the Tracks," in Chinese. They resided in streets running parallel to the River Sungari (in Chinese: the Songhuajiang) or leading down do it. Especially in the early period, fewer Chinese were seen on Pristan's nearby main avenue, the glittering Kitaiskaia ulitsa (Chinese Street), or in the comfortable residential quarter, Novyi gorod (hereafter New Town; Chinese name: Nangang, "South Hill"). Only a few years later, the Chinese would become the ethnic majority in Harbin, though thanks to the presence of Russian schools, churches, newspapers, hospitals, and theatres, the Russian residents would continue to regard the city as essentially Russian – which will be one of the themes of this book.

In December 1917 the small Bolshevik faction in Harbin received orders from Vladimir Lenin in Petrograd to take charge of the city.[10] Harbin's Bolsheviks proceeded to arrest key officials of the tsarist administration and to demand the replacement of others. The long-serving manager of the CER, General Dmitrii L. Khorvat (1859–1937), responded by calling in Chinese troops, who entered Harbin to quash the attempted takeover. Thereafter, the CER and its headquarters in Harbin were cut off from Bolshevik Russia, while maintaining close links with the White government in Siberia. In the summer of 1919 a strike broke out on the railway, which lasted for two months. Khorvat was forced to resign in March 1920 and soon left Harbin for Peking. In a particularly heavy blow to the status of Russians in China, their extra-territorial rights were abolished in September 1920. After the regime in Moscow declared tsarist passports invalid, the Chinese authorities took the Russians in Harbin under their jurisdiction.

Harbin had once been a distant colonial outpost of Russia; after 1918, it was flooded with refugees fleeing from Russia's revolution and civil war. Their arrival caused a sharp rise in unemployment and urban crime. In the early 1920s, the Russian population in Harbin reached an all-time peak of more than 185,000 and Harbin had become one of the world centres of the Russian emigration along with cities like Berlin, Paris, Prague, Belgrade, and Sofia.[11] Many of these refugees then moved to other cities in China, re-emigrated to other countries, or returned to Soviet Russia. By 1929, Harbin was home to only about 57,000 Russians (almost equally divided between émigrés and those in possession of a Soviet passport), as against nearly a hundred thousand Chinese and fewer than six thousand persons of other nationalities.[12]

In October 1920 the Manchurian warlord Zhang Zuolin (1875–1928) turned the CER alienation zone into the Special Region of the Three Eastern Provinces, with a head office in Harbin. From his seat of power in Mukden, present-day Shenyang, he was able to maintain independence from the weak central government in Peking. In September 1924 the Soviet government and Zhang Zuolin's regime signed the Mukden Agreement, which restricted employment on the CER to subjects of the Soviet Union and China. Émigrés would lose their jobs unless they took a Soviet or Chinese passport. In October, Zhang sacked and imprisoned the émigré engineer Boris V. Ostroumov (1879–1944), Khorvat's successor as manager of the CER, an official who by all accounts had displayed mercurial energy since being appointed in April 1921.[13] This was the final move in a complex political game in which Soviet agents had approached Ostroumov and other senior figures in the émigré leadership of the CER, convincing them of the need to join forces so as to prevent a Chinese takeover of the railway.[14] Harbin's special status as a mixed city, strengthened by the presence of foreign consulates, enabled a Russian-dominated municipal council to function until 1926. Its replacement by a new council, on which Chinese held forty of fifty seats,[15] marked the definitive end of Russian authority in Harbin, which dated back to 1898.

In 1928, the political situation in Manchuria changed again after Zhang Zuolin was assassinated by his former Japanese sponsors. His

son and successor Zhang Xueliang (1901–2001) raided the Soviet Consulate in Harbin in May 1929 in an attempt to take control of the railway. The Soviet Union responded by invading northern Manchuria.
Soviet troops, who crossed over from the bordering Transbaikal province, massacred rural settlements of Cossacks and Old Believers in the
Three Rivers area (Trekhrech'e; Chinese: Sanhe qu), the basin of the
tributaries of the Argun River in Inner Mongolia. About 10,000 inhabitants of the border region and of the largest town Hailar, Cossacks and
Russians, fled from these atrocities to Harbin.[16] When Zhang Xueliang
accepted defeat in December 1929, the previous arrangements regarding the railway were restored and employees with Soviet passports,
whom Zhang had fired and temporarily replaced with émigrés, were
able to resume their work with the CER.[17]

On 18 September 1931 the Japanese military staged an incident in the
vicinity of Mukden, to provide cause for the invasion of Manchuria.
Japan's Kwantung Army quickly swept through the region but did not
enter Harbin until 6 February 1932. The last emperor of the fallen Qing
dynasty, Puyi (1906–1967), was enthroned as puppet ruler of the new
state of Manchukuo, founded on 1 March.

The Japanese regime soon initiated measures to bring the Russians
under its control. A dedicated Bureau for the Affairs of Russian Emigrants in the Manchurian Empire (known by its Russian abbreviation
BREM) was established in December 1934. Russian fascists, active in
Harbin since 1925 and organized as a political party since 1931, received
the support of the Japanese authorities and were appointed to senior
positions within BREM. The bureau collected information and compiled intelligence files on every Russian in Manchukuo; meanwhile, the
Japanese imposed strict censorship on the Russian press (which now
had to refer to Japan as "Nippon"). They also ended the autonomy of
Russian schools and churches, and through the secret police engaged in
extortion, blackmail, and kidnapping for ransom.[18]

Many Russian émigrés soon left Manchukuo, moving on to Shanghai
or Tientsin (Tianjin). After the Soviet Union sold the railway to Japan in
March 1935, more than 20,000 holders of Soviet passports were repatriated collectively to Soviet Russia between April and June; those who
chose to remain behind became émigrés or allowed their Soviet papers
to lapse over the following decade.[19] Ostensibly, the Soviet Union had
arranged the return of its citizens to protect them from Japanese persecution. In reality, within two years, the returnees were accused of
spying for Japan and other foreign powers. In September 1937, Joseph
Stalin's henchman, Nikolai Ezhov, the Commissar for State Security,
issued an order for the liquidation of "Harbinites," who included all

the Russians from China.[20] That year and the next, the NKVD arrested between 42,000 and 49,000 "Harbinites" in Soviet Russia; between 28,000 and 31,000 of them were executed.[21] By 1937, fewer than 34,000 Russians were living in Harbin, still outnumbering the growing Japanese community. By this time, Harbin's Chinese outnumbered the Russians by a factor of ten.[22]

In August 1945, Soviet troops invaded Manchuria, hastening Japan's defeat in the Second World War. They entered Harbin to the cheers of their former compatriots, about 10,000 of whom, however, were soon deported to the Soviet Union, to be executed or imprisoned in Siberian labour camps.[23] Random arrests and the looting of property took place all over Manchuria as it was "liberated" by Soviet forces. Survivors of these Stalinist purges on Chinese soil counted themselves fortunate to pass under the rule of the Chinese Communist Party, who took over Harbin from the Red Army in April 1946, yet for many of them the year of Soviet control had proved decisive. In 1947 and 1948, some Harbin Russians joined the voluntary return of Russians from China, about 6,000 from the country as a whole. On arrival in Soviet Russia, they were usually arrested.

After the Communists came to power over China in 1949, the remaining Russians in Harbin were made to realize that they had overstayed their welcome. A year after Stalin's death in 1953, the Soviet Union launched a massive campaign to repatriate them. Across China, about 100,000 people repatriated to Soviet Russia between 1954 and 1960.[24] Boarding the trains of the former CER (renamed the North Manchurian Railway by the Japanese, and later the Chinese Changchun Railway by the Republic of China in 1945; the railway passed to full Chinese control in February 1950), they prepared to atone for their émigré past by settling in uncultivated parts of Siberia and Kazakhstan – the destinations assigned to them by the Soviet government. Others departed around the same time for Australia and South America. For Harbin's Jews, the founding of the State of Israel in 1948 offered another option.[25]

The severing of relations between the Soviet Union and the People's Republic of China (PRC) in 1960 made the last Russians in China the target of persistent attacks. By 1967, all but 150 Russians had left Harbin, the last departures triggered by the outbreak of the Cultural Revolution.[26] Less than a dozen elderly Russians still lived there by the end of the twentieth century. None of them are alive today. In this way the collective story of the Russian presence in Harbin, and the life stories of the individual Russians there, passed from the realm of experience into that of history.

Aims and Method

While this book is indebted to the cumulative contribution made by the large body of historical writing on Harbin and Manchuria in several languages, it takes its cue from the only sustained analysis of Russian-Chinese relations in the region so far, that incorporated into R.K.I. Quested's *"Matey" Imperialists? The Tsarist Russians in Manchuria, 1895–1917*. The publication of this monograph in 1982 opened an almost uncharted field; it also set standards that have seldom been matched in subsequent research.[27] Though she focused on international and diplomatic history, Quested also wrote about the frequent intercourse between Chinese and Russian officials and their families in the upper tiers of Harbin society, the alienation and mutual suspicion between the respective middle classes, and the tendency toward racial animosity among the lower.[28]

This study concurs that the two sides generally had little knowledge or interest in each other. However, there was another strong feature to Quested's work: a conviction that individual cases of engagement with the other side are also worth studying, both on their own account and for what they may reveal about the communities in question. This approach sees no need to construct Harbin as a site of interethnic harmony in order to justify its interest in cross-cultural relations. It allows for occasional comparison between Harbin and other locations in which interactions between Chinese and Westerners took place: certainly Shanghai, but also the border towns Kiakhta and Maimachen (Chinese: Maimaicheng), where, not wholly unlike the later situation in Harbin and Fujiadian, Russians and Chinese lived in close interdependency, isolated from metropolitan Russia and China. In the Russian Far East, by the 1890s, Vladivostok, Khabarovsk, and Blagoveshchensk also had large Chinese populations. Some aspects of Russian-Chinese relations in Harbin come into clearer perspective when we compare them with relations between Chinese and Japanese in southern Manchuria; other parallels take us out of the China framework altogether.

By "Russians" I will usually mean *Rossiiane*, the inhabitants of Harbin with roots in the Russian empire, who spoke or understood Russian. Likewise, "Chinese" refers to the broad category of *Zhongguo ren*, rather than signifying only Han Chinese people. As the first chapter will demonstrate, both the Russian and the Chinese sides encompassed many other ethnicities. Geographically, Harbin Russians remained in emigration even after taking Soviet passports, as many of them did in 1925, although in legal terms they were no longer émigrés at that point.

Moreover, the legal status of many remained undetermined for years after 1925 while their applications for Soviet citizenship were being reviewed; others switched from being Soviets to émigrés once Manchuria came under Japanese rule.

The method of inquiry will be analytical rather than chronological, but it will also be important to show how perceptions of self and other changed over time. And time flowed differently for different groups of people: by the early 1920s, some of Harbin's Russians had lived among the Chinese for about two decades, whereas for those recently arrived in the city after the revolution, China was an entirely new world. The following chapters will advance from 1898, when Harbin was founded, to the 1950s, highlighting different aspects in the history of Russian-Chinese relations in the city during that half-century. The point of departure is the first encounter between Russian and Chinese settlers in Manchuria and the first crisis they faced, the Boxer Uprising of 1900. The main objective is to show how people in Harbin – mostly, Russians and Chinese – interacted with and thought about people of different ethnic origins, languages, and religions across the entire spectrum of their common life in the city. The reciprocal images they had of one another were partly ideological: some Russians thought in terms of the "yellow peril" and their country's civilizing mission in the East; Chinese cultural isolationism was coloured by mounting nationalism. More prosaically, this book also draws a detailed picture of daily contact between people of different ethnicities. And to understand how people perceived others, it is necessary to understand how they perceived themselves.

A double-track historical biography by Alan Bullock (1914–2004), published in 1993, modernized the ancient idea of "parallel lives."[29] In the book you are reading, the parallel lives are those of a city, Harbin, and of a person, the physician Baron Roger Budberg. The scholar of Chinese art Wu Hung introduces another historiographical experiment by underscoring the tensions generated by "the juxtaposition of the two narratives."[30] The writer Grace Paley (1922–2007) puts it best: "To get the story told you have to tell two stories. The second comes rising up next to the first, or sometimes comes rising up inside it, and it's the telling of the two together that makes the story."[31]

Historians argue about the best methods to truthfully describe the past (and some non-historians will say there is no way of achieving that goal). Following the life of a person reflects the unpredictability of history as the story of the individuals who lived through it. Their present becomes "the past" for us, and while we are bound to miss much because we are not privy to the full archive of their lives and thoughts, we have the advantage of knowing more than they did about the larger frame in which they acted. Therefore, we can place their singular experience – insofar as we can understand it – in a context as broad as we may wish to extend it. One can go a step further, however, and this strategy is essayed here: by separating the narrative of an individual's life in the city from the general story, we may see better where the two intersect and where they clash. Although both are inevitably tales we tell (and all histories are tales, told in words), we may discover how knowledge gleaned from a single case challenges conclusions from an aggregate of cases, and how the particular story stretches the range of possibilities. The life story at the centre of the book's even-numbered chapters 2, 4, and 6 is not meant to be representative. Rather, it was an exception, from which nonetheless much may be learned. The odd-numbered and even-numbered chapters run as parallel strands until merging in chapter 7. The final chapter reflects on the legacy of the Russian-Chinese encounter in Harbin; the epilogue situates the general and the particular histories (the macro and the micro levels of history) in relation to each other while expanding the frame of analysis to the scale we now often refer to as global.

As I have written on Harbin before, I need to alert readers that this book replicates none of my previous publications. Those are listed in the bibliography and may be read as separate contributions on their subjects.[32] In a much altered form, parts of the book draw on my DPhil thesis at the University of Oxford, which was supervised between 1999 and 2003 by the late Professor Glen Dudbridge (1938–2017) and Professor G.S. Smith. Overall, then, this project has taken twenty years to complete. Carrying it in my mind for all this time, even when taking leave of it to do easier things, has kept me thinking about the many different ways of writing history.[33]

For the eventual outcome, I am deeply grateful to persons who honoured me by their confidence: to the late Victor Popoff (1927–2013), Baron Budberg's grandson, who graciously answered my questions and showed me his photograph albums during three memorable days of conversation at his home in Seraing, near Liège, Belgium, in summer 2005, and to his wife Marie Louise Popoff and daughter Myriam Popoff, for their warm hospitality; to Dagmar Raczynski in Chile and all the members of the Raczynski family, whom I met in Riga in 2012, for allowing me to read and use the unpublished correspondence and memoirs, without which this book would have been so much the poorer; and to Ute and Michael Köhler in Germany for sending me additional photographs. I could not have done without the support of family and friends, the encouragement and advice of the late Rosemary

Quested (1923–2012), the generous help of Olga Bakich in Toronto, Ji Fenghui and Dan Ben-Canaan in Harbin, Georgijs Dunajevs and Frank Kraushaar in Riga, Toomas Hiio in Tartu, and Pavel Ratmanov in Khabarovsk. After some false detours in the search for a publisher, my friendship with Olga Bakich led me to the University of Toronto Press, where I found the perfect editor in Stephen Shapiro. I acknowledge the diligent work of my research assistant in Tel Aviv, Sergey Bronshtein, and grants from the Israel Science Foundation and the Chiang Ching-kuo Foundation for International Scholarly Exchange.

Being a study of a frontier region, this book is situated at the margins of what is usually understood as Russian and Chinese history. In order to make the work accessible to a broader audience, some concepts and events that will be familiar to specialists have been explained. In the bibliography, titles of sources in Russian and Chinese are translated into English. Dates usually follow the Gregorian calendar, indicating O.S. (Old Style) whenever sources refer to the Julian calendar, which lagged twelve days behind the former in the nineteenth century and thirteen days in the twentieth, until the adoption of the Gregorian system in Russia on (a day that for the rest of the world was) 14 February 1918. As in this introduction, endnote references to sources that are included in the bibliography will be given in abridged form and a full citation used only for sources of lesser relevance to the book's subject, which the bibliography omits. Translations are my own throughout, unless indicated otherwise, while transcriptions from Chinese follow the Hanyu pinyin system and those from Russian the modified Library of Congress system. Chinese place names such as Peking and Tientsin, however, are spelled here in that way for the period before the establishment of the People's Republic of China, whereas Harbin is spelled so everywhere except in transcriptions from Chinese, where it becomes Ha'erbin, and from Russian, where it becomes Kharbin.

1

Of Ethnicity and Identity

At the end of the nineteenth century and the beginning of the twentieth, populations of various ethnic and geographical origins met in Manchuria. These were more than simply Russian colonists, on one side, and colonized Chinese, on the other. It is imperative to recognize the presence of many other actors on the scene as well as the diversity within each of the main parties to the encounter. Let us begin with a sketch of Manchuria as the Russians found it.

Manchuria before Harbin

The Manchus and Qing Policy

From the inception of the Manchu dynasty's rule over China in 1644 to its demise in 1911, Manchuria was the locus of contending and often opposing perceptions. The Qing emperors saw it as the sacred ancestral land of the Manchu people. Roots-finding missions had been sent to the Changbai Mountains in what is now Jilin province since the days of the Kangxi emperor, who reigned from 1662 to 1722. His grandson, the Qianlong emperor, who ruled China for six decades as well, from 1736 to 1795, celebrated the Qing's myth of origins in a Manchu poem, "Ode to Mukden," dedicated to the city then known in Chinese as Shengjing and now as Shenyang.[1] Beginning from Kangxi in 1668, Qing emperors attempted to block Han Chinese settlement in Manchuria to prevent the spread of Han influence in the land from which China had been conquered.

Maintaining strict control over valuable resources in Manchuria, including the ginseng root, used in Chinese medicine, and freshwater pearls, was also economically important.[2] Additional considerations behind the settlement ban were the need to maintain a buffer zone along China's borders with Russia and Korea and, possibly, to preserve a bolt-hole in the event that the Qing fell from power in Peking. Manchu identification with Manchuria weakened over the Qing's long rule, yet the court did not open the region to Han Chinese settlement until 1878.[3] The official ban, nominally in force for two centuries, had never been effective; the Chinese population of Manchuria was steadily rising.[4] Nonetheless, the removal of the ban led to an increase in Chinese migration, for it was accompanied by a new policy of encouraging settlement in approved areas through land grants, loans, and rewards. Not until 1908 was Manchuria administered like the rest of China within the Great Wall: the three eastern provinces were formed in 1907 and 1908, and the military administration was replaced by a civilian one. This late acknowledgment by the Qing of the flow of migrants into Manchuria, and changes in policy so as to direct the migration process and extract revenues from it, had a parallel in tsarist Russia: the resettlement of peasants in the Asian parts of empire, Siberia and the Far East, only became state policy in the 1900s, although the independent movement of people to those regions had begun much earlier.[5]

During the time when it was maintained as an imperial reserve, Manchuria was also a place of exile. Isolation and a severe climate made it a suitable dumping ground for the Qing empire's criminals and disgraced officials, just as Siberia was for the tsars. Before the conquest of Xinjiang in the Far West was completed in the mid-eighteenth century, Heilongjiang in the extreme northeast was considered the harshest destination within the penal system.[6] However strong the Manchu rulers' sentimental ties to Manchuria were, when pushed to the wall by imperialist foreign powers, they preferred to make far-reaching concessions on the periphery rather than yield to foreigners a smaller foothold in China proper. Accordingly, by the treaties of Aigun in 1858 and Peking in 1860, the Qing agreed to Russian annexation of about 932,400 square kilometres north of the Amur River and east of the Ussuri. These lands were incorporated into Russia's newly founded Amur and Maritime (Primorye) provinces. In 1884 the Governor Generalship of the Priamur was established, comprising these two provinces and the Transbaikal. Chinese historians would later describe the territory Russia had gained from the Qing as two and a half times the size of England, or more than the combined area of Jilin and Heilongjiang.

While assertions of the Qing historical ties to the northeast served as a counterargument to Russian claims to the Amur basin, the limited Manchu presence on the ground reduced the court's special relationship with Manchuria to the realm of rhetoric. Indeed, by the seventeenth century most of the Manchu population had left Manchuria for the comforts of life in the capital, Peking, or for service in Qing garrisons around the empire. The "eight banners" system, which had been developed before the Manchus conquered China, divided the Manchu army, and the Chinese, Mongols, and others who joined it, into detachments known as banners; originally, there were four "plain" banners (yellow, white, red, and blue), to which four "bordered" ones were added. Bannermen served the Qing Empire as hereditary soldiers. Accordingly, the Russians who came across them and wrote on the subject called them "the Chinese Cossacks." Until the revolution of 1911 (final abolition of the banner system came as late as 1924), Manchus still held most administrative positions in the old Qing garrison towns.[7] Even so, by the late nineteenth century, ordinary Manchus in Manchuria represented a social group in decline. Most of them lived along the banks of the Mudan River (Mudanjiang, traditionally known as Hu'erha; a right tributary of the Sungari) and the right bank of the Sungari.[8] With little education to prepare them for another occupation, especially after Manchuria's switch to civilian administration, many bannermen became impoverished.[9] At the start of the twentieth century, facing a crisis in its former way of life, the Manchu population in Heilongjiang began to transition from military service to agriculture.[10]

Frontier Tribes

The relationship between the Manchus and the other ethnic groups native to Manchuria had characteristics of its own. The Qing incorporated the tribes, which at the time were known collectively as the Solon (Chinese: Suolun) or the Daur (Chinese: Dawoer), into special hunting banners. The tribes enjoyed relative autonomy under the Qing in return for submitting furs and ginseng to the imperial court.[11] The Daur, who were close to the Mongols in terms of language and culture, mainly inhabited the Nonni river basin in Heilongjiang between Qiqihar and Mergen (today's Nenjiang).[12] Many of the Orochen (also Oroqen; Chinese: Elunchun) joined the hunting banners, but scattered groups remained in the Khingan Mountains south of the Amur and Argun rivers.[13]

The cession of land to Russia in 1860 disrupted the tribute system on which the native peoples' relations to the Qing Empire had been based. Some of the Orochen, Hezhe, and Giliaks came under Russian rule.[14] The Giliaks, known today as Nivkhi, came to Russian attention mainly as the native inhabitants of northern Sakhalin. The Hezhe, whom the Chinese also called Yupi dazi, meaning "Fishskin Tatars," and whom

Russians knew first as Gol'dy, and later as Nanaitsy, were split in two by the new river borders. The Orochen in Heilongjiang adopted Russian clothing and food along with Russian names.[15] Under pressure from both empires, the indigenous people of Manchuria declined by the early twentieth century, but they continued crossing the borders of Russia and China.

Mongols and Koreans

The tracks of the Chinese Eastern Railway passed through Hailar, the main station of the western branch, and reached the Russian frontier at a station the Russians named Manchuria (as an indication of how foreign the name "Manchuria" was to the Chinese, they transcribed it as Manzhouli, which is how the present-day border city is still called). At its other extremity, from Vladivostok in Russia's Maritime province, the railway began its long run through Manchuria at Pogranichnaia (Russian for Border Station; the current Chinese name, Suifenhe, is borrowed from the nearby river). At these two ends of the track, the Russians encountered sizeable non-Chinese populations. In Hailar they lived in proximity to the local Mongols. A person who was born in this area – "close to the Gobi Desert" – remembered the Mongols and said he could journey for miles inside the country without meeting "a single Chinese." He also recalled an amazing "profusion of flowers" growing wild in the spring, fields alive with "all kinds of insects" and birds, the rivers nearby and the mountains of the Khingan Range, which he used to climb – all very unlike urban Harbin.[16]

Here the Russians also saw herds of camels and sheep and, out in the steppe, felt-covered Mongolian yurts. Such contacts as took place in Hailar continued the long history of Russian-Mongolian trade, also conducted in Urga (now Ulaanbaatar) and Kiakhta in eastern Siberia. Kiakhta, a town south of Lake Baikal on the Russian border with Outer Mongolia (a protectorate of Qing China), had been the centre of the tea trade between China and Russia from its foundation in 1727. Mongol-speaking peoples were also part of the multi-ethnic Russian empire: the Buryat Mongols, who inhabited both sides of Lake Baikal, were one of the largest ethnic groups in Siberia. Pressed by Russian colonizers in the late nineteenth and early twentieth centuries, and fleeing Bolshevism after 1917, many Russian Buryats immigrated to Mongolia and Manchuria.[17]

Russian peasants had more contact with the sedentary Koreans than with the nomadic Mongols. The Ussuri region in the south of Russia's Maritime province saw an influx of Korean migrants after floods and famines beset northern Korea in the late 1860s. Many of them settled along the right (Russian) bank of Suifen River. Unlike Chinese labour migrants, who arrived on their own and returned to China regularly, the Koreans had arrived with their families and with the intention of staying as agricultural settlers. Also unlike the Chinese, they were naturalized as Russian subjects (in stages after 1891) and received the right to own land. After the 1870s, Koreans also crossed the Tumen River border to settle in the part of Jilin province then known as Jiandao or Kando (now the Yanbian Autonomous Prefecture) and in southeastern Heilongjiang. Another wave of Korean migrants entered Manchuria after Japan annexed Korea in 1910.[18]

Chinese Settlers and Immigrants

The conflicting images of Manchuria – a sacred place of origin; a territory banned to Chinese settlers yet the destination of exiles; a border defence zone; a political periphery – represented only part of the picture. This was how Manchuria was seen by the government and court. It took a combination of Russian aggression on the frontier and the need to meet the financial exigencies of the Taiping Rebellion for the Qing state finally to permit Chinese settlement in Manchuria. But Manchuria had attracted peasants from China's densely populated northern provinces even before the settlement ban was lifted. By 1842 there were more than 1,665,000 Han Chinese in Manchuria, largely concentrated in the region's south. The Chinese presence had doubled by 1872 and reached more than 5 million by 1890, making up the clear ethnic majority in Manchuria.[19] After 1860, settlement fanned out into northern Manchuria and pioneer land cultivation replaced the traditional patterns of Chinese agriculture.[20] Natural disasters in China gave incentive to this process. Between 1876 and 1879, drought and famine killed between 9 and 13 million people in northern China. In 1876 alone, as many as 900,000 migrants arrived in Manchuria.[21]

After the late 1890s, the employment offered by the Russians on railway-building projects brought about a boom in Chinese immigration. The arrival of Chinese settlers transformed Manchuria linguistically and culturally as well as ethnically.[22] Over 95 per cent of all new migrants in Manchuria in the late nineteenth century came from two provinces: Zhili (the name of Hebei until 1928) and Shandong.[23] Heilongjiang alone received over 4 million settlers between 1900 and 1930, by which time almost half the province's population consisted of immigrants who had arrived there since 1918.[24] The large majority of immigrants to Manchuria were men; most were unmarried, and the others had left their families behind. Moreover, most of them had not come to stay, preferring "seasonal" or "circular" migration. After one to four years of work in Manchuria, at least two thirds of them returned to their home villages. Even during their time in the northeast, they regularly travelled back to spend the winter months and celebrate the Chinese New Year in the places they had come from.

Thus, the main population groups that Russians encountered in Manchuria and the Manchurian borderlands were a large majority of Han Chinese; Manchus; nomadic peoples, spread both along the borders and in the territories ceded to Russia in 1860; and Mongols and Koreans, respectively in eastern Inner Mongolia and the Ussuri region. An immigrant Japanese community in Manchuria would gradually form as well, encouraged by Japan's military victory against Russia in 1905. What, then, was the "ethnic profile" on the Russian side?

Arrival of the Russians

Cossacks

The origins of the Cossacks are disputed, but they included Turkic and other Asian components next to the Russian. Rather than a separate ethnic group, the Cossacks were a Russian-speaking and Orthodox military caste within the tsarist estate system. After the sixteenth century, Cossacks spearheaded the Russian expansion into Siberia. Following the Treaty of Aigun in 1858, the Governor General of Eastern Siberia, Nikolai N. Murav'ev (1809–1881), freshly named Count Murav'ev-Amurskii in recognition of his achievements in enlarging the realm of the tsar, moved Cossacks from their home parts east of Lake Baikal to new settlements along the Amur and Ussuri rivers. By 1862, these Cossack villages numbered around one hundred: placed at an average of 25 kilometres apart, they served as border posts as well as bridgeheads for civilian Russian colonization. About 16,000 Transbaikal Cossacks arrived in the Amur and Maritime provinces with their families by 1862. In 1860 the Amur Cossack Host was created, and by that decade's end a first wave of peasant settlement had brought the number of Cossack and civilian villages to 193.[25] Four new towns, among them the port of Vladivostok, were founded in the Russian Far East.

The Cossacks' role in Manchuria attracted some criticism. An article published in 1904 by an exiled revolutionary, who had explored the Argun River, is a veritable "J'accuse." Written under a pseudonym, embracing unusually pro-Chinese positions, and carried by the Western-leaning journal *Vestnik Evropy* (Herald of Europe) in Saint Petersburg, it was based on three years spent among "the Cossacks and peasants of the Shilka and Argun regions."[26] The Cossacks' attitude toward Chinese and Mongols in this border area was epitomized for the author by the term *tvar'* (beast, creature), which Cossacks applied to their neighbours. Cossacks would shoot at the Chinese across the Argun for no better reason than to test a new gun. In the summer of 1900, when Russia occupied Manchuria during the Boxer Uprising, they indulged in the random extermination of Chinese civilians. The author bitterly called such acts "tuition fees for the lessons in humanity and civilization, which we have administered to the yellow-faced barbarians."[27]

Thirty years later, an anthropologist documented peaceful material exchanges between Cossacks and the Reindeer Evenki (a small nomadic group, who had crossed into China from the Russian Far East in the late nineteenth century) in the same border region, calling their relations "an example of culture contact without conflict."[28] And in fact, the Cossacks could be accused of becoming too much like the natives just as easily as they could be accused of mistreating them. The explorer and Russian nationalist Nikolai M. Przhevalsky (1839–1888), writing on Mongolia in 1880, warned that "assimilation is going in an undesirable direction here. It is the Cossacks who adopt the language and customs of their non-Russian neighbours, passing onto them nothing of their own. The Cossack at home shows off in a Chinese coat, speaks Mongolian or Kirghiz, prefers tea to any other food, and the nomads' dairy food. Even his physiognomy has degenerated and more often than not resembles his ethnic neighbour."[29]

Ukrainians and Other Russians

The Ukrainians were one of the largest ethnicities in the late tsarist empire. However, their separate identity became submerged in the Russian. Alexander II banned the Ukrainian language in Russia in the Ems Edict of 1876 (so called after the spa town Bad Ems on the Rhine, where the tsar was then taking the waters). Under the Russification policies of his successor, Alexander III, this prohibition was eased but not cancelled.[30] In contrast to the tightly knit groups of Cossacks and Russian sectarian believers in Manchuria, who gathered around military or spiritual leaders and were cognizant of their particularity within Russian society, Ukrainians had become "to all intents and purposes Russian," as one historian put it, perhaps as early as the end of the eighteenth century.[31]

Ukrainians were attracted to the Russian Far East and migrated there in the last quarter of the nineteenth century; it was often they who subsequently reached Manchuria.[32] Ukrainian nationalism found political expression in Harbin during the Russian Civil War, and the memory of the independent Ukrainian republic, founded in 1918 but divided between Bolshevik Russia and Poland by 1921, lingered among émigrés though it was suppressed in Ukraine itself. The Manchukuo regime revived the Ukrainian House and the Ukrainian National Colony in Harbin. Nonetheless, the latter association counted only three hundred members in Manchuria in the 1930s.[33] Most ethnic Ukrainians in Manchuria either considered themselves Russian or registered as Russians for practical reasons.

Many other nationalities were represented in Harbin and along the CER line in Manchuria: in more marginal numbers, tsarist subjects included Georgians, Armenians, Tatars, Lithuanians, Poles, Latvians, and Baltic Germans, to mention only some. Besides language, religion was a main component in the self-identification of Harbin's Russian nationals; except for the large Jewish and the small Turkic-Tatar communities, all the rest were Christians.[34] The tensions and confessional differences among the Russian Orthodox, Polish Roman Catholics, and German Lutherans (there were also a handful of Russian Catholics) were all but invisible to the Chinese.

Similarly, Europeans in Harbin had only a vague idea about relations among Han Chinese, Manchus, Mongols, and Koreans. The common wisdom was that Harbin's Chinese "came from Chefoo" (Zhifu, now part of Yantai), a port in northern Shandong. Besides migrants from Shandong and Hebei, however, Harbin also had people from Jiangsu, Zhejiang, Hubei, and Guangdong; they often settled on different city streets, belonged to different native-place associations, and spoke different dialects; they even tended to enter different occupations.[35] Even within the largest community of Shandong migrants, counties of origin were central to people's relationships and careers.

Sectarians and the Crisis of 1900

The Russians who had rejected the reform of the Russian Church by Patriarch Nikon in 1654, when native ritual was replaced by that of the Greek Church, became known as Old Believers. The Russian state also referred to them as schismatics (*raskol'niki*), a term used until 1905 for all religious dissenters within Russian Christianity. Blaming the tsars for corrupting the true faith, and escaping the state's persecution, Old Believers fled to remote frontiers of the empire or, like the English dissenters who journeyed to North America after the Act of Uniformity in 1662, crossed those frontiers in search of religious freedom. By the late nineteenth century, there were around 10 million Old Believers in Russia.[36] Some of them settled along the Baltic coast, while others made their way to the Amur. The two main sects of Russian Spiritual Christianity, the Molokans and the Dukhobors, founded villages in the Amur province after 1859. The edict on religious toleration, which Nicholas II issued in April 1905, introduced the distinction between Old Believers and sectarians while ending discrimination against both groups by the state and the Orthodox Church.

In contrast to the pejorative images generally associated with adherents to heterodox beliefs (in China, such groups have been regarded as potential rebels and feared by both dynastic courts and the Communist government), in late tsarist Russia Old Believers were admired for their industriousness and moral fortitude.[37] The Governor General of the Priamur in the 1890s wrote in the same positive tone about the hard-working, non-drinking sectarians in the Transbaikal and Amur provinces.[38] However, attitudes toward Old Believers and sectarians differed across segments of Russian society and were open to revision.

During the Boxer Uprising in Manchuria, the Qing military opened fire on Russian ships in the Amur River. Then on 2 July 1900 by the Russian calendar (15 July N.S.), they attacked the border town of Blagoveshchensk from the village of Sakhalian on the opposite bank of the Amur with cannon, small arms, and grenades. The total population of Blagoveshchensk in 1900 was about 40,000, including some 4,000 Chinese. In response to the shelling, on 4 July 1900 (O.S.), the town's Chinese were rounded up and ordered at bayonet point to swim to the other shore. The operation was repeated on 6 and 8 July (O.S.), resulting in between 2,000 and 4,000 deaths.[39] As the author of the Aigun gazetteer was to write in 1920:

> Far off on the opposite bank, the Russians were forcing countless of our compatriots [*Huaqiao*] to gather at the riverside, and the noise made the earth tremble. Looking carefully, you could catch a glimpse of the Russian soldiers, each grasping knives and axes, slashing to the left and hacking to the right; of dissected bodies and crushed bones, among earth-shaking noise and sounds of wailing. The severely wounded died on the shore, while those whose injuries were lighter died in the river; those who were not wounded leapt into the water and were drowned, and the river was overflowing with human bones. Some eighty men managed, with the last resources of their strength, to keep afloat; stark naked, they were in too much of a stupor to be able to utter a word.[40]

This gazetteer further relates the drowning of 5,000 Chinese in the Amur and the massacre of 7,000 defenceless peasants in the "sixty-four villages," a Qing enclave on Russian territory, safeguarded under the terms of the Treaty of Aigun of 1858, that was populated by Manchu, Daur, and Han Chinese peasants. Both figures for the 1900 deaths are exaggerated, but the "sixty-four villages" beyond the Zeya River (at the confluence of which with the Amur the Russian town Blagoveshchensk is located) were indeed the first to be wiped out.

A wave of indiscriminate killings of Chinese and everyone who looked Chinese swept through the Amur province.[41] Fear of the Boxers had unleashed mass hysteria, which fed on rumours and activated existing perceptions that the "yellow races," above all the Chinese, were an imminent threat to Russia – a frontier version of the "yellow peril."[42] The siege of Blagoveshchensk lasted nineteen days, but despite all the anxiety endured, Russian civilian losses during the summer of 1900 proved limited. The Russian population of Harbin fled after an attack on the town on 13 July, a date that Russians subsequently commemorated with annual ceremonies and a public holiday. Thus, in July 1903, Harbin's first newspaper, the Russian-language *Harbin Herald*, reported that the holiday's events included street performances by Chinese jugglers.[43] On the twentieth anniversary of the Boxer attack in July 1920, a steel cross was erected in Harbin's Old Cemetery in "eternal memory" of the city's Russian defenders.[44] By contrast, the drownings in Blagoveshchensk were forgotten, though a shocking account, based on the archives, was published anonymously in *Herald of Europe* in 1910.[45] In Soviet Russia, the story of the drownings was silenced. In China as well, it vanished from official discourse by the 1920s, to be evoked again half a century later during the Sino-Soviet rift.[46]

One Russian summary of the incident in Blagoveshchensk, published after the Russo-Japanese War, put the blame on Molokans. According to the author, A. Sokolova, Molokans ran about the town in a frenzy, inciting people to do away with the Chinese and setting an example through indiscriminate murder and looting. The Molokans supposedly exploited the situation to get rid of Chinese merchants to whom they had become indebted.[47] The Molokans were the largest non-Orthodox denomination among the Russians in Amur province, which had become their main centre by the 1900s. They vigorously pursued commercial activities in Blagoveshchensk and were resented for their wealth.[48]

Sokolova presented the Russians in town as the protectors of Chinese against Molokan atrocities. One Chinese merchant allegedly spent two

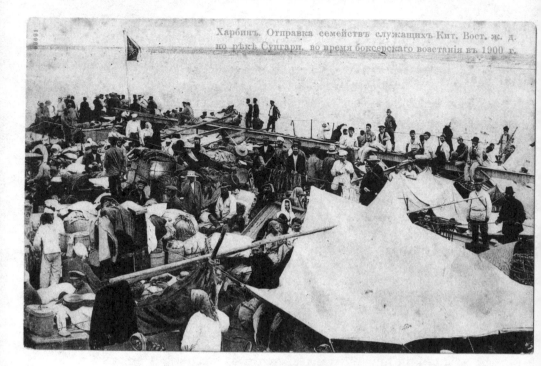

Харбинъ. Отправка семействъ служащихъ Кит. Вост. ж. д. по рѣкѣ Сунгари, во время боксерскаго возстанія въ 1900 г.

1.1. "The families of Chinese Eastern Railway employees evacuate
Harbin by the Sungari River during the Boxer Uprising."
Postcard, author's collection.

days hiding in the lavatory of Governor Gribskii's house; the governor himself brought him food.[49] Yet it is Lieutenant-General Konstantin N. Gribskii (1845–1918), the military governor of Amur province and commander of the Amur Cossacks, who is widely reputed to have ordered the round-up. Other Russian voices tried to absolve their side by blaming the victims. The founding director of the Oriental Institute in Vladivostok and teacher of future Harbin sinologists, the Mongolist Aleksei M. Pozdneev (1851–1920), wrote in a report to the tsar:

> The local Russian authorities displayed all possible measures of humanity … It was impossible to leave the Chinese on the left bank of the Amur since most of them had been part of the conspiracy and naturally sympathized with their compatriots … The location chosen for having them wade across the river was entirely suitable … It is not our fault if the Chinese began shooting at their own people, spreading a panic among them which then led to the totally unpredictable disaster.[50]

An official investigation of the treatment of the Chinese population soon began, at which point more convincing explanations were needed. The exiled revolutionary Lev G. Deich (1855–1941), then living in Blagoveshchensk, turned the denunciation of the "bloody days" on the Amur into a personal campaign. While venting his hatred of the tsarist regime, Deich must have seen the drowning of the Chinese through the prism of an aspect of ordinary Russian violence more familiar to him: the pogroms against Jews, his own people.[51] Some Russians, though, insinuated that Cossacks had been the main culprits.[52]

The image of enlightened imperialism could be better sustained if the enforcement of authority over the natives was attributed to segments of Russian society that were themselves the internal "other." Thus, in narratives of the events in Blagoveshchensk that acknowledged that something had gone wrong, it was sectarians who had incited violence against the Chinese and Cossacks who had drowned them in the river, while European Russians lamented these events. A British traveller who had left Blagoveshchensk two weeks before the massacre was told by "no less than five eye-witnesses" that "General Gribsky … sent word to the Cossacks that they were to turn all the Chinese out of the town and make them cross the river. Unhappily the order was given to men who could not be trusted to act humanely. The Cossacks, who were little better than savages, threw themselves upon the helpless Chinese – among whom there were fortunately very few women and children."[53] In 1901, the economist and theorist of colonization Aleksandr A. Kaufman (1864–1919) reported on the general embarrassment among Blagoveshchensk residents about the massacre of the previous year and repeated the rumour that blamed the violence against the Chinese in their town on Molokans. This rumour lasted long enough to be woven into the bestselling crime novel *Amur Wolves*, published pseudonymously in Blagoveshchensk in 1912.[54]

Reports from Blagoveshchensk had rather little to say about the people living in the opposite village. Sakhalian, on the right bank of the Amur, was distinctly visible from the Russian side of the river until 20 July 1900 (O.S.), when the Russian army's Cossacks burnt it to the ground.[55] One recollection featured the Orochen: unperturbed by the general panic, they had moved freely between the Russian and the Chinese riverbanks, lending help to both sides. "Nashi vsem pomogai!" (Us help all!), is how one of them reportedly phrased this in pidgin, addressing a Russian gold miner.[56] Several other villages on the Chinese bank were razed by the Russian military, and the bodies of their inhabitants were added to the numerous corpses that, many days after the massacre, could still be seen and smelled in the Amur.[57]

The Han Chinese were a minority in this northern part of Heilongji-ang. Sakhalian was a Manchu place name, meaning "Great Black River," which was also the Manchu name of the Amur River (Sahalian Ula). The same meaning is preserved in the Chinese name Heilongjiang, used for both province and river, and in modern Heihe, the city that replaced Aigun (Chinese: Aihui), the northernmost Qing town and garrison, twenty miles downstream from Blagoveshchensk.[58] Russian troops razed Aigun on 22 July 1900 (O.S.). The tsarist army went on to occupy northern Manchuria. On 30 July, military governor Gribskii issued an order declaring that in "the former Chinese town Aigun and Sakhalian," all settlement of Trans-Zeya Manchus (former inhabitants of the "sixty-four villages") and other Qing subjects was henceforth forbidden. This effectively both nullified some of the terms of the Treaty of Aigun and erased the town in which it had been signed.[59] Because the population of Aigun did return after the Russians left the town in ruins, the Manchu language (practically extinct today) survived there long enough for the ethnographer Sergei Shirokogoroff (1887–1939) to conduct an important field study in 1915. As he wrote, "in the Aigun district the Manchu peas-ants were beyond the immediate Chinese influence and preserved the original character of their culture so purely that, during my visits there, I found even today some old men and women who did not wish to speak Chinese and strictly practised the Manchu *fe doro* [old way]."[60]

Ethnic Diversity and the Question of Identity

The apprearance of Russians in China's northeast, beginning with the bloodless territorial gains of 1860 and culminating in the confrontation of 1900, had consequences for the lives of all the peoples inhabiting the region. Natives and other minority groups were either engulfed by the expanding Russian empire or obliged to secure an alternative for their former tributary relations with Qing China. The banner system had been disintegrating for a long time, and the impotence of the Qing army had been demonstrated by its defeat in the war with Japan in 1895. However, the death knell of the Manchu military tradition and the social caste the banners represented was sounded in the summer of 1900 with the fall of the Manchu garrisons of Aigun and Qiqihar. The life and death of Shou Shan, the military governor of Heilongjiang province at the time of the Boxer Uprising, illustrate the nuances of identity among the uniform-looking foe, whom the Russians observed from the riverbank in besieged Blagoveshchensk.

Born in Aigun in 1860, Shou Shan was the son of Fumingga (Chinese: Fuming'a), who was governor of Jiangsu province during the Taiping

Rebellion and later governor of Jilin from 1866 to 1870. The father's adopted Manchu name is misleading: an exception among the military commanders of Manchuria in the late Qing, he was of Han Chinese rather than Manchu or Mongol origin. Shou Shan was a seventh-generation descendant of the Ming dynasty minister of war, Yuan Chonghuan, a general who had driven back the encroaching Manchus in Liaodong; at the famous battle of Ningyuan, in February 1626, his troops inflicted deadly wounds on Nurhachi, the founder of the Manchu state. Court intrigues, however, led to a false charge against Yuan of being in league with the enemy, and in 1630 he was executed as a traitor, cut to pieces in the Peking marketplace. Yuan's son afterwards joined the Manchus.[61] The invaders had incorporated vast numbers of Chinese into their military system, so that by the time of their conquest of China, the original Manchu eight banners had become "a dwindling minority" within the army. The Han Chinese Plain White Banner, of which Shou Shan was a hereditary member, was established in 1642.[62]

In the eighteenth century the Qing demobilized large numbers of the Han Chinese bannermen (Hanjun), but this policy was not applied in Manchuria.[63] In 1894, Shou Shan left Peking, where he had held minor hereditary posts for the previous six years, to fight in the Sino-Japanese War in Fengtian. His younger brother was killed and he himself was wounded in battle. Upon his return, following a brief appointment to Kaifeng in central China, he was promoted to brigade-general (*fudu-tong*; also translated as military lieutenant-governor) of his hometown, Aigun.[64] A native of the Amur border, he had been to Blagoveshchensk and apparently had some knowledge of Russian.[65]

In January 1900 Shou Shan was appointed military governor of Heilongjiang. In July of that year, ambiguous messages from Peking, where the Boxer Uprising against foreigners was by then in full swing, communicated to him and the governors of Jilin and Fengtian the court's desire for an attack on the Russians. The military engagement, begun with the shelling of Blagoveshchensk, was swiftly decided in favour of the enemy. After the destruction of Aigun, Shou Shan proposed an immediate ceasefire. As this belated attempt to prevent the occupation of the Heilongjiang capital Qiqihar and with it the entire province was met with no answer, on 28 August Shou Shan was forced to comply with the Russian ultimatum and surrender Qiqihar to the army of Major General Pavel Rennenkampf. On the same day, he carried out what he had been taught was the duty of a defeated commander. A detailed, if not entirely reliable, later account by Shou's daughter-in-law describes the general's attempts to kill his whole family before taking his own life and supports the version that Shou swallowed gold in an attempt to induce death. He then ordered his son to shoot him; a subordinate carried out this command.[66] By the time the Russians entered the city, the coffin with Shou Shan's body was being carried south from Qiqihar on its way to Inner Mongolia, the homeland of his Mongol wife.

Shou Shan's political testament was an eve-of-death call for the Qing government to intensify Chinese settlement of Heilongjiang as the only way to repel the foreign threat.[67] Was Shou more "Manchu," or more "Chinese"? It has been a premise of this chapter that in order to understand the Russian or Chinese view of the opposite side, we needed first to appreciate the diversity within both groups and then try to explain how they saw themselves. Identity does not have to mirror ethnicity (the latter term, in English, dates from the 1950s), and Shou Shan was born a bannerman and died as one. Among Qing-era Manchu and Han Chinese members of the banner system, this sense of belonging was stronger than any ethnic differences, despite the hierarchy that put Manchus on top.[68]

Other senior bannermen of both Manchu and Han origins committed suicide once they grasped the scope and implications of the Boxers' defeat.[69] Pushed to the borders of Mongolia, Jin Chang, the former *fudutong* of Mukden, who had ordered the execution of Christian missionaries, went on fighting the Russians at the head of a small army. His follower Shou Chang, the last survivor, was captured by the Russians in March 1901 and taken to Port Arthur, and then farther on to Vladivostok and Irkutsk, where he committed suicide.[70] Cheng Dequan (1860–1930), a Han Chinese official from Sichuan, whom Shou Shan had entrusted with the task of concluding a truce with the Russians, leapt into the river rather than serve as puppet governor of Heilongjiang under Russian control; rescued, he too was taken prisoner, but was soon liberated. In 1904, Cheng became the first non-bannerman Chinese to be appointed *fudutong* (in Qiqihar), and then, in 1906, the first Han official to hold the post of military governor of Heilongjiang.[71]

In Russian-occupied Manchuria, in the years between the Boxers' defeat and the Russo-Japanese War, the choice facing China's elite military commanders was at least as old as the seventeenth-century "Ming-Qing cataclysm," when Ming loyalists mounted a prolonged resistance, persevering, often to the death, in their refusal to serve the new dynasty. The military governor of Jilin in 1900, Chang Shun (1839–1904), chose not to resist the Russian army and personally welcomed it into the provincial capital.[72] Chang Shun, who came from Buteha (now Zhalantun, northwest of Qiqihar), was of Daur origin and a member of the Plain White Banner. Newly founded Harbin was located in Jilin province; the

Russians gratefully remembered the governor's conduct and later sent delegates to his funeral. A Harbin newspaper, unaware of the ethnic nuances of the case, described "the Chinese ceremony" of transferring Chang Shun's coffin from Jilin to Mukden.[73]

As we look at the ethnic and religious diversity on the Russian side of the Manchurian encounter, another conclusion emerges. The Russian government had been settling Cossack families along the Argun, Amur, and Ussuri rivers since the 1860s and meant for them to occupy that land permanently. Similarly, the promise of religious freedom encouraged Old Believers, who joined the Cossacks in crossing to the Three Rivers area beyond the Chinese bank of the Argun, to regard that corner of Manchuria as their new home. Molokans (numerous enough in Harbin to have their own house of prayer and graveyard) may have felt the same, although too little is known about them to be sure.[74] By contrast, the bulk of Russian newcomers in Manchuria from the beginning of the CER construction project had no intention of settling down. Descriptions of these early arrivals speak of young men in search of a quick buck – a motif in Harbin's emerging image of a Wild East.[75] Elsewhere in the world, colonists tended to form ties with the new land only at later stages of settlement, drawing on the relationship that pioneers had established with the native population. It is rare for colonizers to be faced with a parallel migrant society, as was the case in Manchuria. Most Chinese migrants, also predominantly male and single, moved back and forth between northern China and Manchuria without settling in the latter.[76] Those who did remain were often natives of the same village or bearers of the same surname. They built "sheds" (*wopeng*), collective farming settlements that allowed them to maintain their home customs while limiting communication with other settler groups, let alone foreigners.[77]

Russian demand for mass labour rose constantly after construction work began on the CER and was met by a stream of migrant workers. Chinese "coolies," hired in the northern ports of Tientsin and Chefoo, provided 70 to 90 per cent of the manual labour. There were 49,000 Chinese workers in Russian employ in June 1899, 75,000 in 1900. The Sino-Russian military confrontation during by the Boxer Uprising of 1900 brought only a brief decline in recruitment. At the peak of construction, the CER employed around 130,000 Chinese workers.[78] The coolies' apparent indifference to national pride and colonial exploitation earned them the contempt of Western observers, who invariably thought in nationalistic terms.[79] The Russians, too, concluded that the ordinary Chinese would be content so long as he had enough to eat and that it did not matter to him who filled his rice bowl.[80] They were tempted, moreover, to respond to the coolies' apparent attitude as an encouragement to colonization.

In rural China in the late nineteenth and early twentieth centuries, nationalism in the sense of allegiance to the abstract notion of the state had not yet taken root. The Chinese, who poured into Manchuria, partly in response to the foreigners' offer of higher wages, did possess a sense of local identity, tied to their home villages and counties, though "identity" in the Western sense was not part of their vocabulary. Their form of self-identification could be easily reconciled with serving the opponents of China in the international arena. It was epitomized in the migrants' transplantation of their Shandong villages onto Manchurian soil.[81] Their home ties were all-important and were stronger than those that bound Russian settlers to their own localities of origin. The Russians identified more with their country and with the Russian army when it waged war in the name of the tsar. Because they expected the Chinese to display their allegiance in the same way, they could not tolerate their presence in wartime Blagoveshchensk.[82]

The memoirist previously mentioned in connection with her version of the events in Blagoveshchensk in 1900, A. Sokolova, had travelled to Harbin with a group of new Russian settlers and officers' wives. Sailing up the Amur and the Sungari from Khabarovsk, their steamship stopped first at Lahasusu (today's Tongjiang), where the two rivers converged, and then at Sanxing (today's Yilan), where the passengers had time to visit a Buddhist temple and the local cemetery, as well as the well-attended tomb of "a Chinese saint." At the cemetery, they saw "log-coffins, placed on the ground beneath the trees, some of them slightly covered with earth. Some graves had been dug up; Chinese dogs and pigs wander freely through the cemetery, snatch the dead out and eat them."

The risk that, through the hogs, deceased townsmen might enter the food chain, did not appear to disturb their neighbours and relatives. Sokolova reported that her queries about this possibility were brushed away in Sanxing with the words, in pidgin: "We eat them, they eat us – it's all the same." By the end of this visit by Harbin's pioneers, the local dogs and pigs were not the only ones to take their pick of the scattered remains. "Soon we returned to the steamship without further adventure, and how great was our surprise when we found out that one passenger had carried off a deceased man's head from the cemetery. Everyone protested, asking him to throw it overboard, but he stubbornly repeated: I need it for my research, which is why I am going to Manchuria."[83] The young passenger was a science student. The "adventure" referred to obliquely had taken place two days earlier at Lahasusu, when a mischievous Russian youth tried to steal a Chinese statuette, "a little horned god, beautifully made out of bronze," from the local temple.[84] The account of the resulting uproar of the natives (more likely Hezhe than "Chinese"), whose fishing boats set out in futile pursuit of the foreign steamship, reads like a parody of the colonial encounter. The fury abated only when a resourceful Russian lady threw a basketful of shining beads down from the deck and diverted the enemy's attention "at the very last moment."

The Russian steamship's final stop was the port of Harbin. There, the wife of the manager of the town's new brickworks, a friend of the author's, was driven to nervous exhaustion for reasons reminiscent of their outing in Sanxing:

> Constantly in motion, penetrating everywhere, the sand began to drive Mme Roganova to despair; it seemed to her that the [Manchurian] gale was blowing around the factory the desiccated dung and refuse, which through years and generations had accumulated on the spot where the abandoned Chinese village stood. Mme Roganova's imagination gradually heightened this picture: in the bread and soup, no matter what she ate, she seemed to sense a revolting smell; even in the air she began to detect the putrid smell of the Chinese dead. What further induced this unhealthy state was the fact Mme Roganova had often observed Chinese funerals, and, on her walks near the factory, would sometimes see a Chinese hand, or a leg, or a whole head with or without a queue.[85]

The real encounter occurs *here*, in the details of everyday life within the same physical space. The Chinese did share their living quarters with pigs, a tradition so ancient as to be reflected in the written character for "home" or "family." During the Boxer campaign and the Russo-Japanese War, Russian soldiers in Manchuria refused pork because they believed that pigs fed on the Chinese dead.[86] Smell was an issue in reference to living Chinese bodies, not only to cemeteries. Specifically, the Chinese poor were associated with the stench of garlic.[87]

As is well known, burying the dead was among the most elaborate and profoundly charged rites in Chinese culture.[88] Graves were sited in conformity with the demands of geomancy (*feng shui*). Contrary to other religious traditions, the Chinese did not emphasize immediate interment of the dead; rather, filial piety and the belief that the spirits of uncared-for ancestors would transform themselves into malevolent ("hungry" or "lonely") ghosts, a peril to their descendants, dictated the need for proper burial. The neglect of the dead, which the two Russian women observed in turn-of-the-century Manchuria, therefore deserves our attention, and those scattered corpses in Sanxing and Harbin (sights

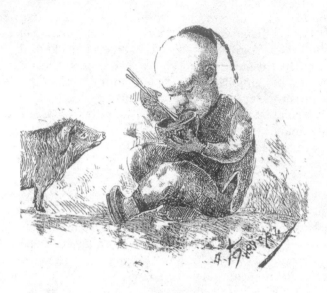

1.2. Drawing by P. Brier. Postcard about 1905. Author's collection.

that Sokolova was not the only one to record) should not be dismissed as figments of an exoticizing European imagination.[89] An often admiring report on the Chinese way of life in Kwantung (Guandong), the Russian leasehold in the southern part of the Liaodong Peninsula from 1899 to 1905, which included Port Arthur and Dal'nii, described the importance of burial rites for the local population, while mentioning that the new Russian administration had relocated Chinese cemeteries farther from the cities and instructed the Chinese "to bury corpses deeper in the ground."[90] In China, death was less sanitized and concealed than it was in Russia – certainly in European Russia, by which the tsarist empire wished to represent itself in the Far East. We must go beyond pointing out the obvious: that descriptions of the "disgusting ways" of the Chinese helped justify the imposition of Western civilization, as personified by Sokolova and her fellow settlers. One step toward an explanation of her accounts of Sanxing and Harbin would be to treat them as distinct cases.

The first "Chinese cemetery" Sokolova described may not have been in use by the Han, but by native people. The leader of a Russian expedition to Manchuria in the summer of 1895, which travelled up the

Sungari with the steamer *Telegraf,* noted that the population of Lahasusu and the next river port Fujin was almost exclusively Gold (Hezhe).[91] The ethnographer and historian Owen Lattimore (1900–1989) saw the Gold inhabitants in Sanxing in 1930; he called the town "the old meeting point of Gold and Manchu."[92] In the brand-new Russian town of Harbin, Prince Khilkov's brickworks was constructed on the site of a Chinese village, whose inhabitants had been evacuated when the land was incorporated into the CER right of way. If the ground had previously served for burial, Mme Roganova's unpleasant findings in the vicinity were hardly surprising.[93]

In northern China, the corpses of small children were deliberately placed in open fields, where stray dogs and other animals fed on them. The most distinguished writer of the northeast, Xiao Hong (pen-name of Zhang Naiying, 1911–1942), alluded to this custom in the title of her best-known novel, *The Field of Life and Death* (1935).[94] An American physician in Shandong in the 1880s, Robert Coltman (1862–1931), noted that parents whose children died young considered them possessed by an evil spirit; their corpses therefore posed a danger to the family, which had to be forestalled by making the spirit enter an animal's body.[95] Unwanted babies, usually female, were also left in the fields and ravines, and Russians in Manchuria were troubled to discover them being devoured by animals.[96]

A perspective on Sokolova's disturbing impressions – one that, of all the attempts at interpretation suggested so far, seems to tally best with what is known of the Chinese migrant society in Manchuria – brings us back to the main concerns of this chapter. A Russian railway surveyor in Ninguta (today's Ning'an, in southeast Heilongjiang) in 1898 had this to say about the Chinese in Manchuria:

> For every Chinese who arrives here, the accumulation of money represents the alpha and omega of his activities. Each of them, even a colonist who has moved here with his entire household, dreams of taking his duly acquired savings back to his native land and the sacredly revered tombs of his ancestors, there to build a new life on the money he has earned in the foreign country. If not fated to return to his native land in his lifetime, he does not relinquish hope of moving there as a dead man and stipulates in his will that he should be buried nowhere but in his family cemetery. Because of this, many Chinese who died in Ninguta are not committed to the earth there, but their bodies, in wooden case-coffins, often painted in bright colours and covered with engravings, are carried out to so-called burial vaults, where the dead patiently await the time when relatives may arrive to transport them to the family cemetery, that place of rest of their

fathers and forefathers. But many have to wait for quite a long time; some of the deceased remain there for several years, and it is easy to imagine what atmosphere surrounds that terrible place, where hundreds of uninterred corpses are allowed to decompose.[97]

The beginning of the above paragraph could also describe the motives of many Russian settlers in Manchuria. Yet it is evident what picture of the Chinese such customs were likely to evoke among Russians less interested in uncovering the reasons behind them. Poverty too could prevent definitive interment and may have been the reason why the corpses Sokolova saw in Sanxing, if indeed they were Han Chinese, received only temporary burial (Chinese: *fucuo*) in coffins laid above ground.[98] Among migrant workers in Manchuria and the Russian Far East, who lived away from their families, ancestral graves, and temples, the task of conveying the dead body home would have fallen to relatives of the deceased, his comrades or fellow villagers, and collectively to the native-place association to which he belonged.[99] These associations maintained coffin repositories across Manchuria. Migrants' coffins were still being transported through the Great Wall in the 1930s, while those lying uninterred in Harbin's Chinese cemeteries prompted the fearful curiosity of Russian children.[100]

Incomprehensible as it was to Europeans, the notion that entrusting a dead person's remains to "a foreign land" would constitute a greater injury than leaving them above ground alerts us to a common characteristic of the emerging Russian and Han Chinese societies in Manchuria. There were others for whom Manchuria was home: Manchus, Mongols, and native people, in particular. But Harbin, the centre of Russian settlement after the completion of the CER in 1903, became the setting for two clusters of sojourners. For both, home was elsewhere. And even as they began separately to build connections to the new place where they lived, each struggled to make sense of the other.

2

Beginnings

The beginnings were slow and long. From the manor house on the bank of the Memel River, invisible paths stretched back to other times and distant lands, and these, so they had heard, were also *Vaterland*. In due course they would perhaps travel there, to see that other fatherland, the old homeland, with their own eyes. They lived in Russia, but their *Heimat*, the place they knew best and called home, was Courland and their language was German. People around them also spoke other languages: Lithuanian, Yiddish, and Polish. As soon as one travelled north, one heard more Latvian and Russian. They were eight children: the four sons and four daughters of Baron Alexander Budberg, who was born in Mitau (by its Latvian name, Jelgava), the capital seat of the Governorate of Courland, in 1834, and Alexandrine, born as Countess Anrep-Elmpt in 1837 on her family estate of Schwitten (now Svitene parish in southern Latvia). The parents were second cousins, sharing a grandmother, but the Budbergs were Lutheran and the Anrep-Elmpts Catholic. They would compromise by raising their sons as Lutherans and their daughters as Catholics. Roger, born in January 1867, was their fourth child.

Like each of his siblings, he had a much longer given name: Andreas Alexander Rotgert Maria, Baron von Budberg-Bönninghausen. There was little consistency in the spelling, or indeed the placement order, in the name of the Courland branch of the family: his relatives also wrote "Böninghausen" or, when using the Cyrillic script, Beningsgauzen or Benninggauzen; they might call themselves Budberg-Bönninghausen one day and Bönninghausen-Budberg on another. Budberg and Bönninghausen were villages in the former County of Mark on the Lower Rhine, a part of the Duchy of Westphalia, now the state of North Rhine–Westphalia in the west of Germany, to which their family traced its origins in the fourteenth century. In the second half of the sixteenth century, Roger Budberg's ancestors came to the Baltic littoral, where German settlement had already begun with the medieval Teutonic Order.

His father was ready to spare him one of the two tees in the name he originally bestowed on his son by calling him Rogert, instead of Rotgert. The son liberated himself from the last of those Teutonic relics by adopting "Roger" as his first name in German. With the addition of the obligatory patronymic, this became "Rozher Aleksandrovich" in Russian. In both languages he used his baron's title and hyphenated surname. The surname could be shortened to "Budberg" on all but the most formal occasions, the German "von" was always dropped in Russian, and the *Baron* could be converted to *Freiherr* in communications with Germany, yet the title could never be forgotten – at least, as long as one was among Europeans. Nevertheless, in his fortieth year, in a faraway place, he would become known, more simply, as "Doctor Bu," in Chinese.[1]

Family

Theirs was a great family. Through their paternal grandmother Baroness Amalie Stockhorner von Starein (1813–1884), who in 1834 married Baron Andreas Budberg (1796–1855), the ancestry of Roger Budberg and his siblings could be traced to an eighteenth-century Duke of Bavaria – a patron of the arts in Mannheim and Munich, who commissioned work from Schiller and Mozart – as well as the nobility of many European courts.[2] Since its founding in 1561, the Duchy of Courland and Semigallia had been in the hands of German nobles, who managed its affairs independently of the Polish-Lithuanian Commonwealth, to which they were formally subordinated. Livland province (Lifliandskaia guberniia, the Governorate of Livland),[3] with its capital, Riga, had been part of the Russian empire since 1710, when Peter the Great wrested it from Sweden in the Great Northern War. In 1795, following the third partition of Poland, Courland too entered the empire as Kurzemskaia guberniia. Thereafter, the Budberg name would resonate in Russia as well as in the Baltic lands.

Baltic German nobles in Russian service customarily used the Russian equivalents or approximations of their first names. Major-General Baron Andrei Iakovlevich Budberg (Andreas Eberhard von Budberg, 1750–1812) became ambassador to Stockholm in 1796, the final year of the reign of Catherine the Great, in whose court he had long served. He remained in diplomatic service during the brief reign of Paul I (who was assassinated) and the ascension of Alexander I (r. 1801–25), reaching the pinnacle of his career as Minister of Foreign Affairs from 1806 to 1807.[4] His short term in that office ended with Russia's defeat by Napoleon; it had also included overseeing the dispatch of a large diplomatic mission to China, which failed to reach the court in Peking, as well as a project, which also did not attain fruition, of addressing the lack of interpreters in the Russian foreign service by initiating extensive training in Oriental languages in Kazan, Tiflis, and Irkutsk (where the minister wanted Chinese and Manchu to be taught).[5]

There were more diplomats among the Budbergs. Baron Andrei Fedorovich (Andreas Ludwig Karl Theodor von Budberg, 1817–1881) was an ambassador of Alexander II (r. 1855–81) to Berlin, Vienna, and Paris, until a row with another Baltic baron during his final posting in 1868 obliged him to challenge his rival to a duel and afterwards resign from service for this breach of discipline.[6] While serving in Berlin in the early 1850s, Ambassador Budberg played a small part in devising Russian plans to establish relations with Japan.[7] In the early twentieth century, under the last tsar, Nicholas II (r. 1894–1917), the former ambassador's son became the last Budberg diplomat: Baron Fedor Andreevich (Theodor Paul Andreas, 1851–1916) spent most of his life on missions abroad and died in Spain shortly after being relieved of his post as Russian ambassador.[8] His brother Baron Aleksandr Andreevich Budberg (Alexander Paul Andreas, 1853–1914) headed the Imperial Chancellery for Receipt of Petitions in Saint Petersburg after 1893 and was later a member of the State Council.[9]

None of these men were closely related to Roger Budberg, although he certainly knew their names: Alexander I's foreign minister was a great-grand-uncle, and Alexander II's ambassador was the son of the same minister's daughter, who had married a Budberg cousin. The above-mentioned brothers Theodor (Fedor) and Alexander were Roger's third cousins. More closely related was his grand-uncle, Cavalry General Baron Alexander Theodor Budberg (aka Aleksandr Ivanovich, 1797–1876), who was admired in the family not so much for his military prowess in Turkey, Persia, Poland, and the Caucasus as for marrying at the age of fifty-six a seventeen-year-old beauty and heiress, Annette Fuhrmann, rumoured to have been an illegitimate daughter of Alexander II, with whom he then had seven children.[10]

Other Barons Budberg chose the army as a career. The military gallery of the Hermitage Museum in Saint Petersburg honours the heroes of the resistance to Napoleon's invasion. On the wall to the left of the monumental portrait of Alexander I on his white steed, there is a portrait of "Baron K.V. Budberg the 2nd, Major General" (1775–1829).[11] The last of the many Budbergs who both attained high honours in the military and served in senior office – if merely for a month and two days as Minister of War in Admiral Alexander Kolchak's (1874–1920) White government during the Civil War in Siberia in 1919 – was General Baron Aleksei Pavlovich Budberg (1869–1945), a distant kinsman from an Estland branch of the Budberg family tree.

This General Budberg left Siberia for Vladivostok in the Russian Far East and from there journeyed to a safer haven in Harbin, Manchuria, in October 1919. In 1923 he joined his eldest son, Peter, in California.[12] Peter, who had first heard Chinese on the streets of Vladivostok and Harbin, stopped using his title soon after reaching the United States and retranscribed his name. As Peter A. Boodberg (1903–1972) he became a professor of Chinese philology at the University of California, Berkeley.[13] The Lithuanian-born émigré Czesław Miłosz (1911–2004), who wrote poetry in Polish while teaching Slavic literatures at the same university, evoked the memory of Boodberg in "A Magic Mountain" (1975), a poem about Berkeley and academic exile, in which he restored his colleague's surname to its original spelling with some quiet wonder at the transformation of a displaced scion of Baltic German aristocrats into an American scholar of ancient China: "Budberg: a familiar name in my childhood./They were prominent in our region,/This Russian family, descendants of German Balts ..."[14] Today the professor and his father the general are – in different circles – the best-known Budbergs of the twentieth century, a distinction they share with an émigré Russian adventuress, suspected Soviet spy, translator of Russian literature, and British grande dame, who, however, only bore the Budberg name as the relic of a brief marriage.[15]

Theirs was a great family on their mother's side as well, and the Counts Anrep-Elmpt claimed no less a connection to the Baltic. Originally from the German Rhineland like the Budbergs, the Anreps came to Russia by way of Sweden in the sixteenth century. Among Roger's immediate maternal ancestors, another roster of military men began with his great-grandfather, Heinrich Reinhold von Anrep (1760–1807), a graduate of the most prestigious educational institution in tsarist Russia, the Imperial Corps of Pages in Saint Petersburg. He was a Lieutenant-General of the Infantry when he fell in the battle of Mohrungen (East Prussia, now Poland) against Napoleon's army.[16] His eldest son, Cavalry General Joseph Carl von Anrep (1796–1860), was also educated at the Corps of Pages. He added "Elmpt" to the family name in 1853 to preserve the title of the Counts von Elmpt, which his wife Cecilia (1812–1892), the daughter and granddaughter of tsarist generals, was the last to bear. Count Anrep-Elmpt fought in the Crimean War and died in Saint Petersburg, reportedly of his battle wounds. His wife then moved to Burgau Castle near Düren in the Rhineland, which had belonged to her family since the fifteenth century. Thirty years after the Count's death, she was buried there in the castle garden.[17] When he was in his fifties, Roger recalled how he used to write to his beloved maternal grandmother daily or even twice a day from the Baltic. He told his sister that his spiritual bond with their grandmother had influenced his whole life.[18]

The eldest brother of Roger Budberg's mother was the cavalry officer Count Reinhold Anrep-Elmpt (1834–1888), another alumnus of the Corps of Pages, turned world traveller and explorer. Uncle Raimond, as Roger and his siblings called him, was seldom to be found in the Baltic homeland after he embarked on his expeditions in 1870; he communicated with his mother and wife by post. Called back to Riga from Australia after the death of his brother, Joseph Alexander (1844–1880), he spent some difficult months at home between 1881 and 1882,[19] only to set out again for Australian shores. By the following summer he had returned to Europe; he began his last world tour from Leipzig in 1887.[20] According to one colourful family version, he died of the plague en route (his favourite niece Antoinette said in her memoirs that his body was thrown overboard for fear of infection); according to another, of tropical fever in Siam or Burma.[21] Roger was then twenty-one. Although nowhere in his writings does Roger mention him, he must have known the four books in which his uncle described his travels: Anrep-Elmpt gave at least two of the four to his sister Alexandrine.

If Roger read the last of them, handsomely printed and bound in Leipzig in 1887, perhaps he noticed some original observations and opinions in the chapter about China, which could have surfaced in memory when he too reached that country. Entering Chinese waters for the first time through the estuary of the Pearl River, Anrep-Elmpt noted with approval that China was not in too much of a haste to accept "the tempting poison of European civilization." Although critical of the prostitution in Canton, he felt that the usual Western reports on Chinese dirt only reflected the density of the population (the average Chinese was not clean, but did keep his bedroom and kitchen in scrupulous cleanliness); and he wrote that a brief visit to that southern city would leave a foreigner with the wrong impression of China. That impression would change considerably for the better once the visitor became familiar with the character of the Chinese people and their many good qualities. Anrep-Elmpt called for a pluralistic outlook on the mores and values of non-European nations, and he saw China as the victim of prejudice disseminated by missionaries and sailors. In truth, he wrote, even the Chinese way of smoking would have been healthier than our own, if only their tobacco tasted better. Donations were being collected in Europe to save Chinese orphans and avert alleged child-killing, yet infanticide was rarer here than in our own civilized countries, and one could say the same about the comparative levels of criminality (only in the treaty ports, which Westerners had forced China to open, was a police force needed). The Chinese taxation system was actually superior to the European one, while stories about polygamy were exaggerated – most Chinese men had a single wife. All things considered, in no other country had he encountered such warm family relations and so little unhappiness. To gain another opportunity "to study the particularities of the Chinese race," he would share the second deck with Chinese passengers as he continued his voyage aboard an American steamship from Hong Kong to Yokohama.[22]

Home

Home was there, on the banks of the river Mēmele (Memel in German; Nemunėlis in Lithuanian), about 20 kilometres southeast of Bauska Castle, which itself was 60 kilometres south of Riga. Years later, this river would serve as a border between Latvia and Lithuania after both had gained their independence from the Russian empire and driven back a Bolshevik incursion. Courland and Semigallia, which made up the Governorate of Courland under the tsars, became the regions of Kurzeme and Zemgale in the Latvian Republic; the land south of the Mēmele was initially transferred to Lithuania before passing back to Latvia in the border adjustments of 1921. Today the state border here follows the course of the Lithuanian river Mūsa.

Physical traces of their home are all but gone: only the name of the village, Budberga, in Panemune parish of Bauska region in southern-most Latvia, the memories of elderly residents, the restored nineteenth-century church, and the ruins of the family cemetery still harbour the spirits of the barons, keeping them from vanishing entirely from the land. On an October day in 2008, I walked up to the cemetery in what is now Budberga Park. The gravestone of Alexander Budberg, Roger's father, was the only one that could still be detected above ground. Time had separated it from its headstone, and it had lost the tall marble cross that originally towered above it.[23] After brushing aside the autumn leaves I could make out the dates, 6 December 1834 to 6 May 1906.

Alexander Budberg's own father Andreas acquired this manor in 1834, the year of his marriage and of the birth of his first son. They called it Gemauert (Walled) Poniemon in German and Murovanyi Ponemun in Russian. Both variants referred to the river's Lithuanian name, Nemunėlis. Located at the northern tip of Ponevezhskii *uezd* (the county named after the town now called Panevėžys in Lithuania), in Kovenskaia guberniia (the Governorate of Kovno, established in 1843, which had its capital seat in Kaunas, or Kovno/Kowno in Russian and Polish), it was too small to be recorded on most maps. Alexander's younger brothers, Andreas (1836–1916; Roger's much respected "Uncle André") and Joseph, were the first of the Budbergs to be born in the manor. In 1849, Alexander's maternal aunt Luise drowned while bathing in the Memel and was laid to rest in Poniemon; so was Alexander's father in 1855.[24] Alexander himself must have been the last of the family to be buried there, at the dawn of a new century. Of Roger's seven siblings, all but one came into the world, like him, in Poniemon: Joseph, his eldest brother, in May 1862; his brother Gotthard in June 1863 and sister Marie in September 1864; so also his younger sisters Cecile in April 1868 and Antoinette in March 1870, and brother Wilhelm in November 1871.[25] Only the youngest of the children, Alexandrine, was born in the manor north of Riga, the Magnushof, which was the family's second home, in September 1874.[26]

Ironically, Budberga officially received this name only after it no longer belonged to the Budbergs. In December 1890, Baroness Alexandrine, mother of the eight, requested to have Murovanyi Ponemun (with its population of 139 people) renamed Budberg and united with the adjacent village (population 109), which was already informally known by this name. She proposed that the joint locality be classified administratively as *mestechko*: literally, "little place," a term often used for small towns with a Jewish majority. The authorities in Kovno turned down her request, pointing out, among other reasons for their decision, that it would enable Jews to legally settle in the village. Undaunted, the baroness appealed to the State Senate, but that governing body, too, rejected her argument that it would be best to concentrate the area's Jews in one locality, "little place Budberg."[27] Budberga village was recognized by the Latvian Republic in the 1920s, after the baronial estate was nationalized.

In 2008, when the local resident Andrejs Žemaitis took me and the Latvian sinologist Kaspars Eihmanis to the manor cemetery, he approached a village woman to ask her to point out the tomb of "the Moor" for us. With an air of having shown the spot to visitors before, she led us confidently to a heavy slab of rock, a few metres higher up the slope, under which she said the Moor lay. This was the black servant, about whom I had already heard from the first person of Budberga origin with whom I had spoken, in Riga in 2004. My informant's grandmother had told her that the servant's name was Abdulla; the Budbergs had

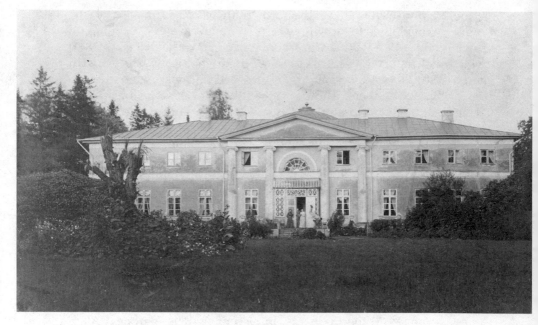

2.1. Gemauert Poniemon, the Budberg family manor. Photograph,
before 1900. Raczynski family album, Chile.

married him to a Latvian woman. When she herself went to school in
Budberga, one of her classmates was a dark-skinned girl – a descendant of the Moor.[28] In the Žemaitis house I saw a photograph of the
Budberga schoolchildren in 1938, which included a brother and sister
of that same background. Valentina Žemaite, Andrejs's wife, believed
that the Moor had fathered about seventeen children in the neighbourhood. Later that day, the oldest inhabitant of the village, Kārlis Āzis,
would estimate their number more conservatively at between twelve
and fourteen.[29]

In the park, on the hill leading up to the cemetery, only the dilapidated
mausoleum bearing the German inscription "Ruhe" (Peace) at the top
of its front wall still stands. The entrance to it has been cemented over,
but at the time of my first visit an opening above ground still allowed
a glimpse into the dark debris within. This mausoleum had been built
by the manor's first owners, the Barons Grotthuss. Kārlis Āzis, born in
1923 to a family that has lived in this village for two centuries, unhesitat-
ingly gave the year of its construction as 1823. In 1925, Latvian ethnographers recorded stories here about the cruel "Grotūzis," who "about

a hundred years ago" had harnessed local girls to draw his carriage to the water source. It was said that he died a horrible death and that his body had been bound with ropes before it was lowered into the vault.[30]

Members of the Budberg family have preserved photographs of the Poniemon manor. In the round main hall, a glass cupola let daylight in and the stars were visible at night; huge exotic plants resembling American agaves, next to a banana tree and a cactus, grew in pots along walls decorated with enormous tapestries, one showing a tree with branches and leaves, the other a heraldic tree, the branches and leaves of which represented the names of people. There was also a large park, where their father planted eight trees with his own hands, a new tree every time a child was born.[31] The servants had been recruited from the barons' former serfs (the serfs in Estland, Courland, and Livland were emancipated in the 1810s, decades before those in Russia); there was a Russian chef, called Ivan, with his kitchen staff, and an old Estonian coachman. But the baron's children were not allowed to talk to them, and they were also forbidden to speak during meals – almost the only time of day that they saw their mother.

They grew up with parents who had little in common. Their mother, the formidable worldly aristocrat, must have felt hemmed in in Poniemon. While there, she hosted grand dinner receptions, accompanied by dancing and fireworks; there were always guests in the house, and some, like a number of painters from Munich, spent months at the manor. She painted well herself. Often she would go away, whether to stay in Riga, make one of her calls to the court in Saint Petersburg, travel in Italy, or spend "the season" at Bad Ems, a favoured destination for the Russian nobility by the Rhine in Germany, when the three monarchs, Franz Joseph of Austria, Wilhelm I of Germany (godfather of her son Wilhelm), and Alexander II of Russia (godfather of her daughter Alexandrine) were all present. During such absences, Aunt Lonny, the wife of Uncle Raimond the explorer, took their mother's place.

This was just as well, because she would not punish them the way their mother did when she caught them making mischief: by hitting a child on his fingertips, after sticking needles in them; or by burning a child with the wax used to seal letters. Or by making us stand in the corner, for two hours, on a special plank that kept our feet turned in opposite directions until we memorized a fable by Krylov in Russian or La Fontaine in French. Mother only spoke to us in French. When she summoned us to her bedroom or to father's, it meant we would be beaten with the leather whip or the steel whip, which was worse. I remember being slapped with mother's ringed hand when I made mistakes in my prayers. We were not allowed to cry, as we were punished even harder for crying and we had to kiss the whip after being beaten, wrote Antoinette.[32]

They saw their father even less. He had no time for them, between managing his properties and performing his duties as justice of the peace. When not busy with these tasks, he prepared the genealogical tables that were meant to put in long-needed order the hopelessly entangled branches of the Budberg-Bönninghausen family tree, or he devoted himself to his hobbies: numismatics, archaeology, and chemical experiments. A man of varied interests, he had travelled in Europe, visiting Germany, Belgium, England, and Scotland, with a predilection for Italy and the south of France.[33] On the only occasion that his wife asked him to give Wilhelm a beating (being in a hurry for a ball, she had no time to do so herself), he broke the birch after she left the room and, on her return, pretended to have administered the punishment; only the child's laughter gave him away. The children were first put in the care of wet nurses, then passed on to Russian nannies until about the age of five. Their next "stations" as they grew older were with a French *bonne supérieure*, an English *nurse*, and a German *Gouvernante*.

In 1889, shortly before she attempted to unite Poniemon with the village that served it, Alexandrine Budberg opened a private agricultural institute on the manor's property, offering a two-year course in farming and housekeeping to women of all nationalities aged sixteen to thirty. With a small subsidy from the government, she invested much of her private fortune in the school, which was a novelty in Russia and even attracted international attention.[34] Locally, it created tensions with the village. The baroness inspired fear among the villagers, who criticized her for wasting too much money on her constant travels, old Kārlis Āzis said.[35] He had only good words about Baron Alexander. His grandparents told him the baron would doff his hat first even when encountering the poorest peasants. Although the villagers were forbidden to enter the manor grounds unless summoned for work there, when the baron saw local women gathering edible grass on his fields, he instructed his bailiff not to chase them away. Āzis's grandfather, a goldsmith, made the baron's coffin in 1906.

Life was freer for the children in Magnushof near Riga. It was located on the northern bank of the Stindsee, where the lake flowed into the Düna as that great river made its way to the sea. Just as in Poniemon, they lived here by the water, with an abundance of fish instead of the crabs that populated the Memel, and plenty of birds and wild game in the surrounding forest. One cannot repeat today the exact route by which they used to reach that other, happier home of their childhood. Steamboats no longer carry passengers from Riga on the river Daugava (the Düna, in German; the Russian Dvina, which flows for more than 1,000 kilometres from Russia through Belarus to Latvia and into the Baltic sea). After sailing about 7 kilometres north, they would dock at the port of Mīlgrāvis (former Mühlgraben), which is now used by large cargo ships. Using more modern forms of transport, one can cross the Daugava and continue another 4 kilometres north along a highway winding along the shore of Lake Ķīšezers, still the haven of fishermen, until one reaches Mangali, a part of the Riga metropolis now associated mainly with the brand name of a Latvian mineral water.

Local history buffs have identified a wooden house here as "the Mangali manor," and it does seem to match the place that Roger's sister Antoinette described in her memoirs. However, to dispel that illusion, one need only read the memoirs of Joseph A. Raczynski (1914–1999), the family chronicler, about visits he and his mother made to Magnushof and Poniemon during their trip to Latvia in 1937. At that time, Magnushof already lay in ruins, and Antoinette shed a tear at the sight.[36]

Studies

What did the future hold in store for Roger? What could he become? Growing up, he would have looked to the people nearest to him for inspiration or for a simple roster of possibilities. When he was nine, he probably heard about the death of his uncle, Joseph Budberg (1843–1876), near Fort Vernyi, the capital of Semirechie province near the Chinese border (now Almaty in Kazakhstan) – the unfortunate conclusion of a military career, which so many other Barons Budberg had chosen.[37] But both joining the army and entering the tsarist diplomatic service were less appealing by the 1880s than they had been during the height of the Romanov dynasty. In 1881, Alexander II was assassinated by a member of the People's Will movement; after the mid-1880s, his successor Alexander III pursued a policy of Russifying the Baltic Germans, which aroused their antagonism.[38] Even so, Roger's parents sent his brother Wilhelm, four years his junior, to an elite military college in Saint Petersburg.

Another direction that some family members had taken was academic study. And here too, there was a well-trodden path that led young men from the Baltic provinces to the University of Dorpat in the Governorate of Livland. The town of Dorpat had been renamed Iur'ev under Alexander III, and since 1917 it has borne the Estonian name Tartu (Dorpat and Tartu will be used interchangeably in this book). Tartu has long been famous for its academic tradition, which can be traced back to its university's founding under Swedish rule in 1632. Under the tsars, teaching at the university continued in German, long the language of culture and education in the region, until the government ordered a switch to Russian in 1895. The University of Dorpat was the beloved alma mater of Baltic German aristocrats, as well as commoners. However, especially after the 1890s, they had to share its classrooms – if not actually rub shoulders – with Russians, Poles, Jews, Estonians, and Latvians. Roger Budberg's father had graduated from the still autonomous, German-managed Dorpat in both law and chemistry, the latter being a less traditional choice.

Roger was a gifted and unruly child. The best athlete, who could swim across the Daugava on a bet, or climb a greased pole in a competition in which everyone else failed, he was also a reluctant and late learner. For his primary education, he was sent to a private German boarding school in Doblen (Dobele, in today's central Latvia), probably the first time he had to live away from home.[39] When he reached twelve, he was admitted to the Governorate Gymnasium in Riga, the well-respected classical high school on Castle Square (now Pils laukums) in the Old Town, which his father had attended.[40] Joseph went to the same gymnasium, graduating in 1882; when Roger enrolled there in 1879, their brother Gotthard was sent to another Riga school, the Realschule. Antoinette remembered that their mother kept a large apartment on Riga's Bastion Boulevard. The children went to watch punishments and executions "on a large square very near to Castle Square and our house"; following one such outing, Roger tried to re-enact the hanging scene for his siblings, including the climax of the hanged man's tongue sticking out, and was saved by the governess, who fortunately happened to enter their room.[41]

After two years the Governorate Gymnasium expelled him, perhaps for pranks of that sort, or for poor achievement, which his teacher noted in the class diary.[42] Budberg never mentioned his Riga schooling, omitting it even from the CV he submitted to Dorpat University.[43] It took a special teacher, a baroness who knew his parents, saw his potential, and believed in him, for Roger to apply himself to his studies. When he was fifteen, he joined a private school for boys, which the baroness (a member of one of the most ancient Baltic German families in Livland, who was known to everyone as Aunt Locca) ran in Adiamünde, today's Skulte, 50 kilometres northeast of Riga.[44] And in the summer of 1884 he was again able to enter a gymnasium, now in Goldingen (Kuldiga), in western Latvia.

In this small, picturesque town on the river Venta (the oldest town and capital of the Duchy of Courland from its creation until the transition to Russian rule in 1795), he spent another three and a half years at his studies, graduating in the winter of 1887.[45] He may have enjoyed more freedom there than ever before. His final grades were still mediocre: he managed only a "sufficient" in German while getting "good" in both Russian language and literature and Russian history. His behaviour and diligence were generally deemed "very good," yet "interest in taught subjects" lagged behind as "sufficient."[46]

In January 1888, when he was twenty-one years old, he lost no time enrolling in Dorpat University. Initially he followed in the footsteps of his father and elder brother by entering the Law Faculty. The university register for 1889 shows Joseph and Rotgert Budberg living together at rented accommodations on 10 Market Street (Marktstrasse, today's Turu Street), by the river Embach (Estonian: Emajõgi).[47] However, Joseph, who had enrolled in 1883, accepted a challenge to a duel in February 1888, in the course of which he wounded his adversary, who later died. Joseph was then suspended from the university. In a second duel near Dorpat, in May 1890, he again wounded a man and soon left town to twice stand trial, in Riga and Saint Petersburg. After appealing to the tsar, he served only four months in prison instead of three years. Having graduated from Dorpat despite these events, he could begin a long career as a judge in provincial Russia.[48] Roger continued to live at the same address at least until 1892, by which time he was a second-year student of medicine.

His switch to medicine, despite the good grades he had earned in the Law Faculty, was not acceptable to his parents.[49] Late in life, he would recall that they cut off their support and that he suffered badly from hunger during his medical studies.[50] While destitution was certainly uncommon for a member of his class, so too was becoming a doctor. According to his sister's memoirs, as a practising physician in Dorpat, he often treated patients without charge since it was unheard of for a baron to request payment for his services.[51]

Once he graduated, "Dr" would join "Baron" in becoming essential to his self-definition. Meanwhile, like his father and Joseph, he joined the Curonia fraternity, which united students of Courland origin – one of the many fraternities that were a central feature of student life. He also joined the Dorpat Society for Nature Research.[52] The main source on this period, his papers in the university archives, mentions his medical work during the cholera epidemics of 1892 and 1893.[53] This first but not last encounter with the terrors of epidemic disease took him east of Dorpat, to the Chudskoe (Estonian: Peipsi) Lake region between Estland and Russia. In May 1897, together with other assistants of his academic supervisor, the German director of the university's surgery clinic Wilhelm Koch (1842–1919), he provided urgent medical assistance to casualties of a railway disaster at Bockenhof. A military train had derailed at that station on the Baltic railway line, south of Dorpat; fifty-eight people had died and many were injured. Budberg received the tsarist order of St Stanislaus, third grade, which was probably awarded to all the junior physicians who participated in this effort.[54]

If he had close attachments or important relationships in Dorpat, this biographer has not uncovered them. His sister Antoinette, however, recalled a particular preoccupation of his student years – redeeming fallen women. Roger spent a good deal of his scant resources in the name of this chivalric cause, buying the girls from brothel owners, although his fellow students mocked him.[55]

After obtaining his diploma in 1895, he specialized in gynaecology and midwifery; in 1897 and 1898 he worked as an assistant in the university's women's clinic.[56] One gets an idea of his large practice and the kinds of patients he treated from a report, written in the winter of 1898, in which he noted that he had disinfected the umbilical cord (by means of alcohol, a method he favoured) in "two hundred cases, quite among the poorest and almost without exception very unclean class of the population."[57] An announcement he placed in the principal Estonian newspaper, *Postimees* (The Postman), informed the public of his daily reception hours at Alexanderstrasse 28 and his willingness to travel out and deliver babies in the countryside.[58] Budberg probably had some knowledge of Estonian, perhaps even the Tartu dialect of South Estonian spoken in the villages, although, in the town of Tartu, there was also a pidgin that enabled communication between Estonians and Germans.[59] He is on record as reaching out to Estonians, through a six-page medical essay (which may have been translated on his behalf), published in a popular calendar in 1902, offering advice and instructions for women on pregnancy, childbirth, and care of the newborn.[60]

In May 1902, Budberg defended his doctoral dissertation, which he had submitted the previous year – a study of the large intestine as it related to the development of the foetus. He dedicated it to the memory of his maternal grandmother, with love to his parents. He also thanked his supervisor, Wilhelm Koch, for "many years of fatherly friendship." After another spell as an assistant at the women's clinic, between May 1901 and October 1902, the University Senate awarded him the title of Privatdozent in January 1903.[61] Specialized articles by Budberg appeared in German and Russian medical journals. They dealt with such questions as how best to extract the placenta – also the subject of his inaugural lecture in the Dorpat University women's clinic in March 1903, where he described a method he had devised and performed on as many as 3,000 women in childbirth since 1898 – and how to treat the remains of the umbilical cord after birth (he recommended that midwives use green soap as a disinfectant).[62]

In May 1903, a curious announcement appeared in the same Estonian daily: a wet nurse for a three-week-old baby girl was being sought, with the contact person indicated as Dr Baron Budberg, now living at another rented apartment in Tartu (12 Suurturg; in German: Grosser Markt).[63] In June he began employment as house physician for a Count and Countess Tolstoy in the Russian interior, where he remained until mid-October. He wrote to Antoinette that he hoped to use the opportunity to improve his Russian and find time for his "literary work."[64] It is unclear quite what he meant by the latter and why he wished to raise his Russian above the good functional level he already possessed. One could speculate on whether he needed to go away then (perhaps it was just a lucrative appointment). He was thirty-seven and had built up a library and a modest art collection.[65] Would he stay on in Tartu as a physician, a university teacher, perhaps also an amateur writer? Would he move his private practice to Riga, marry a woman of his standing, and do his part in securing the continuation of the Budberg line? Once before, his restless nature had surfaced and he had sought radical change in the midst of what appears to have been a steady career climb in the Baltic environment that was so familiar to him. Although he had travelled abroad on only one occasion (to Germany, after his grandmother's death in 1893), in October 1899 he applied to join a mission of the Russian Red Cross to the Transvaal.[66] But the war with Japan in Manchuria turned him in another direction, which must have been unexpected for him as well as a surprise for those who knew him.

To China

War broke out on 28 January 1904 (10 February, by the Gregorian calendar used outside Russia), two days after Admiral Togo attacked the Russian fleet at Port Arthur, Manchuria. Within two weeks, Roger Budberg was named plenipotentiary and senior physician to the floating hospitals of the Russian Red Cross on the rivers Amur and Sungari (by their Chinese names: Heilongjiang and Songhuajiang).[67] That was how he suddenly found himself in China. In these late days of empire, members of the Russian and Baltic German nobility continued to move within the same circles; thus, the telegram informing the university rector in Dorpat of Baron Budberg's appointment bore the signature of a relative, Vasilii Anrep (1852–1927), a professor of medicine and pioneer anaesthesiologist. Anrep was a member of the Executive Committee in the Main Directorate of the Russian Red Cross Society. In that capacity he received a telegram from Baroness Budberg, née Countess Anrep-Elmpt, on 16 April. Using Russian rather than German but deliberately addressing the professor by their shared surname, she wrote to inquire whether "medical personnel have been sent to my son for [equipment of] the floating hospitals."[68] Anrep replied that this had been done.

Despite this reassuring answer from the Russian branch of the family, all was not well, and the sparse information on Budberg's wartime service suggests that conflict between him and his superiors began to brew at an early stage. Contrary to the version of his war record that was later included in his published memoirs and repeated by his sister, he did not reach Manchuria as a member of the Baltic medical brigade equipped for the Russian Red Cross by Empress Maria Fedorovna (1867–1928), mother of the reigning Tsar Nicholas II. He was already there before the arrival of "Her Majesty's flying column," which was also known as "the column of Professor Zoege" after the famous Dorpat surgeon who headed it.[69] Budberg was ordered to report to Sretensk, a port on the Shilka River in the Transbaikal province, which since 1900 had been the terminus of the Trans-Siberian Railway.[70] In peacetime, peasant and Cossack settlers bound for the Amur province or Manchuria sailed downriver on steamers and barges from Sretensk. In late March, a nurse named Else Riemer wrote a telegram from Tartu in a mixture of German and Russian, expressing her urgent wish to volunteer for "the detachment of barge lazarettos under the management of Baron Budberg." She was told that no such detachment was being formed.[71] Budberg's larger ambitions for establishing lazarettos were overruled by the Chief Plenipotentiary of the Russian Red Cross with the Maritime and Amur armies, Prince Boris Vasil'chikov (1860–1931).[72]

Despite these setbacks, Budberg apparently had his way: in June the Baltic German press told readers that he had arrived in Blagoveshchensk on the 14th to oversee the journey of five barges to Harbin.[73] But then, in July, a Russian newspaper in Riga reported that he had died of typhus in Manchuria.[74] As the news spread across the Baltic, there followed an outpouring of praise for all the good work Budberg had done as a physician in Tartu, especially in treating the town's poor. The interest in him in the Estonian press reflected his prestige in Tartu, notwithstanding the ethnic tensions between Estonians and the Baltic German nobility. It took almost a month for the rumour to be squelched by a letter from Budberg himself, who conveyed his greetings to the readers of *Postimees* in Tartu. A Tallinn weekly reported that far from being dead, Baron Budberg had established his floating hospitals so efficiently that he had earned a congratulatory cable from the sister of the tsar, Grand Duchess Xenia Aleksandrovna (1875–1960).[75]

An American medical observer of the Russo-Japanese War left a description of the Russian floating hospitals along with a verdict on their efficacy:

Beside hospital trains, I should also mention the flotilla of hospital boats built by the [Russian] Government and partly by the Red Cross for the evacuation of the sick and wounded from Harbin, by the Sungari river to the Amur, to be distributed along that mighty stream to Khabaroff [Khabarovsk], Blagovestchensk, and Chita. These boats are flat, two-decked barges, with a capacity of about 130 beds, towed by tugs. The scheme was a failure. Owing to the variable stage of water in the Sungari in summer, from flood to complete dryness, the travel up and down the river is very uncertain, many days being spent on sand banks. In winter, the boats, bound up in ice, become too cold to be habitable. They have been abandoned.[76]

An internal report by the Russian Red Cross in late 1904 presented the scheme in a more favourable light: granted that the idea of evacuating wounded men on boats and barges over long distances had proved absurdly inefficient, the barges were still put to good use once they were turned into stationary hospitals. Moored opposite the town of Harbin, along the "entirely deserted" left bank of the Sungari, they were soon converted to accommodate convalescing officers. Prince Vasil'chikov had initially rejected the model for equipping the barges, which Budberg, together with an engineer named Kochendörffer, had devised in Sretensk. That model was accepted, however, after the author of this report was appointed full-time plenipotentiary of the Red Cross in Harbin.[77]

Medical assistance to the troops was not the only aspect of warfare in which Japan had proved better prepared (as even the above-cited Russian report acknowledged). Painful retreats followed the battles at Liaoyang in late August 1904 and at Shahe, south of Mukden, in October of the same year. Russia was losing the war. Heads rolled: the defeat at Shahe led to the recall of Admiral Evgenii Alekseev (1843–1917), who had been named the tsar's viceroy in the Far East in August 1903. The Russian Baltic fleet, with forty-two ships and a crew of 12,000 men, sailed from the port of Liepāja (German: Libau) in Courland in October 1904 only to be destroyed in May 1905 at the Tsushima Strait between Korea and Japan after its delayed arrival. In January 1905, the Russian fortress at Port Arthur surrendered after a Japanese siege of five months. In an atmosphere of intensifying public dissatisfaction with the war's progress, Budberg lodged a complaint against what he argued was mismanagement of funds by the Russian Red Cross. He accused Vasil'chikov of personal corruption but proved unable to pursue the matter, probably because of the prince's connections at the tsar's court.[78]

Apparently in connection with this complaint, Budberg returned briefly to European Russia: after reporting to Saint Petersburg he passed through Poniemon, to leave again for Manchuria in February 1905. He had brought a Chinese boy with him, whom he called Sjödro (the first syllable in this transcription perhaps standing for *xiao*, little), and left him behind in the care of his father.[79] There were precedents for such imports. The Budbergs' black servant, "the Moor" Abdallah, had reached Europe after Baron Tettow, a German diplomat, purchased him as a child in a slave market in either Sudan or Egypt. He escaped from the baron, returned to his African homeland, learned that his siblings of the Faraj clan wanted to kill him for becoming Christian, escaped again via Cairo by joining a travelling theatre troupe from Tiflis (now Tbilisi in Georgia), and wandered through Russia with it before being noticed in Riga by Roger's mother. She brought him to Poniemon and had him married against his will to a fifteen-year-old girl from Schwitten, who had become pregnant by a count. The couple would have another sixteen children after the count's first. Six of them were raised by Antoinette and her husband Sigismund Raczynski (1861–1937); two sisters were taken to Rome by Marie in the 1900s.[80] Roger may have acted similarly in China, buying a child to be his servant or perhaps his adoptive son. His father wrote that Sjödro "belonged" to him.

Roger wrote weekly to his father after his second departure. However, a letter from "Liugan" (probably, Liaoyang) in late August was followed by protracted silence, which led the old baron to fear for his son's life: on 6 December he wondered, in a letter to Antoinette, whether Rogert's "love for taking excursions, which he tied to his ethnographic studies, might not have landed him in the hands of robbers or *Choncusen*" (from the Russian *khunkhuz*, a calque of the Chinese *hong huzi*, literally redbeards: the common term for Manchurian bandits). On 14 November, a general strike in Russia paralysed the postal services, and only in early January 1906 did Roger's next message get through, a telegram from Kuanchengzi, the railway station near Changchun in Jilin. He asked his father to send Sjödro to him: starting from Riga, the boy was to collect a microscope, clothes, and more of Roger's belongings in Dorpat, and then continue on to Saint Petersburg, where Kochendörffer would provide him with travel money.[81] He was expedited accordingly, reaching the engineer, Roger's recent associate in the equipping of barges in Sretensk, who then alerted Baron Alexander that it would presently be too risky to let little Sjödro travel on his own through turbulent Siberia. The father replied that since Rogert "missed his boy so much," he would appreciate it if Kochendörffer kept Sjödro with him until the opportunity should arise to send him to Manchuria. Writing about this to Antoinette, Alexander Budberg (then in the last months of his life) added that he had accepted the suggestion of a Dr Kramer, a friend of his son's in Dorpat, to have Rogert's apartment there cleared out and the remaining furniture sent over to Poniemon: for in each of his letters home, the father said, Rogert has insisted that he did not wish to return to the Baltic and would make his future in China.

In what must have been the autumn of 1904, he met in Mukden his second cousin, the railway engineer Prince Paul Lieven (1875–1963), who headed a field lazaretto of the Red Cross representing the Governorate of Livland. Budberg persuaded him to leave the Red Cross railcar for a day's stroll in Mukden and a night in a Chinese tavern. He then displayed an ability to enjoy sleeping on the *kang*, the heated brick bed common in north China, that left his younger relative incredulous, all the more so as Lieven was unable to handle the chopsticks offered him at breakfast.[82] Budberg's own acculturation, after only half a year in China, had been remarkably quick.

Antoinette would recount that in her brother's second term of service in Manchuria in 1905, he was placed under the command of General Rennenkampf, a Baltic German and, of course, a relative. The general told Roger he would leave him free to do his own work as long as Roger did not meddle in his. Paul Georg (by his Russian name, Pavel Karlovich) Rennenkampf (1854–1918) was commander of the Transbaikal Cossack Regiment. An account based on information from Budberg himself, in the publisher's introduction to his memoirs, says that on the advice of General Otto Richter (1830–1908) he had transferred as a physician from the Red Cross to the Fourth East Siberian Rifle Regiment and then to the Third.[83] Both sources describe a special arrangement that freed him from his duties in the last months of the war, thus affording him the leisure to explore China. As a gynaecologist, Budberg would probably have been of little use on the battlefield. According to the same publisher's introduction (which does not mention Rennenkampf), Major-General Pavel K. Dombrovskii (1848–after 1917) allowed Budberg to move from the Russian army base to a Chinese town; and Lieutenant-General Nikolai I. Ivanov (1851–1919) permitted him to stay on in Manchuria rather than return to Saint Petersburg when he was summoned there for the second time. The town in which he settled "in complete isolation from Europeans" and began studying Chinese was then called Fenghua. Russians knew it by the local Chinese dialectal

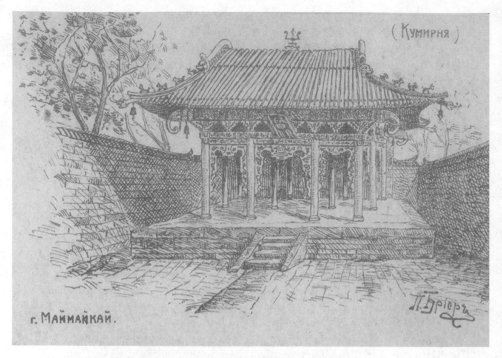

2.2. A temple in Maimaikai. Drawing by P. Brier. Postcard about 1905.
Author's collection.

appellation, Maimaigai (Trade Town); today this is the county town of
Lishu, administered by Siping City in Jilin province.[84] Budberg would
recall fondly the hours he spent among peasant children during the war
in Manchuria as he wandered through Chinese villages on his walks.[85]

The defeat of the Russian army in the decisive Battle of Mukden in
February 1905 led to the resignation of General Aleksei Kuropatkin
(1848–1925) as supreme commander of the Russian land and naval
forces in East Asia. The war ended in early September (late August, by
the Russian calendar), and the revolutionary unrest, which had been on
the rise since a suppressed demonstration in Saint Petersburg in January ("Bloody Sunday"), soon forced the tsar to sign the October Mani-
festo, which granted limited powers to a new parliament, the State
Duma. Baron Alexander Budberg, the distant relation of the family
who headed the Chancellery of Petitions, was part of the select group
of State Council members who advised the monarch on this epoch-
making document.[86] It did help quell the revolution by December.

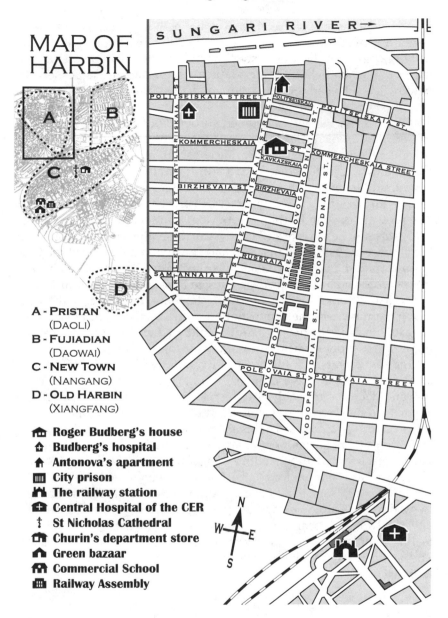

MAP OF HARBIN

A - PRISTAN
   (DAOLI)
B - FUJIADIAN
   (DAOWAI)
C - NEW TOWN
   (NANGANG)
D - OLD HARBIN
   (XIANGFANG)

🏠 Roger Budberg's house
⛪ Budberg's hospital
🏠 Antonova's apartment
▥ City prison
🏚 The railway station
✚ Central Hospital of the CER
✝ St Nicholas Cathedral
🏠 Churin's department store
🏠 Green bazaar
🏠 Commercial School
🏛 Railway Assembly

2.3. Harbin in Roger Budberg's time, indicating the main streets and places
mentioned in this book. Map created by the Riga artist Reinis Gailītis
on the basis of the map in S.M. Fomenko, *Sputnik po Dal'nemu Vostoku*
(A Companion to the Far East) (Shanghai: Russkoe knigoizdatel'stvo
i tipografiia v Shankhae, 1919).

In faraway Saratov on the Volga River, rebellious peasants had meanwhile destroyed the estate of Uncle André Budberg's young wife Marie, née Princess Kugusheva. The shock waves of the revolution were also felt in Poniemon, where Roger's father, one of the few Baltic German landowners who had chosen to remain on their estates, had to deal with robbers, bandit gangs, and, while his wife was vacationing in Rome, a political strike among the women students of her school. A casualty of the times, which Alexander Budberg mentioned in a letter to his daughter Cecile, was the "beautiful castle" of "the poor Budberg from Wannamois," a former chief district administrator in Estland.[87] After an assault on Magnushof, his youngest daughter Alexandrine, who lived there with her brother Gotthard, fled to a Riga hotel for two weeks.[88] The pressing issue in Harbin, where Roger Budberg was living by late 1905, was not the railway strike, nor was it the mysterious fires that (in the absence of castles and manors) had consumed buildings of the CER administration, but the challenge of transporting 100,000 demobilized troops, who had just lost the war, back to Russia from Manchuria.[89]

The list of persons in the Far East who were decorated by the Russian government for their contribution to the war effort in 1904 (a very long list, considering the poor results) did not include Roger Budberg's name.[90] An application he submitted on the eve of the war for the position of professor at his home university was turned down.[91] The appointment might have brought him back to Dorpat; the failure of his candidacy and probably also the rejection of his wartime complaint against his superiors must have sealed his decision to stay in China. In the first surviving postcard to his sister from Harbin, dated 23 July 1906 (O.S.), he described the new apartment he had just moved into that morning: it had "a bedroom with a plank *kang*, where I can be Chinese." There was also "a room for Sjödro," who by then must have made the perilous voyage from Saint Petersburg, "and eventually for the others." In his next postcard, two days later, he explained why he no longer had any need for European luxury: "For myself, however, I am Chinese, feeling completely at ease on my plank *kang* and with my chopsticks."[92] The next natural step for him toward becoming more fully Chinese was to find a Chinese wife.

3

Intermediaries and Channels of Communication

Arriving from various parts of their countries to meet in Manchuria, Russians and Chinese (including members of the many ethnicities affiliated with the two nations) could not communicate with each other at first. Early attempts to question peasants on the name of their village resulted in bewildered responses and the alleged appearance on Russian maps of places called "Budunde," after the Chinese for "don't understand" (*budongde*).[1] Even if this story was apocryphal, the Russians were in dire need of interpreters: to collect precise geographical data and deliver intelligence during the Russo-Japanese War, to recruit and supervise workers for railway construction, and to facilitate daily contacts with the local population. There were too few Russians who could do the job, and Chinese interpreters were cheaper to hire, so the latter became essential intermediaries for Russian military officers, engineers, merchants, and administrators.

Interpreters, Brokers, and Compradors

Some bold claims have been made about Chinese interpreters in Russian service and their supposedly nefarious impact. Rosemary Quested was inclined to see Russia's continued dependence on them as one of the causes of its ultimate failure as a colonizer in Manchuria.[2] Interpreters' ostentatious behaviour and corruption are said to have fuelled anti-Russian sentiment, encouraging the tendency of the Chinese population to aid the Japanese side during the Russo-Japanese War.[3] Some interpreters were suspect in the eyes of their Russian employers because of their links to the most popular religious sect in northeastern China from the mid-nineteenth century to the republican period, the *Zaili hui*, which was heavily involved in the persecution of Christians during the Boxer Uprising.[4] To train a cohort of more reliable interpreters, the Russian administration in the Kwantung leasehold opened two four-year schools for Chinese pupils, but the military defeat in 1905 signalled the end of these efforts.[5]

Typically, the Chinese who translated for the Russians in Manchuria have been accused of extorting money from their masters while using them as protection when bullying their own people.[6] Some such allegations had a basis in fact, but they also reflect an image of the native interpreter that could well be universal. In a colonial setting, interpreters were also guides and informers – a role that dislodged them from the society into which they were born, even while they were prevented from fully entering the one they served.[7] Public opinion in the late Qing period labelled Chinese who engaged in contact with foreigners as *Hanjian* (traitors to the Han nation), and interpreters were included in this category.[8] Acting on this conviction, the Boxers killed Chinese interpreters in Manchuria as collaborators; no wonder that those who could escaped together with the Russians.[9] At the end of the Russo-Japanese War, interpreters were tried and punished by both the Japanese and the Chinese authorities.[10]

The Russians had no pleasant memories of their protégés: Vladimir F. Liuba (1861?–1928), himself a trained interpreter from Chinese and Manchu, who was the tsarist Consul General in Harbin between 1907 and 1909, reported on "the Chinese interpreters, recruited God knows where and with what past [behind them] ... who, abusing the confidence placed in them, were cooking underhand their shady deals with the railway contracts, managing all kinds of gambling dens, etc."[11] Liuba surmised that the Russians in Manchuria needed to learn Chinese, and he developed projects to advance that aim.[12] Baron Petr N. Wrangel (1878–1928), a leader of the White Army and, later, of the Russian military emigration, has left a portrait of a Chinese interpreter from the time of his service in the Russo-Japanese War. The brave but "mean, cunning and exceedingly greedy Andrei" – the Russian name he used – "deeply despised the Chinese population, from which he himself emerged and, using his position as an interpreter, took every opportunity to mercilessly swindle and cheat his compatriots, who in turn hated him utterly for this." Andrei's dream, according to Baron Wrangel, was to open a brothel in Vladivostok.[13] That may have been so, but accusing interpreters of making "shady deals" with contractors during the period of railway construction was also an attempt to divert attention from Russian corruption.[14]

Where did the interpreters come from? Who had they been before an often rudimentary knowledge of Russian qualified them for their new occupation? The Russians did not have a clue, and in this sense

Consul Liuba's words, cited above, are revealing. Working relations with the interpreters were more complex than the simple pattern of master and employee that could be maintained with coolies. Possessing the language of communication gave the interpreter greater leverage than most other Chinese in Manchuria could boast of vis-à-vis the foreigners. Especially in the initial period of contact, colonialists everywhere depended on native interpreters and middlemen, and the resulting frustration was not limited to Manchuria. A prominent official in Russian Turkestan (territory that, unlike Manchuria, had been added to the Russian empire) complained in 1913 that "a wall made of native administrators, traders, and translators" separated the Russians from their subjects during the first decades of rule: "we looked through the eyes, heard with the ears, and thought with the cunning, grasping minds of this live wall."[15]

In Manchuria, too, the interpreters were the closest at hand and the easiest to blame for every setback. At each interpreter's shoulder there came to hover the spectre of a *khunkhuz* – the omnipresent Manchurian bandit. That same word served the Russians to label all suspicious-looking and hard-to-classify Chinese who came their way. Much like interpreters, "bandits" could be used as scapegoats for the railway's inefficiency and corruption.[16] The crafty interpreter and the dreaded *khunkhuz* had another thing in common: both had stepped out of the frame of Chinese society, renouncing such typical roles as peasant, coolie, or soldier. The point here is not to deny the motive habitually ascribed to the interpreters, that of mercenary greed. It is to suggest that some of these ambitious men (there is no evidence of Chinese women taking up the occupation) were animated by additional interests and that they perceived their proficiency in Russian as a chance to rise above their station. In a different context, a historian called "this [linguistic] accomplishment … the essential passport and temptation to changing who and what they were."[17] Even coolies and peasants could have such aspirations, and also act out of cultural curiosity.

Arriving as intruders in a traditional society, the Russians offered those willing to seize it an opportunity to acquire new knowledge. With all the attendant problems of colonialism, the representatives of Russia in Manchuria brought modern ways to that periphery of China. Keen as they were to adopt the material trappings of the new culture, interpreters were much quicker than their contemporaries to assimilate foreign dress, tastes, and manners.[18] Later in Harbin, as we shall see, many things Russian became part of the texture of Chinese daily life. Interpreters along with compradors – another important type of intermediary, to be discussed immediately below – may have been the first to respond to the inexorable trend of Harbin's and Manchuria's Westernization.

A historian gives the following snapshot of comprador conduct in early twentieth-century Shanghai:

> When in the company of Caucasian colleagues, they donned mandarin costumes and affected a refined courtesy and studio-names to pretend to a measure of culture; when in a Chinese milieu, they wore Western clothes, assumed Christian names, displayed Western habits ... The compradore's home was a Western-style house appointed with both Chinese and European furniture and objets d'art, but he ate Chinese food. Some of them embraced Christianity but at the same time practised Confucian ethics.[19]

In Manchuria, the Russians' need for interpreters and brokers opened opportunities for Chinese entrepreneurs. A comprador would buy agricultural produce from peasants, who were reluctant to deal directly with foreigners, and then resell it to the Russians, making a profit for himself in the process. At a higher economic level and playing for considerably larger stakes, a broker serving as an official in the Chinese administration would negotiate complex deals for the Russians involving real estate or coal mines. A person such as this travelled the uncertain continuum between the positively perceived roles of negotiator and intermediary and the negative ones of collaborator and double-dealer. Zhou Mian, an official in Qiqihar and Harbin, was intimately involved in diplomatic and financial operations with the Russians from the 1890s to 1905, when his own plotting, Russian mistrust of his activities, and denunciations to the Peking court from the Qing administration in Manchuria led to his downfall.[20]

However, compradors in Manchuria differed from those who worked with the seaborne foreigners in China's treaty ports inasmuch as they operated in a border region with a long-standing tradition of shifting loyalties. The rapidly growing Russian towns, founded after the annexation of the Amur and the Maritime provinces, attracted Chinese migrants in search of a livelihood. In 1893, Khabarovsk authorities reported only 307 Chinese out of a total population of 6,353; but the first Russian national census of 1897 counted 3,652 Chinese inhabitants in Khabarovsk out of a total of 14,971. The population of Vladivostok in 1900 was about 37,600, of whom 12,800 were Chinese.[21] By October 1900, the Chinese were back in Blagoveshchensk, where according to an official report their number had reached 1,427.[22] All three towns had Chinese quarters, in which most of the Chinese migrants and long-term residents concentrated. Because of their determination to take the money they earned in Russia back to China, their living in closed male communes, and their success in displacing Russians from manual jobs by being ready to work for lower salaries and longer hours, they became the target of animosity and sporadic violence. Overcoming any Russian prejudice against them, at least two prominent financial brokers emerged from the ranks of the Chinese in Khabarovsk and Vladivostok.

Ji Fengtai, better known as Nikolai Ivanovich Tifontai, was the first to demonstrate just how high one could rise.[23] He was born in either 1849 or 1853 and came from Shandong's Huang County; according to one Chinese version of his life story, his father brought him to Vladivostok soon after the Russian port opened in 1860.[24] A Russian memoir dates Tifontai's arrival in Khabarovka to 1873, describing him as a low-paid interpreter as of 1877.[25] However, he was already acquiring real estate and trading in furs, and he soon became a name to be reckoned with in mercantile circles. In 1894 he briefly returned to his original occupation, serving as an interpreter for Russia in diplomatic negotiations on the Chinese border. The following year he joined the Russian expedition into Manchuria from Khabarovsk aboard the steamer *Telegraf*; when the ship docked at Lahasusu, he presented a samovar to the local Chinese official.[26] As long as he could move between the two countries, his financial schemes flourished. By the 1900s, Tifontai's coal mines and mills, and his chain of shops on both sides of the border, had made him a millionaire. A travelling British officer, who also commented on the great demand for Chinese interpreters to enter Russian service, noticed that he was the main contractor of the CER prior to the Boxer Uprising.[27] In addition, Tifontai brewed the best beer in Khabarovsk; the brewery he built in 1903 was still in operation a century later.

In his first petition to become a Russian subject in 1885, Tifontai claimed that having left China as a youth, he had "grown completely distant from the life and customs of [his] former native land" and that, after twelve years in Khabarovka, he regarded the Russian empire as his "second motherland" (*Rodina*). It is hard to read too much into these statements, which were of the sort that applicants were expected to make (more than 160 petitions from Chinese subjects to be naturalized in tsarist Russia have been documented).[28] Tifontai's request was granted only in 1893, the same year that Khabarovka was upgraded to Khabarovsk, after he had been christened into the Orthodox faith and cut off his queue (a step he had tried to avoid).[29] A Russian travel account from 1904 describes a Chinese named Nikolai Ivanovich, who entered the author's rail wagon while on a business trip to Harbin. This man said in fluent Russian that he had been a Russian subject since 1893. Now his daughter was studying at a Russian gymnasium and his son at a technical high school. He also spoke of the tsar as "our sovereign." The author commented that "the ties of this Chinaman to Russia had strengthened through his children, who found a second fatherland [*otechestvo*] in it."[30]

Tifontai enriched himself once again, just as he had during the Boxer troubles, by becoming the Russian army's main contractor during the Russo-Japanese War. He also gathered intelligence for Russia in Manchuria, besides organizing and financing a Chinese detachment of *khunkhuz* horsemen and former soldiers, which fought on the Russian side in the last two months of the war.[31] By 1905 he may well have thought of himself as a Russian patriot, and in any event he would have been under pressure to prove himself one. For his role in the war, the Japanese sentenced Tifontai (in absentia) to decapitation as a Russian spy. This distinction did not spare him the fate of colonial middlemen: to be mistrusted by all sides. The most famous Russian novel about the Russo-Japanese War, *Port Arthur*, published in the 1940s, portrayed him as a devious double agent; he has been called a treasonous comprador in China.[32]

Russia's defeat brought Tifontai to the brink of financial ruin. Besides all his property in southern Manchuria, he lost the lavish European residence he kept in Port Arthur. Converted into a Yamato hotel of the South Manchuria Railway in 1908, it survives to the present day (with the ornamental third floor flattened during renovation in 1977) as a shabby-looking hotel of the People's Liberation Army. A plaque, put up by Dalian Municipality in 2002, does not mention Ji Fengtai, saying only that the building was constructed in 1903 and, as a hotel, provided the venue for the 1927 wedding of the Japanese-raised Qing princess and spy, Kawashima Yoshiko (1906?–1948); the puppet emperor Puyi stayed there in 1931.[33]

A share of Tifontai's fortune went into the construction of theatres in Harbin, Dal'nii, and Port Arthur.[34] The one in Harbin, which closed down by 1910, was on Vodoprovodnaia (Waterworks) Street (today's Zhaolinjie), the part of Pristan' (Daoli) quarter where most of Harbin's Chinese lived.[35] Chinese plays were staged in these theatres, and one may speculate that, despite the complete break with his Chinese identity, which he declared in applications to the Russian authorities, Ji Fengtai himself occasionally attended performances at them before fleeing Manchuria. When he died in Saint Petersburg in January 1910, he was still fighting to obtain compensation for his wartime losses from the Russian government. His body was sent by the railway to Harbin,[36] probably to continue the prescribed journey to his native place in Shandong, although his final resting place is unknown. One of his several wives, a Chinese woman in Khabarovsk, who spoke no Russian, was legally recognized as his widow by the Russian state. His son Vladimir Nikolaevich Tifontai married a Russian and settled in Moscow. His daughter Vera, who studied in Saint Petersburg, immigrated to Britain.[37]

Almost a generation after Tifontai began his rise in Khabarovka, Vladivostok saw the rise of Zhang Tingge, who arrived there at the age of twenty-one in 1896.[38] Drawing on his ability to master Russian and his roots in Shandong's Ye County, he landed a job in a firm founded and run in Vladivostok by fellow countymen. On the firm's behalf, Zhang supplied the needs of the Russian army before and during the war with Japan; like Tifontai, he also amassed a private fortune as a contractor. But he did not stay in Russia. In 1912, Zhang transferred the Shuanghesheng firm ("Sonkhoshin," as Russians knew it) to Harbin. New profits from transporting flour to Europe via the Trans-Siberian Railway during the First World War enabled him to liquidate his Vladivostok base by 1919 and become Harbin's most prominent industrialist. Besides flour mills, Zhang owned a tannery (reputed the largest in China when he founded it in 1920) and a cooking oil plant, both equipped with advanced European technology, as well as a brewery near Peking.

A member of the Russian-dominated Harbin municipal council since 1918, in 1926 Zhang capitalized on the council's refusal to make Chinese (rather than Russian) the official language of debate; this led to the establishment of a new council, of which Zhang was elected the chairman. Zhang's later career included the private financing of General Ma Zhanshan's (1885–1950) anti-Japanese army in 1931. Nonetheless, he went on to assume official posts under the Japanese occupation. When the Red Army captured Harbin in 1945, Zhang's Russian once again proved useful to him; he served under the Soviets as the acting city mayor, a position he kept until the end of that year. Having survived the first waves of political attacks against him in the PRC, Zhang died in 1954, shortly after a fire ravaged his flour mill.

Tifontai's apparent assimilation into Russian society was an exception. Zhang Tingge's success was unusual as well; that said, he was not the only Chinese to exploit the economic advantages that contact with the Russians could offer as long as their political power lasted. It is possible to view this pattern either as a way of reconciling collaboration with tacit resistance or as self-interested opportunism. Pragmatism is a neutral and therefore more appropriate term, one that also helps us understand some Chinese responses to the challenges of modern education.

Education and Elites in Contact

The Russians in Harbin before the change of regime in their home country were representatives of the tsar's empire. Temporary sojourners rather than fully fledged colonists, they did not come with "a mission to civilize"; rather, they attempted to accommodate their newly founded city within the frame of Russian statehood.

Attracting Chinese students was never an objective of the Russian schools, geared as they were to serving the community's own needs. When the first elementary school opened in Harbin in December 1898, there were only eleven Russian children to be taught, so Chinese pupils "aged from about twelve to twenty years" were taken in separately. Thirty-two of them attended the school during that first year, which turned out to be their last, since in the second year the CER stopped paying their tuition. The school's principal recorded their "amazing" diligence and high motivation as well as the ease with which they learned Russian. The moment was unique, as the growth of Harbin's Russian population soon overwhelmed its fledgling education system.[39]

The next experiment in mixed education had to wait until 1906, when four Chinese boys entered Harbin's new Commercial School. Intended for the children of the CER's Russian employees, who were accepted from the age of nine, the Commercial School consisted of two adjacent but separate establishments: a boys' school, founded on 26 February 1906, and a school for girls, founded on 18 September (dates in O.S.). In 1907 the Commercial School for Boys introduced Chinese as an obligatory subject. Despite a petition of protest from the pupils' parents, this policy was maintained, making this school, reputed to be the best in Harbin, the only one in the city until as late as 1929 to insist on a six-year Chinese language course for Russian pupils.[40] The detailed memoirs of Mikhail Hintze (Russian spelling Gintse, 1900–1992), whose father Alexander Hintze (1856–1919) headed the CER Exploitation Service from 1906 to 1918, show that the senior staff of the railway took Chinese studies seriously. As a young child in Harbin, Mikhail began studying daily with a private tutor, a Chinese *dragoman* (interpreter) of the CER, even before he entered the Commercial School: his father had simply told him that "living in China, [he] needed to know Chinese."[41]

Twenty-two Chinese boys and ten Chinese girls were among 583 male and 364 female graduates when the Commercial School was under Russian management, from its foundation to 1925.[42] All of the Chinese girls and all but two of the boys were admitted in the school year 1911–12 by a top-level agreement between the Governor General of the Three Eastern Provinces Zhao Erxun (1844–1927) and the CER manager, General Dmitrii Khorvat. Hardly any Russian pupils attended Chinese schools: the extreme rarity of the arrival of Russian children aged seven and eight at a school in Fujiadian, in September 1919, comes across in a report on that event in Harbin's Chinese newspaper, which cited the precedent of Russians attending the Peking Imperial College under emperor Kangxi.[43]

Early on, Russian and Chinese elites in Harbin lent their joint support to charitable causes. In January 1904, a Russian-Chinese home for foundlings opened in New Town. A branch in Old Harbin (Chinese: Xiangfang, Incense Lane), in the extreme south of the young town, followed in March.[44] The home was created under the patronage of Camilla Khorvat (1878–1953), wife of the railway manager. It lasted at least until 1918, when donations for its upkeep were solicited from Chinese and Russian merchants in the name of friendship between the two nations.[45] In setting itself this purpose, Khorvat's institution was one of a kind. Orphanages and asylums in Harbin were run by the Russian Orthodox Church, by other religious congregations such as the Jewish, or by Chinese charitable societies, with each institution caring for members of its own community. There were also Polish, Jewish, Georgian, Ukrainian, Korean, and Japanese schools.

Until 1916, all of the nineteen elementary schools that the CER ran in Manchuria catered only to the children of Russian employees, while excluding the Chinese. Schools for Chinese employees began to be opened thereafter, reaching a total of ten along the entire railway line by 1924, and of sixteen by 1926.[46] A Russian school in Harbin might accept individual Chinese pupils, usually from the upper classes. However, mixed Russian-Chinese education at the primary or secondary levels was not essayed even at schools that featured the words "Russian-Chinese" in their names.[47] After 1917, émigré education in Harbin as in other Russian communities in exile aimed at ensuring that the younger generation continued to speak the language of their parents and retained their native ties to Russia and the Russian Orthodox Church. Seen from this perspective, learning the language of the host country became a threat to the preservation of identity. Unlike French in Paris or German in Berlin, the Chinese spoken on the streets of Harbin was not perceived as a language worth acquiring for its own sake. Indeed, in the daily life of "Russian Harbin," hardly any knowledge of Chinese was required.

The extension of the benefits of higher education to a small number of Chinese students remained one of the last means of projecting a positive image of the Russian community after the balance of political power had swung in favour of the Chinese. Having turned from pioneers into émigrés, in the early 1920s the Russians began to redefine their role as carriers of technological progress and prosperity to Manchuria through the Chinese Eastern Railway.[48] The Harbin Polytechnic, which trained railway and electrical engineers, became the centre of Russian professional education. Founded as the Russian-Chinese Technical College on a large tract of land in New Town in 1920, it immediately opened preparatory courses for Chinese candidates.[49] The college was renamed the Russian-Chinese Polytechnic Institute on 2 April 1922, a date celebrated as its foundational moment ever since.[50] As a CER institution, after 1925 it only accepted students from families holding Soviet or Chinese passports, thereby excluding émigrés. The "Russian" component of the institute's name survived until 1928, when it became the Polytechnic Institute of the Special Region of the Eastern Provinces.

With active encouragement from the Polytechnic's joint Sino-Russian management, attendance in its preparatory courses in Russian constantly grew: from a total of only nineteen students in the first two years, the numbers climbed to 351 in 1930–1. What had begun as a one-year course was transformed into a two-year, then a three-year course, by the end of which the Chinese students were expected to attend regular studies.[51] Forty-five had graduated by 1933, just under 10 per cent of the Polytechnic's total number of graduates. The Polytechnic was closed to Russian students from 1935, when the CER was sold to Japan, to 1945. It reopened to admit Soviet and Chinese citizens in 1946, employing Russian teaching staff until the Sino-Soviet rift in 1960.[52] It is now the Harbin Institute of Technology (HIT), one of the highest-ranked universities in China.

In March 1920, Russian academics inaugurated a Faculty of Law in Harbin. It was housed in the Railway Assembly (the Zheleznodorozhnoe sobranie, abbreviated as Zhelsob in Russian), an iconic building on the main avenue of New Town. Only by autumn 1926 did it open a two-year language course to prepare Chinese students for admission. In 1929, the faculty was taken over by the Chinese authorities and the study of Chinese became compulsory in all Russian schools in Manchuria.[53] A separate Chinese stream was then offered to students who were unable to follow lectures in Russian. Despite these measures, the faculty had only nineteen Chinese graduates out of a total of 297 when, along with other Russian schools, it was closed under Japanese rule in 1938.[54]

These young Chinese people were engaged in the dual pursuit of excellence and prestige. From the beginning of the twentieth century, foreign education was the key to social status in China. Some of those who went to study in Japan, the United States, or Europe launched

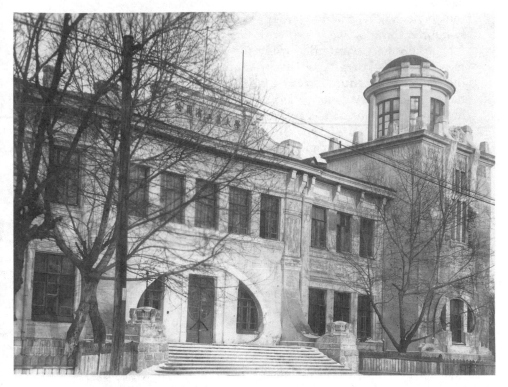

3.1. The Polytechnic Institute. Photograph from the archive of Vladimir
Ablamskii, courtesy of the A.M. Sibiriakov Museum
of Irkutsk City History.

highly successful careers on their return. And many, who could not
travel abroad, regarded the schools run by foreigners in China as the
next best thing. The reputation of Harbin's Russian schools attracted
aspiring Chinese students from throughout the country, but they had
to struggle to get accepted in them. Thus, the first medical school, inaugurated by the Medical Society of the CER Central Hospital in October
1921, had ninety-eight students, but only one of them was Chinese (and
a female at that). These students completed their fourth year of education only to witness the closing of their school in September 1925,
after the change of CER administration. Taking its place was a Chinese-
managed Medical College (the predecessor of today's Harbin Medical
University), founded in August 1926.[55]

Nationally minded historians in China have found it difficult to
explain why Chinese students chose to attend the Faculty of Law and

the Polytechnic when they were run by Russians. Resorting to the time-honoured formula *Zhongxue wei ti, xixue wei yong* ("Chinese learning for the substance, Western learning for use")[56] cannot do justice to the reasons why students spent years studying Russian and then faced the challenges of education in a foreign language as a minority among native speakers. Arguably, the pragmatic concept of "Western learning for use" retains greater relevance for explaining the aims of Deng Jiemin (1890–1926), who in 1918 founded the Donghua (East China) middle school in Harbin and directed it until 1922. Born in Bin County east of Harbin, Deng had started out as a Russian interpreter for the local magistrate at the age of fifteen before going on to study in Tientsin and Tokyo. Whereas Russian was the language Chinese students had to master to attend Harbin's prestigious institutes, pupils in Donghua School were required to learn English.[57] Other Chinese children were placed by parents in foreign mission schools in Manchuria; English was usually the medium of education in these as well.[58] In the early 1920s, when Chinese nationalists protested against the Japanese education system in southern Manchuria, school directors there pointed out that their Japanese-taught classes attracted large numbers of Chinese, who had chosen them of their own volition; moreover, almost one third of the students came from outside the South Manchuria Railway zone, which was under Japanese control.[59]

In 1917, a first batch of students from Liaoning went to Japan on funds remitted from the Boxer indemnity. One of them was Wang Fengrui (1897–1981), who studied transportation engineering in Tokyo. More than 3,500 Chinese students made use of the opportunity to study in Japan between 1924 and 1932; despite obvious animosity toward Japanese militarism, their numbers reached an all-time peak immediately following the Japanese occupation of Manchuria. Typically, Wang later took great care to justify his choice. He wrote that his father despised the Japanese and had objected to his decision but that he had been won over by the argument that one should study China's oppressors. Wang reminisced that he went to Tokyo out of concern for China's need to improve its transportation system. During his time there, he was involved in student protest against Japanese colonialism in southern Manchuria. After further study in the United States and Canada, Wang returned to China as an engineer in his home region.[60]

It was wholly in the nature of such contacts with the foreign that they should give rise to unexpected personal connections. Such was the case with Mordechai Olmert (1908–1998). He was born near Samara on the Volga River and brought to China in 1919. The family lived in a small Russian settlement (*poselok*) adjacent to Qiqihar's CER station. Qiqihar was predominantly a Chinese-speaking town, making it more likely for a curious youngster to pick up the language. Olmert left his parents' home to study at the Harbin Polytechnic in 1927.

Among his fellow students in Harbin, Olmert found twelve young Chinese, graduates of the preparatory courses, which at the time lasted two years. His knowledge of Chinese soon brought him into direct contact with them, and he started earning pocket money by tutoring two groups of young men and women. More than in his engineering studies at the Polytechnic, however, the ardent Zionist Olmert was interested in immigrating to Palestine. British immigration permits were unavailable in Manchuria, so he hoped to obtain one by reaching Europe. To fund his trip, in late 1929 he began teaching Russian in the high school of Shuangcheng, another CER station about 50 kilometres south of Harbin (Shuangcheng is today a district within the Harbin metropolitan area). The adventure lasted a whole year. Fifty years later, in an autobiography written in Israel, Olmert devoted a chapter to this experience. He remembered living as the only foreigner in the Chinese town and returning to Harbin only for school vacations. While he insisted on presenting himself as Jewish, not Russian, he did not notice and may not have been interested to know that some of the people he came across were not quite, or not only, "Chinese." Shuangcheng's population included the descendants of Manchu (as well as Mongol, Han, and other) bannermen, who had been settled there and in nearby Ashihe by a decision of the Qing court between 1815 and 1838.[61]

Olmert did recall long, friendly talks with Yang, a Shandong villager who worked at the school as a caretaker and sent money to his family back home. He described roaming the streets, joining fellow teachers to watch a Chinese theatre performance, and shooting the winning basket in a basketball game against another Chinese school. Concluding the chapter "Shuan-ch'i-fu" in Olmert's memoirs is a photograph titled "with Chinese students at the Harbin Polytechnic." Before he boarded the train leaving Harbin on the last day of 1930, Chinese friends threw a goodbye party for him. One of the three friends appearing in the photograph wears traditional clothes, another a buttoned, uniform-like jacket; the third, standing behind Olmert and resting a hand on his shoulder, is dressed in a suit and tie: an inadvertent silent testimony to change.[62]

One would have liked to hear these Chinese students' memories of their years at the Polytechnic. Would they think back as fondly of the Russian preparatory course? Sun Yunxuan (Sun Yun-suan, 1913–2006), who was born in Shandong's Penglai County, spent two years as one of only two Chinese pupils at the Harbin Commercial School from 1925.

He was then admitted to the Polytechnic through the preparatory courses and graduated at the top of his class in 1934. The first year at the Commercial School he remembered as a nightmare. More than half a century later, he told his biographer that in the most difficult moments he used to think of his father's words – that he should study Russian in order to enter the Polytechnic and win back China's state rights. Once in the Polytechnic, he invented a shorthand method to take notes of the Russian lectures. Looking back on that time, he claimed that he kept working hard because Harbin Russians considered the Chinese dirty and primitive. "I used to tell my fellow Chinese students: let's compare our grades and theirs, and see who will come out on top."[63] Sun later served as Premier (Head of the Executive Yuan) of the Republic of China government in Taiwan between 1978 and 1984.

The thirty children from Liaoning who were admitted to the Commercial School in 1911 were lodged with the families of Russian schoolteachers and high CER officials in order to ease their adaptation.[64] In 1921, one of these Chinese graduates, Li Shaogeng (b. 1896), was appointed to manage relations with the Russians at the magistracy of Binjiang (Fujiadian). Later Li became a minister in the Manchukuo government. His final post, in 1945, was as ambassador of Manchukuo to the collaborationist government established by the Japanese in Nanking (Nanjing); his fate after Japan's surrender remains unclear. So the Russian education that some Chinese received in Harbin led to the emergence of a new professional elite, whose members often had close personal contacts with the Russian community. As they matured during the Republican period, they were also influenced by the growth of Chinese nationalism and anti-foreign feeling in the 1920s. This did not prevent some of them from using their skills in cross-cultural communication to advance their careers under Japanese rule.[65]

Because they could speak and read Russian, these people differed from the older bureaucratic establishment in Harbin, who were the products of the Confucian examination system, which had been in force until 1905. Such older officials, who qualified for their jobs partly through their competence in the composition of classical poetry, gathered for literary improvisations, drinks, and recitals in the garden of Ma Zhongjun (1870–1957), head of the Heilongjiang Railway Diplomatic Bureau (jiaoshe ju) from 1914, and head of the Directorate of City Administration of the Special Region from 1921 until his retirement in 1925. Ma was born in Haicheng (southern Liaoning) to a family that had served the Qing in the Chinese Bordered White Banner. He called the garden, which he had built between 1919 and 1924, Dunyuan (The Garden of Retreat) after two lines from the Book of Changes: "retreat is becoming of a gentleman," and "there is no boredom in retreating from the world." A part of it survives and is now called the Ma Family Garden. Located in the Xiangfang quarter, which the Russians called Old Harbin, it was ready to receive guests by the time Ma retired from public service. After the Japanese occupation, Ma settled there with his large family. Among the pavilions, steles and grottoes, he wrote philosophical poetry in classical Chinese.[66]

The circle that orbited around Ma Zhongjun included Liu Zhe (?–1954), the first rector of the Polytechnic from 1928 to 1938, and Guo Zongxi (1878–1934), the former Harbin circuit intendant (*daotai*), governor of Jilin province, and first supervisor of the CER. Their small literary group was active from 1925 to 1932, its key participants being known as "the nine elders of the Songhua River."[67] Like Ma, these top officials were seasoned by contact with the upper echelons of the Russian administration besides being steeped in Chinese literati culture. They could switch between these worlds as easily as their host, who, before moving into his Confucian scholar's retreat, had occupied a villa in Majiagou (at the time, a settlement by a river of the same name, southeast of New Town; now part of Nangang District), an imitation Italian castle built in 1910. The large domestic staff included a cook who specialized in Western cuisine; there was a tennis court and a Russian-style carriage, Christmas was celebrated with fanfare, and a private teacher taught the Ma children Russian, horseback riding, and dancing.[68]

When, in the early 1920s, Ma Zhongjun had his life's achievements inscribed on an epitaph tablet, to be stored in the garden, he prided himself most upon his success as a negotiator: on a diplomatic mission to Vice-Admiral Alekseev, commander of the Kwantung leasehold in Port Arthur in 1900, he had managed to prevent Russian military operations from spilling over into Fengtian (Liaoning) province.[69] Although Harbin's Europeans were unacquainted with Ma's classical poetry, they remembered him as a prominent Chinese figure who cultivated close social relations with high Russian officials.[70] The connection between membership in that elite and some readiness for cultural accommodation with Russians is attested in Song Xiaolian (1860–1926), a native of Jilin and a negotiator with Russia throughout his career in Manchuria from 1888 to 1923. A predecessor of Ma Zhongjun as the head of the Heilongjiang Diplomatic Bureau and the last military governor of the province under the Qing, Song remained in senior positions after the revolution of 1911 thanks to membership in the so-called Beiyang clique of Yuan Shikai (1859–1916), the northern general who seized power as president in Peking in 1912.

After General Khorvat was compelled to step down as manager of the CER in March 1920, Song Xiaolian was appointed director general of the railway in June. In July the Russian railway guard, an important manifestation of Russia's military presence in Manchuria since 1897, was disbanded, and the Cossacks were replaced by Chinese soldiers. As of September, Russian extraterritorial rights in China were abolished. That same year, the Chinese authorities realized that most Chinese railway workers did not know Russian. Rather than view such knowledge as redundant after the change of power, they created a Russian Language Institute, hired Russian language instructors, and made the study of Russian obligatory for Chinese employees of the CER.[71] Similarly, the Chinese administration in Harbin in the 1920s managed the complex situation in the mixed city by keeping Russians among the police staff and encouraging them to learn colloquial Chinese; at the same time, Chinese police officers were taught some Russian.[72]

Between October and December 1921, Song Xiaolian surveyed the entire railway line between Manzhouli to Suifenhe. Travelling west from Harbin, he noticed that signs on many of the railway stations still bore inscriptions solely in Russian and that a number of station names were only approximately transcribed in Chinese characters. Instead of recommending that the Russian signs be replaced by Chinese ones, he called for new signs to be prepared in both languages. Another observation Song made was that Russian children at CER station schools were unable to speak or write Chinese. As he put it, "because the railway is located on Chinese territory, these Russian pupils certainly should know the Chinese language." While this much was predictable, Song's proposed solution to the problem was less so: "the children of Chinese employees should be taken in [the schools], to enable the exchange of knowledge in the interest of both sides."[73] Song combined his nationalism with his conviction that mixed education would be beneficial, even though Chinese historians have described him largely as a fighter for the recovery of China's territorial and railway rights from the Russian colonialists.[74] Alongside the top Russian officials, Dmitrii Khorvat and his deputy, the engineer Vasilii D. Lachinov (1872–1933), Song was joint chairman of the board of the Harbin Polytechnic.[75]

Song Xiaolian left the northeast in January 1922, soon to end his days in Peking. His efforts to regulate names and signs on the CER line bring to mind a scene from a famous travel book by the first Chinese communist to visit Bolshevik Russia. Qu Qiubai (1899–1935), who had studied Russian in Peking and was to become General Secretary of the Communist Party of China in 1927, found himself stranded in Harbin for almost two months in the winter of 1920 before he could continue his rail journey to Moscow. He described an invitation to a Harbin Russian home, where he was surprised to hear from his hosts that they "had never been to China." Russian life in Harbin, they said, offered them "few chances for contact with Chinese culture." To return to his hostel that evening, Qu hired a Russian coachman, who took a long time to find his address, complaining: "How come you Chinese people all of a sudden don't know the Russian names of Harbin streets?" Qu thought to himself that a coachman "driving on Chinese ground should know the Chinese names of Chinese streets."[76] In 1925, Russian street names in Harbin were officially replaced by Chinese ones, and in a departure from Song Xiaolian's moderate position, a policy of banning Russian signs was introduced.[77] The city's Russian-speaking inhabitants went on using the Russian street names nonetheless.

Sinologists, Sinophiles, and Eurasianists

A Harbin Russian school did not usually equip its graduates with more than a smattering of Chinese language competence or acquaintance with Chinese literary culture. This situation began slowly to change only after China and the Soviet Union reached an agreement on joint management of the CER in 1924. After the study year 1925, Chinese was to be taught in all the elementary schools the railway ran in Harbin and along the CER line; however, this requirement could not yet be enforced in private Russian schools. This educational reform was announced in a CER organ, which that same year made the momentous decision to switch to the new Russian alphabet (introduced by the Bolsheviks and resisted as a symbol of their regime by Russian émigrés worldwide). The writer for the railway's *Economic Bulletin* rued tsarist Russia's failure to train more than a handful of sinologists in Manchuria, demanding instead "that the Chinese masses learn our Russian language."[78]

This author, who is otherwise unknown, underestimated the number of sinologists in Harbin. Also in 1925, the Institute of Oriental and Commercial Studies, newly established by Harbin's Society of Russian Orientalists, proposed to address the lack of knowledge about China. The institute's two faculties, the Oriental-Economic and the Commercial, taught a variety of general subjects (such as law, insurance, and banking) and also offered lecture courses on China, Japan, Korea, Tibet, and Mongolia. In the language classes, emphasis was placed on the acquisition of practical skills in Chinese, Japanese, and English. During the sixteen years of the institute's existence, a time of turbulence in Manchurian politics, it was attended by some 750 students (including many auditors). After 1928, students could join a study circle in Oriental Studies, which had its own museum and library. Chinese was also taught after 1924 at the Oriental Department of Harbin's Faculty of Law under the energetic direction of Sergei N. Usov (1891–1966), the author of several Chinese textbooks. Usov was responsible for the courses in Chinese, which the CER had begun offering to its Russian-speaking employees; the Chinese authorities also appointed him inspector of the Department of Education. The Oriental-Economic Faculty aimed to train sinologists; the Faculty of Law, interpreters and translators.

In 1935 the Japanese authorities moved the Institute of Oriental and Commercial Studies to the Institute of St Vladimir, founded the previous year (not coincidentally, this saint was also the patron of the Russian Fascist Party in Manchukuo). In 1938, the Institute of St Vladimir was reborn as a strictly theological institution and Oriental studies were transferred to the North Manchuria University (founded in 1937), which billed itself as the only institution of higher education for Russians in Manchukuo.[79] When the Polytechnic reopened under Soviet management in 1946, its Oriental-Economic Faculty offered a training program to prepare Russian interpreters for the railway, with intensive Chinese courses and lectures on China's history, ethnography, geography, and economy.[80]

That some members of the Russian community studied China suits the image of Harbin presented in the nostalgic memoirs of former inhabitants – an image that has partly spilled over into historical writing. This is a perception of Harbin not only as the place where Russianness was preserved under adverse circumstances, but also as the setting for a mutually enriching encounter between East and West.[81] To correct this charming misapprehension, the original proportions of Harbin sinology need to be traced.

One task undertaken by the Society of Russian Orientalists, founded in Harbin in 1908, was the creation of a social network. With Harbin as its base, the society maintained branches in other Chinese cities with a Russian presence[82] and extended aid to its members. Many of them were graduates of the Oriental Institute in Vladivostok (founded in 1899) and so had known one another before coming to China. Another organization with nearly the same name and interests, the Harbin branch of the Russian Society of Eastern Studies, was identified with Saint Petersburg, and its members were predominantly of a military background.[83] Their professional careers, which eventually led them to Manchuria, developed along similar lines. Typically, they started out as interpreters during the Russo-Japanese War and later continued in the same capacity on the CER. The establishment of academic institutions in Harbin offered them a chance to move into part-time teaching. To make a living, sinologists doubled as journalists and editors, taught Chinese in Russian schools, or became teachers of Russian to the Chinese.

The organ of the Society of Russian Orientalists, *Vestnik Azii* (Herald of Asia), provided a forum for ongoing research by society members, thus fostering a sense of scholarly community. Most of the journal's articles from 1909 to 1927 (the year the Society of Russian Orientalists was dissolved) were devoted to China at large; Manchuria occupied only fourth place in the number of published articles.[84] It was the Society for the Study of the Manchurian Region (Russian abbreviation: OIMK) that took up the investigation and description of Manchuria, from 1922 to 1928. This scholarly association combined sinology with *kraevedenie*, the Russian term for local studies, and was modelled on the Society for the Study of the Amur Region in Vladivostok. A Museum of Local Studies opened in Harbin in 1923, but it did little to familiarize Manchuria among the general Russian public: the lectures and field trips, offered by enthusiasts who were true pioneers in research on the region, made less of an impact than the continuous erosion of the Russian foothold in northeastern China.

The Society for the Study of the Manchurian Region made no attempt to recruit Chinese members. Aleksei M. Baranov (1865–1927), Head of its Ethnographic Section, argued that the participation of "highly placed" Chinese in the society would ease official restrictions on members' research. This implied that the Chinese could hardly contribute to the research itself. The full membership list of the society in its second year reveals only four Chinese names out of a total of 258.[85] In the absence of translations, the studies published in the society's journal were inaccessible to most Chinese readers.[86]

An exception to this pattern of operating within the Russian-speaking world was the career of Aleksandr V. Spitsyn (1876–1941), another graduate of the Oriental Institute in Vladivostok, who edited the CER's Chinese-language newspaper, *Yuandong bao* (The Far Eastern Paper). Published from 1906 to 1921, it served the CER administration's agenda by promoting a favourable image of Russia in Manchuria. But it also reflected the views of the Chinese writers it employed.[87] Its Russian and Chinese staff deserve separate treatment as intermediaries between the two societies. So do the officials of the CER Department for Relations with the Chinese Authorities, established in 1901, which later financed the publication of *Yuandong bao*. They worked closely with the aforementioned Chinese Diplomatic Bureaux.[88] The Department and the

Bureaux ran the mixed courts, which dealt with all legal issues that arose between Russian and Chinese subjects in the CER zone until Russian extraterritorial rights were cancelled in 1920. In 1921, the Department for Relations with the Chinese Authorities was renamed the Russian-Chinese Secretariat, and from that time until the sale of the railway to Manchukuo it employed equal numbers of bilingual Russian and Chinese staff.

The study of China provided jobs and salaries for specialists as well as a cultural pastime for the educated public. Russian Harbin enjoyed a lively literary scene, and famous theatre troupes and some of the world's premier musicians included it in their Far Eastern tours. Nonetheless, a painful sense of provinciality was endemic among the local intelligentsia, especially when they compared Harbin to other centres of the Russian emigration. From China, it was difficult for them to secure a position in the virtual "Russia abroad," whose life played out on the pages of the émigré press in Europe. Some of Harbin's intellectuals, however, developed a method of turning provinciality into an advantage: beyond the remotest pale of Asian Russia, they could actually claim to be best placed.

The prolific poet and writer Vsevolod N. Ivanov (1888–1971) joined the discussion of Russia's destiny between West and East, Europe and Asia, which a coterie of Russian academics had initiated in Prague in 1921. He did so in a survey of Russian history titled *We: The Cultural-Historical Foundations of Russian Statehood*, which came out with a publisher named The Bamboo Grove in Harbin in 1926.[89] The Prague circle and its followers called their ideology Eurasianism.[90] Its proponents expressed resentment against "the West," by which they meant Europe, where they and their families had found refuge from Bolshevik Russia. They urged Russians to proudly acknowledge the Eastern component of their national identity. In defiance of the standard image of the Mongol yoke, the linguist Prince Nikolai S. Trubetzkoy (1890–1938), who had become a professor of Slavic philology in Vienna, celebrated the "legacy of Genghis Khan" in an essay with that provocative title in 1925. But the Eurasianists stopped short of identifying Russia with Asia. The geographer Petr N. Savitskii (1895–1968) presented the geopolitical tenets of Eurasianism as the belief that Russia was neither Asia nor Europe, but contained both East and West; it was, in fact, best described as Eurasia. Savitskii opened his essay, published in German in Leipzig in 1934, with a statement expressing rivalry with China rather than any wish to join it: "Russia is much more justified than China to call itself 'the Middle State' (Chzhun-go, in Chinese)."[91]

Vsevolod Ivanov, for his part, boldly called himself "Aziat," an Asiatic. Russia, he argued, needed to do more than simply contemplate its Eastern heritage; it ought to look toward the Orient, where that heritage was still alive – toward China, including Manchuria, and Japan. In a public exchange with a Eurasianist in Paris (a scholar of Persia and a former tsarist consul in that country), Ivanov wrote from Jinan in Shandong province that one could not discuss "Asia" from Europe.[92]

Ivanov had settled in Harbin in 1924 after shorter sojourns in Wonsan (then known as Gensan, in Korea), Mukden, Tokyo, and Shanghai. He stayed in Harbin until 1933, when he left Manchukuo for Tientsin. One of his several forays into poetry, *Refugee Poem*, also published by The Bamboo Grove in 1926, opened with painful yearning for Russia and fear of dying in alien China. Nonetheless, after a meditation on ancient Russian history, Ivanov declared that becoming a refugee in China was really a miraculous return to blessed Eastern origins. The final image of the poem was still that of the "yellow-blue Chinese" indifferently passing by and of the poet realizing that a long and inhospitable road lay ahead.[93] Ivanov mastered Chinese, becoming a fluent speaker. In 1936 in Tientsin he edited five richly produced and illustrated issues of a *Vestnik Kitaia* (China Herald), which also carried the title in Chinese *Hua-E yuekan* (Chinese-Russian Monthly). It was launched with the statement that the older generation of the Russian emigration in China, although it had spent almost twenty years in the country, "has managed to encapsulate itself to such an extent that … it has learnt nothing about China, has not noticed it, has passed it by."[94] The editor hoped that the younger generation, in contrast to their parents, would learn Chinese and give Russia more scholars of China than it ever had.

In his journal, Ivanov marvelled at the visual qualities of classical Chinese poetry, which he demonstrated by analysing in the original a Tang poem by Li Bai (701–762). In another essay he compared "the logic of Europe and Asia," finding the latter far superior to the former. A Chinese person, Ivanov argued, enjoyed boundless freedom from the shackles of the preconceptions, which dictate our own behaviour as Westerners and limit our world view. Still, he argued that the Chinese found the Russian world view closest to their own, which was why Russian literature was so influential in China.[95] *China Herald* published excerpts from traditional Chinese literature as well as articles on the Chinese New Year, Chinese philosophy, fortune telling, netherworld currency (samples of the paper money bills, burnt for the use of the deceased, were artfully pasted onto the pages of the journal), and the Jews of Kaifeng; it also introduced readers to the nature, culture, economy, and politics of contemporary China. The journal folded abruptly amid suspicions that it was providing a cover for Soviet espionage, never to supply the promised continuation of a "Chinese novel" by a Russian German author on the life of fisherman Tsin from Chefoo.[96]

In 1926, the same year that Ivanov's two books came out, Nikolai A. Setnitskii (1888–1937) published an essay on the way the Russian philosophers Vladimir S. Solov'ev (1853–1900) and Nikolai F. Fedorov (1829–1903) perceived China. In his final apocalyptic work, *Three Conversations*, written during the Boxer Uprising in 1900, Solov'ev warned of the danger that a united force of China, Japan, and Mongolia posed to Russia and the West. He thereby combined the spectres of pan-Mongolism and the yellow peril.[97] To counter such views, Setnitskii cited Fedorov, his own lifelong mentor, who opposed Russia's joining the European powers to suppress the uprising in China, and who regarded the Chinese cult of ancestors as a moral example. Fedorov went even further than the Chinese in honouring the ancestors, since his teaching of "cosmism" charged the living with the task of resurrecting the dead.[98]

Setnitskii had arrived in Harbin in 1925 as a Soviet citizen, to work in the CER's Economic Department while carrying out "economic espionage" against Japan.[99] Besides editing and publishing Fedorov's works, he wrote on Chinese politics and the soybean trade, subjects he taught at the Polytechnic and the Faculty of Law. An economist and statistician by profession, a philosopher by calling, Setnitskii was not a trained China expert.[100] Rather, like other Russian lecturers at the Faculty of Law, who, as the common turn of phrase had it, "found themselves in China," he became interested in that country because he lived and worked there. These were curious intellectuals committed to thinking and research – a mindset that made China a natural object of their academic inquiry while in Harbin. The faculty published twelve volumes of a scholarly journal in Russian (*Izvestiia Iuridicheskogo Fakul'teta*), which contained many studies on China, above all Chinese law. The authors used European sources, engaging the help of Russian sinologists and the faculty's native-speaking language teachers when they needed to consult Chinese texts. After the sale of the railway to Japan in 1935, Setnitskii returned to Soviet Russia, where he was executed two years later as "a Japanese agent." Vsevolod Ivanov, who repatriated from Shanghai to Khabarovsk in 1945, lived to a ripe old age there as a successful Soviet writer.

Introducing a *Survey of the Economical Geography of China*, which he published in 1925, Ivan I. Serebrennikov (1882–1953), a former minister in the Kolchak government, who became a historian and memoirist during the thirty-three years he spent in Harbin, Peking, and Tientsin, felt the need to apologize: "the author of this work is no expert

Orientalist, he lives in China by accident [*sluchaino*], is here bereft of a scientific environment and therefore begs in advance the reader's indulgence."[101] Yet the biographical "accidents" of spending years in China or of being born there could determine a person's life path. As we shall see in chapter 8, some of the younger generation of Russians in Manchuria justified the hopes placed in them by Ivanov in his introduction to his short-lived journal, the *China Herald*.

The Languages of Communication

When Russians and Chinese did communicate with each other in Harbin, as they had to in various situations of daily life, they often resorted to a pidgin referred to as *moia-tvoia* (literally, "mine-yours"). It was not invented in Harbin, but was brought to Manchuria from the Russian Far East, where it was the language of communication in the second half of the nineteenth century. An earlier pidgin, named for Kiakhta, the border town between Russia and Qing Mongolia, was already current in the eighteenth century. During the Russo-Japanese War, tsarist officers from Saint Petersburg learned to speak in the "Russo-Chinese jargon": "*Shima minza*? I questioned him sternly," reported Baron Wrangel in a wartime letter peppered with the exotic argot; here he was interrogating a suspected *khunkhuz*, whom his Cossacks had just brought in, tied by the queue. A footnote explained to readers of the *Herald of Europe* that the author was asking the bandit for his name.[102]

Making do with a limited vocabulary and a simplified grammar, a Chinese peddler on a Harbin street could offer his wares, while a Russian customer might employ the same language to haggle over the price. In this imagined scene, the customer is consciously distorting his or her language, assuming that the peddler would not understand standard speech. In research on pidgin, speakers of the dominant language who reduce their speech to the essentials while addressing speakers of the subordinate language are described as using "baby-talk," or "foreigner-talk."[103] Not all Russians would use pidgin, and few would do so in conversation with a Chinese person whom they recognized as belonging to a high social class. As for the peddler, he probably would not have been able to speak a grammatically correct Russian, but if he did pick up at least the Russian words for "I" and "you," he was acting out a tacit agreement about the limits of knowledge. In Harbin society, the Chinese, not the Russians, were expected to learn the other's language – or rather *maozi hua*, "hairies' talk," as the Chinese called it, thus identifying a patois that was really a mix of the two languages with the Russians. Cooks and domestics learned this kind of Russian to speak with their masters, and if the masters happened to speak another language, they knew they had to learn that, too. An outsider, the violinist Hellmut Stern (1928–2020), commented on the "arrogance" of Russians' refusal to learn Chinese and on the remarkable linguistic skills of Chinese domestics. (His claim that one of them, in the employ of a Jewish family, ended up speaking Yiddish with a Berdichev accent should, however, be taken with a pinch of salt.) Born in Berlin, Stern lived in Harbin as a Jewish refugee from 1938 to 1949. To get through the education system, he needed good Russian; not being part of the city's Russian society, he also needed spoken Chinese.[104]

While these language relations were convenient for Russians, the Chinese may not have been keen on Russians learning their language. As things stood, they were in the advantageous position of understanding without being understood themselves. By addressing the "native" in an inferior version of Russian, the speaker of that language was, in a way, redressing the linguistic imbalance: "While I still cannot make head or tail of his Chinese, he has somehow managed to learn my Russian – but then look what a primitive Russian it is." These frustrations and consolations were familiar to colonialists anywhere.[105]

When Russians and Chinese spoke *to* each other, one term of address that Russians used was *khodia*. The precise origin of the word is obscure, but it is associated in Russian with the verb *khodit'*, to walk: as a diminutive, it reflected a benign image of itinerant Chinese and street hawkers.[106] However, *khodia* clearly turned into a condescending term from the time when it was interpreted as "friend" and as a "tender form of address" by Russians during the Boxer campaign and the Russo-Japanese War. A note that a Russian general made in his diary while passing through Harbin in the summer of 1918, when Chinese troops were consolidating their control of the CER, attests that the Chinese perceived it as patronizing. The Chinese, Aleksei Budberg wrote, justly answered the old nickname *khodia* with the words in pidgin: "Well now it's you [literally: your] the *khodia*, and I [mine] the captain" (*Nu teper' eto tvoia khodia, a moia kapitana*).[107] In an article on Russian-Chinese relations in Harbin, published in a Nanking journal, the author Mao Hong, who presented himself as a long-time Harbin resident, glossed *khodia* as *huoji* (Chinese: "mate," or "comrade"). He added that, since the days when Russians used that appellation for the Chinese, they had become so much reduced that now it was the Chinese who called them "poor hairies" (*qiong maozi*).[108]

The vocabulary that Russians and Chinese employed to speak *of* each other is indicative of their respective stereotypes. Pejorative terms for the Chinese that had become established in the Russian Far East spilled over the border into Manchuria, but in Harbin their use was attenuated by the need to maintain correct relations with the Chinese, who soon outnumbered the Russians. One example of such derogatory slang was *manza*. It was used when no Chinese person was in hearing range.[109]

Explanations linking *manza* with "Manchu" cannot be sustained: the term entered Russian speech in the 1860s through contact with Han Chinese rather than Manchus in the Russian Far East.[110] A Manchu, moreover, would never identify as *Manzu* before this modern (Chinese) term for the Manchu nationality emerged in the early twentieth century. A British officer who travelled in Manchuria in 1886 reported that Manchus he met called themselves *qiren* (bannermen), whereas the Han migrants, by then the ethnic majority in the region, still thought of themselves as "southerners," *manzi*.[111] If we take the last meaning as the indigenous source of *manza*, the term may not have been conceived as derogatory when it first entered Russian usage in references to Chinese in the Maritime province.[112] It did become a slur well before 1900.

Chinese appellations for the Russians in Manchuria did not lag behind *manza* and *khodia*. Russians were called *lao maozi* ("old hairies") or subsumed under other variations of "foreign devils."[113] They might also be called "big noses" (*da bizi*), as distinct from the "small noses," a term used for the Japanese.[114] Lattimore noticed that Russian soldiers (*soldaty*) were ridiculed as "smelly Tatars" (*sao dazi*), which suggests that some Chinese, like some Russians, thought their opposite numbers stank.[115] Among educated Chinese in the twentieth century, the belief took root that denigrating foreigners in racial terms was their natural right, since China was being exploited by the Western powers. Thus, chauvinist prejudice was aggravated by political impotence, exacting the revenge of the weak. Denigration of the Russians was mild compared to the torrents of racial abuse launched at the Japanese occupants of Manchuria by Chinese propagandists in the 1930s and 1940s.

The bilingual realm of daily life made inroads into the vocabularies of both Russian and Chinese speakers. Every Russian throughout the Far East knew what *fanza* (from *fangzi*, a house), *khunkhuz*, *manza* and, of course, *lamoza* (the "Russified" version of *lao maozi*) meant.[116] In Harbin, these words, appropriated from the Chinese, became more than part of a functional pidgin. Russian speakers employed pidgin words, with an ironic twist, in conversation with one another. Writers of poetry or fiction played with the ambivalent effect, redolent of both familiarity and exoticism, that such words produced on the printed page. The Chinese, too, inserted Russian words into their spoken language even when no Russian was in sight, while customarily employing Russian terms of weight and measurement (such as *pud* and *arshin*) in their own commerce.[117]

Some Russian words were phonetically accommodated into the spoken Chinese of Harbin.[118] Russian *mashina* (car) became *mashen* ("horse spirit"), while *plita* (oven) became *bilida* ("built-in-the-wall"). The St Nicholas Cathedral was appropriated in familiar terms, as *lamatai* ("Lama platform"); Lamaist temples were known across Manchuria. Perhaps the most revealing aspect of the linguistic behaviour of the two communities in Harbin was not so much their tendency to borrow from each other, but the reciprocal attribution, by Russians to Chinese and vice versa, of special linguistic knowledge in cases where, in fact, neither side had any. A number of pidgin words were used with the shared impression that they must have come from the other language. One keyword in this Russian-Chinese pidgin, *shango* (used for approval as in "good," "great"), may have come from the Chinese *shang hao*, although the Chinese suspected it was Russian, and the Russians thought it was Chinese. Linguists call this phenomenon a double illusion. *Khanshin*, used for a popular Chinese alcoholic beverage, is another example, in this case one intimately connected with Harbin history because a distillery (*khanshinnyi zavod*) existed there in 1898 and was the first installation acquired by Russians.[119] But the greater enigma for Harbin's Russian and Chinese populations, to the extent that they were troubled by it, had to do with their city's name.

Among early Russian explanations of the alleged meaning of "Harbin" in Chinese, the one most persistently recurring is *veselaia mogila* ("a happy grave"). As a memoirist of the Boxer Uprising put it, "Harbin – in Russian translation, *a happy grave* – indeed became a grave for many and an unhappy one of course, although previously everybody had really lived there very happily."[120] As late as 1989, a Harbin-born novelist in Russia wrote: "Specialists claim that the [place] name is not Chinese; the characters Ha-er-bin correspond only to its sound and, in translation, yield variable or meaningless reading: 'a high shore' or 'a happy grave' (which is not without reason, in my opinion)."[121] Only "shore" does correspond to the last syllable of "Ha'erbin." Clearly, when Russians tried to ascertain why Harbin (as they thought) meant "happy grave," they worked back from the Chinese. In 1980, however, a Chinese scholar opened a history of the city by demonstrating that "Harbin" could not have meant "grave" in Russian.[122]

A possible reading of the "happy grave" tag for Harbin would be as a mock-Oriental place name, constructed by Russians to compensate for the intractability of the local geography – the threateningly unknown prehistory of the site on which they built their city. British colonialists called the West African coast "the White Man's grave." The sensitivity of some early Russian settlers to traces of Chinese burial sites in

Manchuria has already been mentioned. Writing in the requisite style of the time, the historian Guan Chenghe, who had sifted through the synonyms of "grave" in Russian to show that none of them sounded like "Harbin," concluded that applying that word to the city was an apt reflection of the "criminal tsarist policy in the Far East."[123] Considering the geomantic requirements of grave siting in East Asia, however, the imagined "happy grave" – although manifestly wrong as a translation of "Ha'erbin" – would have made sense. A "happy," or felicitously chosen, burial site was a familiar concept: one example is Fuling, literally Happy Tomb, the Chinese name of Nurhachi's mausoleum outside Mukden.[124]

There was never enough communication between the Russian and Chinese inhabitants of Harbin to prevent the circulation of basic misinterpretations of the city's name, but scholarly accuracy on the matter was in any case secondary to politics. In the 1980s, local historians were determined to keep the origin of the city as far as possible from the problematic legacy of Russian imperialism. Within the limits of pure Chineseness that the northeast could offer, this meant identifying "historical Harbin" with a capital of the Jin dynasty of the Jurchens (1115–1234), the ancestors of the Manchus. Relics of the Jin upper capital Huiningfu were discovered south of Acheng (formerly called Ashihe), about 40 kilometres southeast of Harbin.[125] In the 1990s, the historian Ji Fenghui countered such medievalist theories with an archival discovery that he thought enabled him to trace "Harbin" to a Manchu name for the "flat islets" at the mouth of the Sungari River. In this reading, the toponym survived the speakers who knew its meaning and was passed down to the population the Russians encountered in the late 1890s, who could no longer explain it.[126] Ji became engaged in public debate with another historian, Wang Yulang, who had updated the version of Harbin's Jin dynasty origins by arguing that the Jurchens called Harbin "a swan" (*galouwen*, in their language) and by proposing that the city exploit the touristic appeal of this attractive appellation.[127] Predictably, the Jin dynasty "swan" won over the Qing dynasty "flat islets," the Harbin municipality adopted Wang's exegesis of what "Harbin" really meant, and many businesses in the city took "swan" (Chinese: *tian'e*) for their name.

We have discussed the language that Chinese and Russians in Harbin used when speaking with each other, the terms they employed to speak of each other among themselves, and the intrusion into (or enrichment of) the native vocabularies of both sides by words in the other's language. The Russian-Chinese pidgin never became a Creole.[128] While no author of Chinese or Russian literature in Harbin wrote in the other language, portrayals of the other side in their works remained problematic insofar as "the other" could not be convincingly described as speaking the same language as the author and his or her reading audience. Naturally, one could write for and about one's own community, ignoring its present location within a foreign milieu. At the other extreme, Chinese characters in a Russian short story could be made its unique subject, described in their surroundings and in communication only with fellow Chinese speakers. Some of Harbin's Russian authors attempted to capture such cameos of undisturbed Chinese life. But the more common choice was to allot the other some space in which to express him- or herself within a narrative grounded in the language of the writer and the readers. For Chinese authors, this solution was the only alternative to the predominant mode of ignoring foreigners as subject matter. Two examples of such representation follow.

Through the Ussuri Region (Dersu Uzala), by Vladimir K. Arsen'ev (1872–1930), the description of an expedition into the Sikhote-Alin Mountains in the Maritime province in 1906, was published in Vladivostok in 1921. The writer had visited Harbin, where the sinologist Pavel V. Shkurkin (1868–1943) helped him transcribe the Chinese place names.[129] In 1923, Arsen'ev published a sequel, *Dersu Uzala*, in which he narrated his second Ussuri expedition of 1907. The second book carried a dedication to the memory of Dersu, Arsen'ev's native Gold (Hezhe) guide, who died in 1908 shortly after the author had tried to introduce him to city life in Khabarovsk.[130]

In the book, Dersu spoke Russian-Chinese pidgin – as he must have done in real life. Besides sympathizing with the plight of native peoples, most of whose troubles he ascribed to the Chinese, Arsen'ev was unambiguously committed to promoting the Russian national interest in the Far East: while Dersu represented the allure of life in nature, Russia stood for civilization. Arsen'ev's counterpart in Harbin was the explorer, collector of zoological specimens, and author of popular fiction about the Manchurian taiga, Nikolai A. Baikov (1872–1958). One of the sketches in his collection *In the Mountains and Forests of Manchuria* (1914) featured a Chinese hunter, who said, literally, the following: *Liao-khu blizko khodi, gou-gou chifan'. Shibko plokhoi gospodin est'. Ego kantrami nado.*[131] Between brackets, Baikov supplied translations of *gou-gou* (dog), *chifan'* (to eat) and *kantrami* (to kill), but only readers in Saint Petersburg, where the book was published, would have needed them. Both Arsen'ev and Baikov have been compared to America's James Fenimore Cooper. For readers in Harbin, they were also what Rudyard Kipling was to the British in India: however distant and exotic the environment these writers described was for outsiders, local audiences read their books as stories of the world they inhabited and for which they felt an affinity even if they knew that world badly, often feared it, and longed for their native country, which they idealized.[132]

In Shanghai in 1936 the writer Xiao Hong (whose most famous work, *The Field of Life and Death*, was cited in chapter 1) published a collection of autobiographical sketches titled *Market Street*. Written with the sensitivity and humour that mark the best of her work, *Market Street* was a fictionalized memoir of two years the Hulan-born Xiao Hong spent in Harbin, from summer 1932 to May 1934, when she shared her life with the writer Xiao Jun (1907–1988). In the opening sketch, "The Europa Hotel," the couple is about to be evicted from that establishment, which is run by a "White Russian." We know from Xiao Hong's biography that she had been staying in the hotel for some time prior to Xiao Jun's appearance. She was pregnant with another man's child and unable to pay her rent.[133] Now the hotel manager demands that the two tenants pay an inflated bill, and when they refuse, he orders them to leave. His words are delivered in broken Chinese: *Ni de mingtian banzou, ni de mingtian zou!* (You tomorrow move out. You tomorrow go!).[134] The hot-tempered Xiao Jun (Langhua, as he is called in the book) reacts by brandishing a sword in the manager's face and putting him to flight. Xiao Hong and Xiao Jun continue to resist eviction, although the Russian manager has called in the Chinese police. Not long afterwards, two "foreign women," apparently Gypsy prostitutes who live and entertain clients at the same hotel, surprise the narrator at the head of the stairs. Again, they are unable to speak Chinese: "'Aiya!' One of them pointed to me and said, 'You – very pretty!' … The two of them swished the fronts of their skirts to show them off for me. 'You – very pretty!' I ignored them."[135]

No doubt, Xiao Hong's readers in Shanghai would not have asked themselves this question, but did foreigners in Harbin really address Chinese people in Chinese? Toward the end of the book, fearing arrest by the Japanese, the couple is preparing to leave Harbin and the small flat on Market Street (Birzhevaia ulitsa), where they had moved from Hotel Europa. Xiao Hong needs medical help and visits a free-of-charge Russian clinic – "but my Russian was so poor that I didn't understand much of what the doctor was asking me."[136] The physician would have addressed her in standard Russian, which Xiao Hong and Xiao Jun actually studied while in Harbin,[137] whereas the manager of Hotel Europa spoke to his indigent clients in condescending Russian-Chinese pidgin rather than the unimaginable Chinese that Xiao Hong later attributed to him. Perhaps he said, *Tvoia zavtra ukhodi!* She may have replied to him in the same way. But as there is no guaranteeing the documentary veracity of autobiographical records,[138] it may also be that by putting an inferior language in the mouth of the hotel manager and the women on the stairs, the Chinese writer was presenting the inverted image of her own inept Russian. Her choice in the dilemma of representation (Which of the two speakers of unequal linguistic levels should be assigned the higher position? Will my own or the other's speech seem inarticulate?) would have been the most natural one.

As for the Hotel Europa, literary-minded tourists in present-day Harbin unwittingly head to a renovated Art Deco hotel at Xi shidao-jie no. 10. This is just off the city's main avenue, the Zhongyang dajie, which was formerly called Kitaiskaia (Chinese Street). The hotel uses the same name as appeared in the title of Xiao Hong's sketch (the obsolete transcription of Europe in Chinese as Ouluoba becomes "Europa" in reverse translation), while styling itself "Europaer Hotel" [sic] in Latin letters on the entrance signboard. There is a bust of Xiao Hong in the lobby, and by paying extra, guests may book "Xiao Hong's room" on the third floor.[139] A heritage plaque installed by the city administration marks it as the place where the writer stayed "in 1937," adding that it was constructed "in 1934." In fact, it was designed by the architect Vladimir I. Babii (1909–2003) in 1942.[140] But there have been two hotels by this name in Harbin, at different points in time. The first, a low-end hotel or hostel, where Xiao Hong lived alone and then, for a month, with Xiao Jun until November 1932, was at no. 21 on the same street, which was called Russkaia (Russian). That building no longer exists. As of 1926 (it may have changed hands by 1932), the proprietors of Hotel Evropa were not quite "White Russians," but a Jewish couple.[141]

4

A Chinese-German Flower

In October 1907, when Baron Roger Budberg was forty, he married a girl with the surname Li, who was about to turn fourteen, although she pretended to be a few years older. She came from a Chinese town near Harbin. Her father was dead and her mother had been unable to raise her. It may be, although only circumstantial evidence supports this conjecture, that Budberg took her from a brothel.

For the first time in the short history of Harbin, a respected member of the Russian community had married a Chinese. Even when mixed marriages between Europeans and Asians became more common in Harbin, about twenty years later, it was Russian women who – often as a survival strategy – married Chinese or Japanese men. The couple's daughter was born on 6 March 1909. The unique name she received, Zhong-De-Hua, "Chinese-German Flower," signalled Budberg's wish to merge two (but not three) national identities, deepening the rift between him and Russian society.

Indeed, he reported with pleasure that the Chinese called him "the German Doctor," or "Dr Bu" (Bu daifu).[1] The Russians, however, had nicknamed him *obmanzevshiisia nemets*. The first word was built on "Manza," a derogatory term for the Chinese; and "nemets" means German. Hence, the meaning of the epithet was something like "German-turned-Chink." They also called him *chudak*, an odd fellow,[2] a milder term that still indicated that his "going native" was unacceptable. Having subverted the colonial hierarchy by his marriage, he affirmed it in another sense by taking a child for his bride. Her age would not have raised eyebrows in Chinese society, given that as many as 20 per cent of rural women in the region married at the age of nine.[3] A Chinese man of Budberg's standing in the 1900s would have taken a girl of such background as a concubine, not a lawful wife. Marriage with girls in their teens had precedents in the Budberg family history and they then gave birth more than once before turning twenty. Often, they became young widows.

Budberg readily acknowledged that his "sinicization" made him happy, and for a long time he did not care about his image in Russian eyes. Nevertheless, he was concerned that the Russian state refused to legalize his marriage. In December 1909 he even wrote to the *St Petersburger Herold*, telling readers of this German newspaper in the Russian capital that fate had led him to marry a Chinese woman and asking them for legal advice on how best to arrange the status of his wife and, by then, his daughter, without requiring them to convert to Christianity. The Russian ambassador in Peking had turned him down, for tsarist law did not recognize civil marriages – a policy Budberg criticized as inferior to the Chinese spirit of religious tolerance.[4] Budberg did not mention that the Qing government had just passed China's first nationality law, which granted citizenship only to mixed children born of Chinese fathers, not to those born of Chinese mothers; moreover, women who married foreigners were deprived of their citizenship, and children born to them could only claim Chinese citizenship if their foreign fathers were stateless or did not recognize them.[5] Budberg's legal struggle with Russian officialdom would drag on for years, but the standing of his wife and daughter was in fact as precarious on the Chinese side.

In letters and postcards from Harbin, Roger described his daily life to his sister Antoinette. Since her marriage to Count Raczynski she had lived in her husband's castle of Augustusburg (Polish: Obrzycko), north of Posen (today's Poznań), a part of Poland that had been under Prussian and German rule since the late eighteenth century and was to remain German until the end of the First World War. The great distance was no obstacle for regular correspondence, which only upheavals in international politics and in Budberg's life interrupted; unfortunately, only his side of the correspondence has survived. The city of Harbin, eight years old when Budberg settled there, had an efficient postal system, enabled by the railway, which carried the post, passengers, and merchandise to Manchuria station on the Russian border and from there all the way to Moscow on the Trans-Siberian. In August 1906, as he was busy equipping his new apartment in Pristan', Budberg wrote that his next step would be to subscribe to the telephone network; this service was worth the expense as it already covered Harbin and the Chinese town of Fujiadian and would soon extend to Vladivostok.[6]

Work

He was also getting his private clinic ready to receive patients. A photograph from his first years in Harbin shows Budberg standing in front of the clinic door with an unidentified Chinese person. Behind their backs, a vertical signboard in Chinese, fashioned in a style used by traditional shops, allows sight of the characters "De," for "German" (also meaning "virtue"), and "Bu," the first syllable of his surname; other characters are obscured by the tassel hanging down from the sign. Below, the large characters *daifu* occupy the centre space. The simple character *bu*, just two brushstrokes literally meaning "to divine," was of course used here for transliteration, but does exist as an uncommon and rather exquisite Chinese surname, which Budberg might have found appealing. *Daifu* was not only "doctor" (as distinct from *yisheng*, which simply meant "physician") but also a title of cultural prestige. In ancient China, the combination of the two basic characters, read *dafu*, was a title of nobility. When preceded by another simple character of the sort Budberg surely learned as he began his Chinese studies, the *shi* of "scholar," it designated the Confucian literatus (*shidafu*); in the Qing, *daifu* also became an honorary title, translatable as "gentleman." To be called *daifu* was therefore a respectful form of address, no less than Herr Doktor. No text in German was used on the signboard of Budberg's clinic, however, and it would have been out of place in Harbin, since the clientele were going to be Chinese and Russian. High above the entrance door, a placard in Russian announced that Baron Budberg specialized in female diseases and *akusherstvo* (obstetrics) and would receive patients at this clinic from 9 to 12 and from 3 to 5. The word "Samanskaia," discernible on the sign, was a curious misspelling of Samannaia (now Xiaman jie), one of the small streets turning from Kitaiskaia, named for the material used in constructing the houses on it (Russian *saman*, adobe).[7]

"Akusher," from the French *accoucheur*, was his favourite Russian word to describe what he did, and it conveyed the sense of a male midwife. In present-day medical terms, he was an obstetrician-gynaecologist. His clinic was an immediate success. The flow of patients kept him busy for most of the day, not just the appointed consultation hours. Chinese patients began to come very gradually, as only the elite would consider seeing a foreign doctor, and it would have taken daring or a medical emergency for a woman to expose herself to a Western physician. Nonetheless, in a letter of February 1907 Budberg could report on the first Chinese woman on whom he had operated, the wife of a rich man from outside Harbin. Most of his European patients came from New Town, which made living and setting up a practice in Pristan' a questionable choice, but he liked to be near the Sungari, for he enjoyed going for a swim or sailing out to the river islands.[8] Perhaps he also preferred this area because more Chinese lived there than in the expensive New Town, the administrative centre of the railway.

He did begin commuting to New Town when in January that year he became head physician of the maternity ward at the Central Hospital of the CER, Harbin's oldest and largest, located near the city's railway station. Happily, his good friend Friedrich Raupach (1871–1938), who had been with him in Dorpat as a fellow assistant of Professor Koch, replaced him at the university's women's clinic in 1902, and who later, like Budberg, served in the Russo-Japanese War, was now head surgeon in the same hospital.[9] Two other friends from Dorpat in Harbin were the ophthalmologist Jan Alexander Göldner (1869–after 1944), who had already reached Manchuria as a military physician in 1902 and went by the name Ivan Nikolaevich among the Russians, and the fellow gynaecologist Paul Kramer (1876–1922), who fell into Japanese captivity during the Russo-Japanese War but returned to Manchuria to start working for the CER in 1907.[10] Their careers show that many professionals took the step of settling in Harbin after the war, because of the opportunities it offered. Budberg probably shared this motivation of his medical colleagues, yet he was alone in combining it with a declared love for China.

In June 1907, Budberg accepted an offer from the CER committee on prostitution to take charge of a "hospital for prostitutes" in Pristan'. Located at the corner of Politseiskaia and Artilleriiskaia (Police and Artillery) Streets by the Sungari River, today's Youyi lu and Tongjiang jie in the Daoli district, it was the second hospital ever to be built in Harbin back in autumn 1898. It had two wings, one of them divided into separate wards for men and women with a total capacity of about forty beds, the other consisting of a day clinic and a pharmacy, with two attached apartments for the feldsher and the hospital director. Although known as "the hospital for prostitutes" because the railway taxed the women for the medical care it provided, it treated male syphilis patients as well.[11] In a letter to his brother Joseph, Budberg described this new job as an opportunity for making observations, which he could use in short articles so as to stay in touch with European scholarship.[12] More room for such observations would open up for him once he became physician of the Harbin city prison from 1910 and, soon afterwards, also the physician in charge of the emergency room at the Harbin police station.

With that much work on his hands, he still found time to write: both the letters to Antoinette, who became his main connection to the family (notwithstanding the obligation he said he felt to communicate his thoughts to his mother and siblings, he soon gave up trying to write separately to all of them), and the short articles arising from his newly gained knowledge of China, which he regarded as a continuation of his earlier medical publications in Dorpat. By December 1907 he reported that his first articles had just been printed in Chinese; another, on cholera, was due to be published "in the Chinese newspaper."[13] It has proved impossible to trace these articles (one of them, enclosed with a letter to his sister, was not preserved), nor anything else by him that ever appeared in Chinese. These short pieces were intended to spread medical knowledge among the population in Harbin and Manchuria as well as to make his name known to the educated Chinese public. The other side of his writing was meant to inform the German (although, significantly, not the local Russian) reading audience about China. Because, like everything he wrote, these articles were highly personal, they offer some keys to understanding how he interpreted the culture he admired and how he deployed his other identities: as an ethnic German and member of the border-crossing German nobility, a Russian subject, and a physician of the CER in Manchuria.[14]

As will be seen below, his judgments of Russia were devastating. Nonetheless, as long as the Romanov empire lasted, he was committed to the Baltic German tradition of personal loyalty to the tsar. A letter he sent from Harbin to Saint Petersburg in March 1908 reflects this. Writing in German to Elisabeth Richter (1841–1916) to offer condolences on the death of her husband, the infantry general and member of the State Council, whom Budberg had consulted during his conflict with the management of the Russian Red Cross in the Russo-Japanese War, he mourned the loss that Richter's demise meant for "our imperial house and the Fatherland." While his use of *Heimat* may have referred to the Baltic rather than to Russia, he lauded the statement made by Nicholas II on the death of the high official of Baltic German origin: "How heartfelt are the words of our Emperor, telling you and the world how dearly he loved the deceased, he could not have expressed his respect and his love in a more beautiful way."[15]

Writing on China

On the morning of 26 October 1909 (13 October for the Russians), Budberg was among the dignitaries gathered at the Harbin railway station to welcome the Japanese elder statesman Itō Hirobumi (b. 1841), who had arrived there for a meeting with the Russian Minister of Finance, Vladimir N. Kokovtsov (1853–1943). Budberg then saw Korean patriot An Chunggŭn shoot Itō, the former Governor General of Korea, who had signed the treaty by which Korea became a de facto Japanese protectorate in 1905. As the first physician on the scene, Budberg rushed to assist Itō. With the permission of Kokovtsov, he had the victim carried into the railway car, where he examined his wounds.[16] He remained by Itō's side until all non-Japanese persons were asked to leave the wagon; Itō died minutes later.

In a detailed letter to his sister on that same day, he described the events and his part in them, including an exasperated tirade on the ignorance of the Russian medical staff, who had insisted on obtaining the "first name and patronymic" of a wounded Japanese officer. Budberg tried to get his testimony into print as soon as possible, but it was rejected by several newspapers before being edited in the Berlin *Vossische Zeitung*.[17] His account was probably rejected because he blamed the Russians even in this context.

The longest of Budberg's essays on China launched a series of five articles by him, all marked "from Harbin," in the high-profile geographical journal *Globus* between March and November 1910. *Globus* was published in Brunswick (now Lower Saxony), by the former publishers of the Stuttgart weekly *Das Ausland*, in which the description of Reinhold Anrep-Elmpt's last travels had appeared in 1891. Academically trained China specialists occasionally also wrote for *Globus*: for example, the renowned anthropologist Berthold Laufer (1874–1934) in 1905. Budberg's first article was on the notorious Manchurian bandits.[18]

He began by tracing the origin of the term "Chunchudzen" (*hong huzi*, redbeards) to a Chinese image of Russian Cossacks – in his description, the robber bands of Siberia, who sowed death and destruction along their path of incursion into northern China. Their hair was usually red or brown, contrasting with the black hair of the Chinese, who even now mocked Russians as *maozi*, or *huzi*, both words being references to hair. Only after the Sino-Japanese War in 1895, Budberg contended, did the term *hong huzi* begin to be applied to the discharged Chinese troops, who turned to robbery and kidnapping. The numbers of Chinese seeking work in Manchuria grew markedly with the construction of the Chinese Eastern Railway. The temptations of easy money then led some young men astray, and the "immorality" of the Russians in their treatment of the Chinese contributed to the spread of Chinese banditry. The lucrative deals offered to bandits for their collaboration during the Russo-Japanese War further encouraged "demoralization" and swelled their ranks. Large organized bands of Chinese *hong huzi* now operated in Manchuria, attacking strictly Chinese (rather than Western) targets. In the border regions and in Inner Mongolia, the bandits often joined with Mongols, Russians, and Cossacks; rather than simply extract money from their victims, they took pleasure in killing them.

The main part of the article offered a detailed description of the *hong huzi* who had been captured and imprisoned by the Chinese administration: the forms of punishment and torture used on them during interrogation and in jail, the methods by which they were executed, and the disposal of their corpses. Two photographs accompanied the article, apparently taken in Harbin and showing prisoners put to death by beheading and by strangulation. In asides throughout the text, Budberg acknowledged that a European would be appalled by these manifestations of Chinese cruelty. He asserted, however, that the executions carried out by the Russians during the Boxer Uprising and in the Russo-Japanese War, and even in Europe, were still more terrible. There could be no doubt, he wrote, that "the Russian far outdid the Chinese in brutality; at least, that is the conviction that impresses itself on every European, who here has had the opportunity to observe both nations in their shared life."[19]

By "here" he meant Harbin, and the European observer, who rated the Chinese so much higher than the Russians, was obviously himself. He narrated some of his own experiences – for example, when at an execution ground in Tieling (northeast of Shenyang in today's Liaoning province) during the war in 1904, he followed a group of sixteen prisoners on their way to be executed in Harbin. Having "often accompanied the criminals on their last journey in the hope of finding out the true Chinese perceptions of life after death," he concluded that their belief in the immortality of the soul was deeper than that of Christians.[20] Was he also, however, the other "European" to whom he had referred earlier, who could not suppress a shudder at the cruelty he witnessed? His letters confirm that such sights put his adopted cultural identification to a test: "I have lived so long in China and have become used to thinking in the Chinese way in many respects, and still the thought about what goes on in the courts and on the execution ground makes me ill."[21] In the article, there was tension between his wishing to present a sympathetic account of China and his desire to document in precise and harrowing detail the functioning of a penal system that placed no value on individual life. Perhaps it was because he realized that his description risked encouraging views of Western supremacy and strengthening anti-Chinese stereotypes that he took pains to balance a potentially damning report on Chinese justice with a wholesale condemnation of Russia and its role in the Far East.

He did so through his commentary, beginning with the folk etymology he endorsed for *hong huzi* as a reference to marauding Cossacks in Russian service. (He added the even more far-fetched claim that Chinese fear of the Cossacks had left Manchuria unpopulated.) A senior figure in Harbin, whom he knew and counted as a friend, Saoke Alfred Sze (1877–1958), a graduate of Cornell University who was

Superintendent of Customs in Harbin from 1908 to 1910 and later an ambassador to London and Washington, associated the "redbeards" with the red cloth that Chinese bandits tied "on the muzzles of their guns"; there are many other explanations of the term besides this.[22] Budberg claimed that Russian soldiers joked whenever a procession of convicts passed by them on its solemn way to the execution field: "kho-dia kantrami," they would say, pointing to their throat and using words the Russians thought to be Chinese and the Chinese considered Russian, but that were intelligible to both sides (*khodia*, Budberg explained, originally meant "workmate" in Chinese, and *kan* was "to chop off"). He added that a Russian soldier "stood lower than an animal in relation to the Chinese, but held himself to be a man of high culture."[23]

And in the mouth of a Chinese convict facing execution, he put a tirade against the city the Russians had built: Harbin, shouted the condemned man, was with its easy money-making a cursed place, where young people were dragged into every kind of vice, and the criminals now facing execution were all victims of that corruption. The only way out was to escape Harbin, back to the countryside, where one was poor but at home (*in der eigenen Heimat*). Here and later in the article, Budberg claimed to be reproducing the words of prisoners he had heard uttered when his understanding of spoken Chinese could hardly have been good enough; he mentioned having a guide beside him, and one infers that if he was not simply ascribing his own beliefs to a fictional personage, he was retelling what someone had translated to him on that day. There is a sketch of Budberg on a Russian rather than Chinese execution ground in the outskirts of Gongzhuling, a town between Siping and Changchun in Jilin. It was written by an Austrian reporter who knew Budberg during the Russo-Japanese War and who later mixed fact with fiction in his novella about those events. Here the narrator's friend, the wise and imperturbable physician, "professor" Budberg, acts on his own responsibility to end the suffering of a Chinese coolie, whose Cossack hangman does not know his job. At the end of this execution scene, Budberg reflects on the riddles of the afterlife.[24]

The contradiction between his subject matter and the positive image of China he wished to convey to German readers was abundantly clear to him as he opened his next *Globus* article, on "Chinese Prostitution," by arguing with another imaginary European, who accused China of barbarism on hearing that slavery had been tolerated by Chinese law until a very recent imperial edict abolished it.[25] Going on to describe the sale of daughters into prostitution, Budberg emphasized that the Chinese loved their children and could only be forced to sell them by desperate famine resulting from floods and droughts. The girls were sold through intermediaries to brothels and theatres, whose owners and operators carried the real blame for their misfortune. According to Budberg, this was a view the Chinese people shared; therefore, they would never "throw a stone at" the hapless victims. This description downplayed the extent to which human trafficking was common and socially acceptable in northern China: it did not, in fact, only take place in crisis situations.[26]

Budberg then offered highly specific information on how a woman sold into prostitution could become free from her "owner." If she dared to turn to the local magistrate's office, her complaints would be heard and investigated; if they were found justified, she would be confiscated from the man who had bought her and placed in a refuge for prostitutes. During a three-month stay there she would acquire basic household skills, and her photograph would be exhibited publicly along with those of other inmates. Any honest man wishing to take her for a wife could then approach the administration of the refuge and hear more about her character. If he was ready to pay her price, and she expressed consent, their way to marriage was paved.

This was an accurate description of institutions for the rescue of prostitutes, created by the state in early twentieth-century China and known in many cities as *jiliangsuo* (literally, office for aiding the good).[27] In Peking in 1921, an American scholar noted that the same police-run refuges (which he called the Door of Hope) also housed "young children who were destined to become prostitutes, but who have been rescued from their abductors."[28] Budberg claimed that prostitution in China was especially widespread in places opened for international trade. Using a term to which he frequently resorted when characterizing the effects of foreign incursion on Chinese society, he argued that the population in such towns and cities became *demoralized*, that is, morally degraded. He did point out that despite the unquestionable suffering of the women confined in them, brothels were also important urban locales, where travelling merchants fixed their business meetings, itinerant storytellers collected their tales, and much current information could be obtained. The women sang and performed on an open stage, which was accessible even to the poor, while the well-to-do visitor could admire "the merchandise" without any social opprobrium being attached to his presence. Most Europeans did not so much as suspect that such places existed.

His next three articles in *Globus* were on the conditions of export trade in northern Manchuria, the religious views of the Chinese, and Chinese law. Given that he lamented the harm done to China by foreigners, it is surprising to see him assume the role of an economic adviser to potential German business interests in Manchuria. His article and private letters show that while he was harshly critical of the opening of China by Westerners and the Japanese, he made an exception for Germany. As he put it when writing for *Globus,* compared to other nations, Germans had the advantages of perseverance and the ability to adapt to unfamiliar conditions. He imputed the complete lack of these qualities to the Russians, whom he blamed for ignoring the principles of the Chinese common law and for "demoralizing" the people in Harbin, as rising criminality in the city attested.[29] Budberg recommended to German merchants that they study Chinese, establish contacts with Chinese firms, and exploit the extraordinary promise of the Manchurian corn market by allying with a Chinese bank that had branches all over the northeast; he also suggested that they make use of the extensive network of the French Catholic Mission in Manchuria.

However, in his next article, he sharply criticized the Catholic missionaries. He described them as the agents of a misguided effort to impose a Christian world view on a nation that needed no alternative to its own tolerant and all-encompassing moral system. Adult Chinese converted solely for material reasons – the true victims of the missions were the children they took in, whose innate free spirit they paralysed with the assistance of Chinese nuns, all of whom suffered from degrees of "neurasthenia or hysteria."[30] Extolling the virtues of the Chinese "moral system," Budberg went so far as to say that even the *hong huzi* obeyed an ethical code – they were loyal to friends and respectful to elders, robbing only the wicked and frequently supporting the needy. In this same article, he defended Chinese medicine against accusations of "barbarity" and explained away even such customs as eating the heart of an executed criminal (also mentioned in his first article) by a capacity for "autosuggestion": someone who ate the heart of a brave man in the belief that this would make him just as brave would indeed act courageously in a critical situation. He rephrased here his earlier conclusions about Chinese beliefs to say that, although the Chinese were convinced that the soul was not bound to the body, ever since the days of Confucius they had refused to preoccupy themselves with the afterlife. It followed that the consolations of Christianity had nothing to offer them.

Budberg's final article in *Globus* was titled "Civic and Public Liability in Chinese Popular Life."[31] An echo, perhaps, of his law studies, it was a statement of unqualified admiration for the core principles of Chinese society as he understood them. This society, he believed, was held together by reciprocal ties. Within the great network, extending from relations within the family to those between employer and employee, everyone knew their place. In view of the Chinese concept of mutual responsibility, even the sentencing to death of whole families by imperial order in cases of grave offences by one of their members should be understandable. Foreigners living in China had to become part of this networked society to avoid constant frustration. Russia's failure to accommodate its practices to these unfamiliar cultural conventions was most evident in Harbin when Russians employed Chinese without so much as bothering to find out their names (instead, domestics were renamed "Ivan" and "Andrei") or asking for the guarantee letters, without which no one could get hired in China except by unwitting foreigners. The inevitable outcome was "demoralization" of the Chinese and the shocking rise of criminality in the region dominated by the railway.

Also in 1910, Budberg published an article titled "The Nations in Manchuria" on the front page of a Berlin daily. He signed with a pseudonym: the vehemence of the sentiments he expressed on the conduct of Russians in the region and their image in Chinese eyes was such that he could ill afford to air them openly.[32] He argued that the Chinese were not the closed and xenophobic people they were imagined to be: whoever lived among them without offending their customs and sensibilities would find himself more easily accepted than in many other countries. The Chinese, he wrote, had developed an ability to distinguish between members of different Western nationalities. The article ranked them, from the most popular to the most hated, supposedly in accordance with the Chinese view. It emerged that the favourite European in China was "the German," whom the Chinese esteemed for his quality products such as shotguns and Krupp-made steel saws, and whom they considered "the model of diligence, learning and energy." Next, but at some distance, came "the Englishman" (English products were well regarded, although still seen as inferior to the German). He was closely followed by "the American," whose wool fabrics were appreciated and who was politically more trusted than all the others. "The Frenchman," while "especially unloved" politically, had earned some affection for being better tempered than other foreigners; yet French wines, conserves, and perfumes had found few takers among the Chinese. Finally, there was "the Russian," and what the article had to say about him merits a full translation:

> The Russian ... is in the perception of the Chinese a complete barbarian, who stands deeply below the cultural level of the Chinese people. He possesses in the opinion of the Chinese very little sense of right and morality, and he is taken to be corrupt, lazy, uneducated and uncouth. Yes, the Russian is often good-humoured, and you can then befriend him. But according to the Chinese conviction, one can never count on his "goodness." He

is always to be feared as a strong and raw barbarian. The bloody acts of
violence, perpetrated by the Russians on the Amur during the Boxer war
are still unforgotten here. Wide areas were then systematically depopula-
ted by them. Hardly any Chinese escaped death in the affected regions. The
large mass of Chinese ascribed the gruesome acts of the Russians purely
to brute instinct. The few politically seasoned Chinese are convinced that
the Russian soldiers carried out their work of gruesome destruction on
high command; that it was the plan of the Russians, through methodical
expulsion and extermination of the Chinese in Manchuria, to make space
for Russian colonists. For it is entirely clear to the Russians, that the Chinese are far superior to them as tillers of the soil and merchants. They hope
to keep the feared competition of other nationalities away from Manchuria by undermining peace and order in the land, deliberately cultivating
Chunchusen robber bands.

The map of his allegiances and animosities, couched in terms of "the
perception of the Chinese," had been drawn. He did not make up the
Chinese perceptions, which he underscored and amplified. More than
twenty years later, another admirer of China, the young American
scholar in Manchuria, Owen Lattimore, wrote similarly that "the most
illiterate unskilled workman who speaks a garbled Russian, and for that
reason rates himself high among his fellows, none the less looks down
with moral superiority on all Russians as uncouth creatures entangled
in barbaric misconceptions of all the true values of life and culture";
and he, too, ascribed to the Chinese a "peculiar contempt for Russians
as ... the violent but stupid northern barbarians."[33] Lattimore believed
that the Russians, in turn, "obstinately held on to a conviction of superiority which outfaces even the profound Chinese sense of superiority."[34]
Budberg espoused a strain of Chinese cultural chauvinism that
agreed best with his own positions. He served a state he despised for
reasons that went far beyond its treatment of the Chinese in Manchuria. His derision for his employers normally had to be concealed, but
it found outlets in articles he sent for publication to Germany and in
letters to his sister, in which he frequently said that he hoped to pass
into the service of the Qing empire. The Russians had brought him
to China and to Harbin, but he would live there as a German and a
Chinese.

A Chinese-German Household

Marrying a Chinese woman was essential: it was a part of his plan. In
February 1907, hinting at the opposition with which such designs must

have met in Poniemon, he wrote to Antoinette in Posen that "although the rumours being spread by mother are unfortunately not yet true, I make no secret of the fact that I am purposely looking about for a Chinese life partner and I hope that I will be able to find this cornerstone of a greater work and homely fulfilment."[35] In March he was preparing to report the happy news:

> It looks now almost as if I would soon arrive at the adequate being, which has been my lifelong, ardently wished goal; at an escape from the abhorrent bachelor life I have always hated into a married life based on ideal purpose. Since the death of my grandmother, with whom alone I had the closest exchange of souls, I have found no other intimate support in which to confide the depths of my heart with all its good qualities and its abnormities.[36]

Their maternal grandmother, Countess Cecilia Anrep-Elmpt, died in Germany, aged eighty, when Roger was twenty-five and Antoinette twenty-two. We do not know how he had lived in Dorpat; now he was alone and imagined the woman he would marry as his ultimate entrée into a new life in China.

This was, however, no easy task. As he explained in the same letter, though he was "very sinicized," he was nonetheless a foreigner, to whom a Chinese family would only give a daughter in marriage for more money than he could afford to spend. But as often happened to him in China, he wrote, good fortune had come his way: a Chinese patient whom he had successfully treated, the wife of a rich building contractor in Kuanchengzi, had readily agreed to act as his matchmaker and had just conveyed to him that she and her husband had found him a bride. She had been presented to him as an adopted sister of the patient's husband and as an orphan, whose father

> had been a teacher [a *guanlidi* – i.e., a Chinese living within the Wall, so a very real one], 19 year-old and proficient in the written Chinese language (!!) Girls do not learn reading and writing, only some mandarins' daughters are educated. She is said to be pleasant looking, very diligent and thrifty. They say it was her own wish to marry a European. No bride money will be required, and I should only guarantee that I will stay in China. She is now up in Tientsin and is expected back in four weeks; I should go to Kuanchengzi to see her. If I like her, the wedding could take place right away.

He elaborated on the good deal he had made: he would need to spend no more than a hundred rubles in gold on small gifts to his bride, and another few hundred on the wedding. He explained that he would rather have the wedding in Kuanchengzi than in Harbin, both because it would be less noticed and because his former patient would be able to arrange everything according to Chinese custom. He had not seen a Chinese wedding yet, and he described for his sister how he would have to play host for three days, entertaining the guests, who would come bringing gifts and teasing the bride. Then he and his wife would travel back to Harbin, accompanied by the couple from Kuanchengzi, who would stay with them for a week or two to replace his parents and to encourage the young woman. So he had it all worked out. Only one detail troubled him: his future wife's parents had been Chinese Catholics, but he (a Lutheran) did not wish to record the marriage with the Catholic Church in China. He wrote that this was also unnecessary because his future children "would presumably be Chinese subjects."

He did not even try to hide his impatience. Anticipating likely reactions to his marriage, he said he knew that all hell would break loose in the Baltics ("im Baltenlande") but that he could count on the understanding of his nearest Harbin acquaintances. Sometime in the future, he mused, he and his wife could travel together to his home ("meine Heimat") and meet his dear siblings. He did have some nagging doubts (he asked Antoinette not to pass on the news to the siblings just yet: "if the thing falls through, the contents of this letter would make me a laughing stock"), and he knew that mixed marriages between Europeans and Chinese in Manchuria were very rare. An example, which he mentioned in a subsequent letter in autumn 1907, was a Herr Schoene, the police chief in Baoding, who was very happy with the beautiful Chinese woman he had married.[37] Indeed, Budberg turned to Schoene for advice once his own detailed plans had come to naught: apparently, the family in Kuanchengzi had decided to give their adoptive daughter to "a poor Chinese, rather than a foreigner." It was a decision he was ready to applaud for what it said about the Chinese, for it was evidence that they placed the purity of their race above any pecuniary considerations. Still, this development left him with few prospects, and he summed up his efforts to find a wife as having been a huge expense emotionally and financially.

There were always "hunger years in China, when extremity can force the family to sell the daughter for marriage to a European, but for this purpose," he wrote in August, "I should travel to Tientsin or Peking – here even through buying I can find nothing." He added that a main reason for his persistence was "aristocratic sensitivity ... No other people as the Chinese can offer so much promise for good race through rational cultivation. What's more, there is the spiritual perfecting, in which

I believe with this people, to whom the world shall belong."[38] Writing to Joseph in December, he put it still more defiantly: "Through my studies of Chinese life conditions and so forth, I have become fully sinicized myself ... and so for me now, after having lived long in Chinese families, European married life has become fully incomprehensible, even repulsive." Another reason to marry a Chinese was the contribution his wife would make to his career: he envisioned laying the foundations for the training of midwives, "which the four-hundred-million-strong people so urgently needs."[39]

But by the time of that letter to his eldest brother, his Chinese marriage was no longer a project awaiting eventual realization: he had found what he was looking for, although, because some of his letters from this time are missing, we cannot be certain how this had come about. In two books he wrote in the 1920s, he often spoke of his wife while saying little about her background. In his Russian memoirs, Budberg wrote that as a seven-year-old child during the Boxer Uprising in the summer of 1900, she escaped to the mountains near Ashihe, southeast of Harbin, with her younger brother and sister. Apparently, their mother was still living at the time but could not take care of them. Budberg referred to his wife's brother, who briefly stayed in their Harbin house in 1919, as "a very bad man"; at that time, he described Li burning incense to the spirits of both her parents during the Qingming festival.[40] The siblings were probably born in or near Ashihe, the Chinese name of a district, a town, and a river, which were called Alchuka in Manchu. Ashihe was founded as a Qing garrison in 1729 and was the main town in the region before Harbin was built.[41] When the Russian army occupied it in August 1900, the town had been abandoned; its people returned only at the end of that year, by which time it had been badly damaged by Russian soldiers, who were still stationed there in large numbers.[42] Ashihe remained an important commercial centre, having become a station on the CER line. At about 50 kilometres to the east of Shuangcheng, where Han settlers were already almost twice as numerous as the Manchus by 1903, Ashihe was still predominantly Manchu and was unique in Jilin province in that respect.[43]

In the opening pages of the book he published in Germany in 1923, Budberg spelled his wife's name "Li-jü-dsehön." While Li is one of the most common Han Chinese surnames, the characters behind "jü-dsehön," which jointly make up her first name, are hard to decipher. Once this exotic transcription is collated with another source, which gives the name as Li-Jui-Dshen, and converted into the modern Hanyu Pinyin system, the most likely guess would be Li Ruizhen, meaning Lucky Treasure.[44] Two photographs in the same book carry captions in which the author's wife is also called Baroness Budberg. The first photograph shows her smiling, in a brightly decorated costume of the Chinese theatre, her long black braids trailing down her shoulders, "on a benefit event at the Railway Club" (the Assembly, known as Zhelsob in Russian) – which suggests that, at least in the beginning, the unusual couple was not ostracized. In the second photograph, dated 1909, she is "in Manchu dress," and her hair is made up in the Manchu way (*liang-batou*, "two-branch-head," in Chinese), the tresses twisted around a flat strip of wood or silver, and her expression is frozen. A female companion, perhaps a maid, is standing beside her; the backdrop seems to be the interior of a photographer's studio.

In the Harbin studio of photographer S. Glushenko, the couple posed with Li wearing her Manchu hairdo, with the heavy bar on top, and an embroidered silk dress. On her lap rests a pair of heart-shaped pouches, another Manchu attribute, although one shared with Han Chinese. A ring is visible on her right hand. She is seated in an armchair with Roger standing behind her in suit and tie, his hands resting on the back of the chair (see figure 4.1). Their formal postures and attire suggest that this undated picture may have been taken to celebrate either their engagement or their wedding. They married according to Chinese law, but nothing is known about the wedding itself, which probably took place in early October 1907.[45]

In one of the photographs in the family albums where Li appears, she again wears her actor's costume with long, braided hair. She was often photographed with the Manchu headdress, which was promoted in the court of Empress Cixi (1835–1908) in the 1900s. It was also adopted by Han courtesans in northern China and featured in Peking opera.[46] On one occasion, Li wears pressed flowers in her hair, Manchu-style; on another, she wears the high-platform shoes of a Manchu woman. In other photographs, however, her dress and hair are in accord with Han Chinese practice. A question inevitably arises: having almost married a Catholic convert, did Roger Budberg's elaborate plans for integration through marriage into Chinese society result in matrimony with a Man-chu rather than a Han woman? Though he called her Chinese, he found her appearance somewhat uncommon: "Where the Creole skin colour of my wife, which I find beautiful, comes from, I do not know. One sees it often among the Chinese."[47]

Another photograph, which reached the Museum of Russian Culture in San Francisco in 1970, sent by an informant in Belgium, is inscribed in Russian: "Baron R. Budberg with his wife, a Manchu, at the Chinese cemetery during the plague of 1910–11." Three more photographs and a letter from the informant, former Harbin resident Victor S. Makaroff

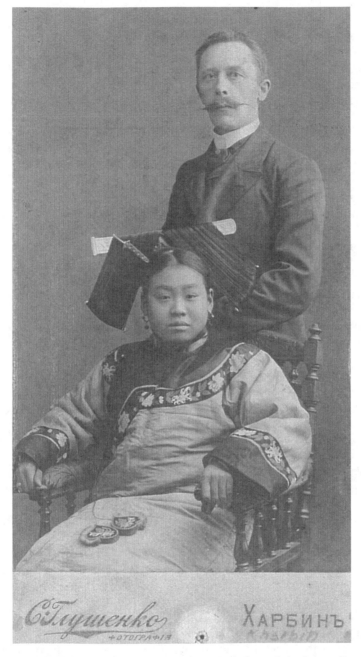

4.1. Roger Budberg and his wife. Photograph made in the studio of S. Glushenko, Harbin. Popoff family album.

(1914–?), were inserted in the museum's copy of Budberg's memoirs, published in Harbin. One of these photographs is captioned: "R.A. Budberg with his Manchu wife of the Bu-ming-li (Manchu: Bumenri) family." This, however, was merely a misinterpretation of the Chinese writing on the tomb of Budberg's wife: *Bu men Li shi* means "woman Li of the Bu family," the character Bu standing for Budberg.[48]

Referring to a former Chief of Police of Fujiadian in 1910, Budberg characterized the Manchus as a stubborn people, lacking in agility and intelligence and repulsed by every novelty.[49] However, the Manchus' conservative position as safeguarders of the empire from the Han Chinese revolutionaries aroused Budberg's respect and admiration, which he expressed in an article he published on "Chinese and Manchus" soon after the revolution of 1911.[50] He made another reference to the Manchu ethnicity – besides identifying as Manchu the clothing of his wife in the photograph reproduced in his German book – when in his memoirs he mentioned that their daughter's old nanny was a Manchu from Hulan, a town northwest of Harbin.[51] And in a late letter to his sister, to be cited below, he expressly identified his wife as Han Chinese *rather than* Manchu.

The boundaries between banner people (both Manchu and Han) and the Han Chinese population were more fluid in Manchuria than anywhere else in Qing China, and they became even more porous toward the end of the nineteenth century.[52] A girl from Ashihe, if that's where she came from, could have been of either Manchu or Han banner origin, or even the daughter of a Han bannerman (Hanjun) and a Manchu woman.[53] Or perhaps she simply liked to dress up as a Manchu. Perhaps it was also her way of signalling that she had become an aristocrat. Some blanks must remain; attempts to fill them in are best formulated as questions, not suppositions. Was the girl Li sold to a brothel, whose inmates took part in theatre performances? This could help explain her easy switching between codes of dress. Did she then reach a refuge for prostitutes, from which Baron Budberg redeemed her after failing to find a Chinese bride by other means and resorting to the same acts of chivalry as he had carried out in the brothels of Dorpat? If this is what happened, and even if he reported it in letters to his sister, it may be no coincidence that these particular letters were not preserved. But here speculation must stop.

Budberg and Li created the first openly mixed European-Chinese household in Harbin. Marriages between Han Chinese and the other East Asian ethnicities that were present in Manchuria were common (only marriages between non-banner Han Chinese and Manchus were prohibited, with some exceptions, until the 1900s), but there were hardly any unions across the racial line that separated Asians from Europeans. Their household also included a Chinese youth, whom Roger Budberg called his "adopted son" (*Pflegesohn*). This boy had been living in the house before he brought in his bride, and Budberg hoped she would not object to his staying on.[54] It is tempting to identify him as the youth appearing alongside Budberg in several photographs in the family albums and to hazard the guess that this was Sjödro, who had been to Ponicmon. There were domestics in the house, whom he occasionally called "my Chinese" in his letters. His child bride was, in the beginning, also like an adopted daughter, and he took charge of her education. A striking photograph shows her, smiling with lips shut, all dressed up with the Manchu hairdo and flower-decorated robe, seated on a *kang* bed with a tray or a writing board set in front of her. A notebook is spread open on it. Behind her, a folded quilt supports what looks like a fashion album, leaning against the wallpaper. On the other wall to her right, vertical scrolls of carefully drawn Chinese characters are pasted. She must have been learning to write (see top image, figure 4.2).[55]

Early on, Budberg acquired wooden Chinese furniture, carved and inlaid with mother of pearl.[56] Photographs taken over the following years show these beautiful pieces as well as his growing collection of Chinese objets d'art: bronze mirrors, figurines of Buddhist and Taoist deities, porcelain vases, and paintings. Budberg was sometimes photographed in the mandarin jacket (*magua*), originally an item of Manchu clothing, which had become common in China during the Qing and was still worn in the republic. This is how he is captured in a late photograph together with his daughter, which is reproduced on the dust jacket of this book. In other pictures he appears to be wearing a gown (without seeing the colours, it is hard to determine whether this is a Chinese gown or that of a medical doctor). Photographs taken outside the privacy of his home show him in European dress.[57]

In autumn 1908 he moved into a large house in the heart of Harbin: originally no. 18 on Kavkazskaia (Caucasus) Street, which became no. 8 when numeration changed in 1924. Chinese artists, who decorated local temples, painted his walls. Budberg described these murals in an article that a German monthly in Riga carried shortly before the First World War.[58] One showed a man falling from a high cliff while a supporting hand stretched out to save him; another, based on "a very well-known story," showed an execution during which the sword broke in two before touching the neck of an innocent victim; in a third mural, a man persecuted by monsters has been delivered from danger by the appearance of white mist, which blocks their path. These iconographic descriptions and the surviving photographs of the murals, which were

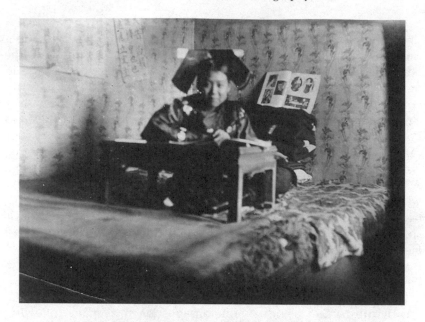

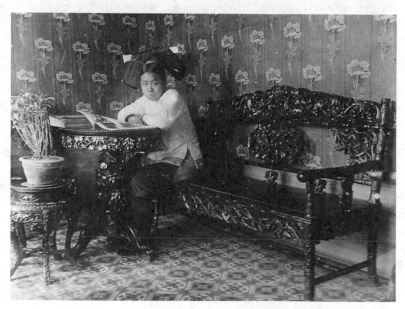

4.2. Li Ruizhen at home. Photographs in Raczynski family album.

taken from distance but allowed the sight of a moustachioed deity and of female figures, suggest a fusion of motifs from the hagiographies of Guanyu (Lord Guan) and Miaoshan, the female avatar of bodhisattva Guanyin.[59] Budberg commented that it was wrong to classify the Chinese as adhering to a specific religion, such as Buddhism or Taoism, since all of them shared a belief in the transmigration of souls. In the same article, he extolled the cornucopia of religious images in a temple he had visited in Hulan. His home in Harbin, too, was decorated with eclectic abundance; the murals were framed by a wooden display cabinet, in front of which he arranged his collection of Chinese art.

When the girl Li entered his home, he did not know her exact age. She claimed to be seventeen (Budberg did not elaborate on whether she said "seventeen" by the Chinese count, which treats a person as one year old at birth – in that case, she really was saying sixteen). He did not believe her and thought she was younger. His "dear little wife" was "not outwardly beautiful: a really flat nose with a round point and blurred features. The eyes are dark brown and so much trust, temperament and liveliness look out of them." In height, she didn't reach his shoulder (and he was not a tall man); she had small but not bound feet, and he admired her lithe, slender hands. Having received no education, she could write some Chinese characters but did not like memorizing new ones. She had little interest in learning German (Budberg intended to engage an older German woman to teach her the language, as well as "handiwork and home economy"), but she was always picking up new expressions in Russian, and her pronunciation of foreign words was perfect. Budberg had told his sister that when he did find a wife, he planned "to keep her away from any social exchange with Europeans," although he "would have nothing against" her socializing with Chinese.[60] After two and a half months of marriage, he wrote that his wife's latest hobby was photography. She was already helping him in the clinic. He liked her and wished he had more time to spend with her, although he also felt that all his free time needed to be devoted to his studies.[61]

He was determined to learn everything he could about China and to quickly improve his skills in the language. As of December 1907, he was still unable to write Chinese but was regularly speaking it. He engaged a private Chinese teacher (a photograph of whom survives) and gained the rest of the knowledge about China for which he thirsted through reading and many excursions to the countryside and talks with the people. With very few exceptions (such as the scientists cited in his last book, *On Life*), what exactly he read cannot be known, for he did not have a habit of quoting and did not mention specific books in his letters. One book to which he did repeatedly refer was the *Analects* of Confucius. His circle of friends appears to have been large despite the suspicion toward him, especially among Russians. A former governor of Kuanchengzi had stayed as a guest in his house (and told Budberg he needed to marry a Chinese woman).[62] There were many more Chinese contacts, such as the already mentioned Sao-ke Alfred Sze, unidentified by name but described in letters as "the current governor," who had lived in the United States, spoke French and German, and approved of Budberg's plan of "becoming naturalized" in China and passing into the Qing service.[63] Once Budberg and Li were married, their house became open to guests and lodgers from all social layers and ethnicities. In a late letter, he recalled (by then, as a nuisance) that fifty to seventy Chinese, families as well as single men, who worked as street vendors, used to live in their cellar.[64]

It is a reflection of Budberg's sociability and frequent gullibility that despite being prone to making the most derogatory generalizations about the character of "nations" and being hostile to Russians in particular, he made friends across class, religious, and ethnic barriers – in later years, even among Russians. Although harshly critical of the missionary enterprise in China, he became friendly with a number of the Catholic fathers in Manchuria; and despite his self-chosen immersion in Chinese life he apparently enjoyed the opportunity to converse with them in German and French. He found missionaries tactful and unpretentious, concluding that "friendship is unharmed by the entirely opposed convictions and aspirations that we follow in China."[65] He felt closest to the small community of German nationals in Harbin; in his estimate, there were between one and two hundred of them in 1909.[66] Two other ethnic groups that, along with the Russians, were regular targets of scorn in his letters to his sister were the Japanese and the Jews. The front page of the issue of the *Berliner Tageblatt* in which his pseudonymous analysis of "the nations in Manchuria" appeared carried news of the annexation of Korea by Japan; commenting on that event in a letter to Antoinette, he called the Japanese "the most horrid people in the world."[67] Apparently, he did not keep Japanese company.

With regard to Jews, he subscribed to the stereotyped views that were prevalent in Russia and Europe in the early twentieth century. His instinctive contempt was both racial and cultural: similar to that sense of superiority which enabled him to speak, parenthetically in a private letter, of "Georgians, Armenians, Persians and whatever other criminal nations there may be,"[68] but also a reflection of the specific role of Jews in German discourse of the late Wilhelmine empire, which certainly reached the Baltic. Championing tradition against modernity and identifying with the virtues of "Germanic culture" automatically made one hostile to the Jews; condemning them was another way of affirming those values.[69] In addition, Budberg embraced the disdain for Jews that was already endemic in Russian society before the Revolution and grew stronger thereafter. So he regarded the many Jewish doctors in Harbin as unscrupulous competitors, while the high visibility of Jews in the local Russian press triggered in him fears of Jewish conspiracy.[70] In the summer of 1910, in one of his unsigned articles in *St. Petersburger Zeitung*, the most influential German-language newspaper in Russia, for which he had written occasionally since the Russo-Japanese War, Budberg lashed out at Jews for their wrongdoing within the Russian administration in Manchuria.[71]

In contrast to his lack of experience with the Japanese, he had been familiar with Jews since childhood. Reminiscing about the spirit of tolerance in which he had been raised (a quality he also repeatedly attributed to Chinese culture), he recalled with admiration a devout Jewish peddler and his daughters whom he got to know in Goldingen; he was fascinated by the interpretations of the Talmud that he heard in their humble home.[72] Sympathetic descriptions of the Jews near Poniemon appeared in the childhood memoirs of his sister Antoinette, which were written after the Second World War and not meant for publication. We shall later see how one of their brothers, assisted by their mother, defied all conventions in bridging the social divide between Jews and German aristocrats.

Roger Budberg's private correspondence as well as his published writings show him to have been an anti-Semite.[73] Since he was able to separate his prejudice against "peoples" from his attitude toward individuals, however, he did employ a Jewish midwife. Almost sixty years later, this woman remembered him gratefully as the "German doctor" who gave her "a lot of practice" in Harbin. Perhaps Budberg hired her because, before arriving in Harbin, she had obtained her diploma in midwifery from the University of Dorpat, or Iur'ev University, as this institution was called by then.

Plague

The Jewish midwife, Esther Komarovskaia, departed for America in 1913, travelling for the fifth and last time on the Trans-Siberian Railway, which had first brought her to China in 1905, and then sailing to the New World by ship from Hamburg. An experience she remembered as a dangerous interlude during her eight happy years in Harbin was "the pest": when "that panic" broke out, she said in a family interview in 1965, she took her son and daughter to the Black Sea. They spent six weeks at the beach in Evpatoria, and visited Poltava, her hometown, as well as Kharkov and Sumy in Ukraine. Only then did they return to Harbin, where her husband worked for the CER.[74]

Plague came to Manchuria in the autumn of 1910, and when it reached Harbin, panic was indeed the right word to describe the people's reaction. In that sense, the atmosphere was comparable to Blagoveshchensk during the Boxer Uprising in 1900.[75] In a city where, as Esther Komarovskaia also commented, Russians and Chinese had to get along with each other because they depended on each other, limited cooperation in daily life was shattered once the epidemic, which Europeans identified as pneumonic plague, proved to choose its victims almost exclusively among the Chinese population. This was because of the terrible sanitary conditions and overcrowding, especially in Fujiadian but also among the Chinese poor in Daoli. The disease killed everyone it touched: up to 8,000 people in Fujiadian and about 1,500 in Harbin (estimates for the whole of Manchuria were as high as 60,000). That almost no Westerners except medical staff were struck provoked Chinese suspicion and increased apprehension of the measures the Russians had adopted to fight the epidemic.[76]

The year before the plague broke out, in the summer of 1909, Budberg was awarded the Order of the Double Dragon. Although not a rare distinction for foreigners in the twilight of the Qing dynasty, it meant much to him, and he made sure to spread the news. In a statement in connection with the award, he emphasized his dedicated study of the Chinese language and culture and notably his intention of "becoming scientifically productive, possibly at a Chinese university in Peking." The honour expressed official recognition of his belief that he could do much for China; it also marked him as a China lover in Russian eyes. As he wrote to his sister in December, "I am hated in Russian circles because in a short time I have won the reputation of one of the best China-knowers."[77] In a book published in Harbin in 1910, a local Russian nationalist pointed to an unnamed Baltic baron, a medical doctor who had married a Chinese woman, as one of only two people among "the whole Russian colony in Harbin" to maintain "close spiritual contact" with the Chinese. Tantalizingly, because the episode is otherwise unknown, this author added that when the same physician initiated a project of regular medical checks for Harbin's Chinese prostitutes, Chinese society "brusquely turned away from him."[78]

In letters from Harbin to his sister, Budberg described the epidemic – the hub around which his life now turned. All the elements of his self-identification as a physician, a non-Russian in Russian service, and a friend and would-be protector of the Chinese people, came to the fore during the plague and were challenged by it. In Augustusburg Castle, however, the letters from the scene of the Black Death in Manchuria were held with gloves, read out loud, and then tossed into the fireplace, although by the time they left Harbin they would have undergone compulsory disinfection by mercuric chloride. Such was the fear of the lethal infection they might have brought with them.[79] Still, Budberg's impressions and experiences during the time of plague were not lost, as in parallel to his intensive medical work, he reported on the epidemic for the reputable *St. Petersburger Zeitung*.

Budberg denounced the Russian administration's plague-fighting as motivated only by its desire to protect its own nationals in Manchuria. The rights of the Chinese population were, he believed, trampled upon in the process. In their repressive policies, the Russians obstinately refused to consider the Chinese character and customs or to acknowledge the potential of collaborating with the Chinese. Unable to adapt to other ways of life, the Russians, as he put it, expected the world to be just like them. He singled out the Harbin newspaper *Novaia zhizn'* (which had Jewish editors) as guilty of incitement against the Chinese. Recognizing that Budberg was the only Russian physician who knew Chinese society and could speak Chinese, the railway administration asked him to help control the plague in Fujiadian, "the Chinese town," where foreigners rarely ventured.[80] He accepted the assignment without pay and, despite his pro-Chinese sentiments, expressed strong criticism of the level of medical care he encountered.[81] This led to confrontation with the local authorities and the influential Fujiadian merchants, causing him to give up his mission of cross-cultural mediation after only a few weeks. He did find time to visit the families of twenty Chinese children, who had been taken out of the Russian elementary school they attended in Harbin because of the plague.[82] For its part, the Fujiadian sanitary committee issued a statement denying that the town had rejected Russian medical assistance: they would have liked to invite Dr Budberg to resume his work in Fujiadian, but given that the feldsher who accompanied him got infected and died, they claimed that the risk was too great. "As he is a foreigner, his death would have weighed on our conscience."[83]

Budberg then switched to Harbin, where he put together a team of four Chinese agents. Their job was to detect the hotbeds of infection by establishing the provenance of the corpses that littered the streets of the city.[84] The bodies had been thrown out secretly by relatives and the proprietors of inns, who feared being taken into forced quarantine if their contact with infected persons became known to the Russian military police. In Fujiadian, which had been cordoned off from Harbin to prevent the spread of the plague into the city, there were scenes of horror that no nightmare could match. Budberg described crowded and unsanitary hospitals turned into death barracks. He took numerous photographs of frozen bodies in the unforgiving Manchurian winter and, once a decision was made to burn the plague victims, of piles of corpses awaiting the flames in ditches. He overheard the Russian sanitary staff cracking gruesome jokes as they dragged the dead by their queues to the cremation pits. Meanwhile, Chinese houses in Harbin were being burnt too, allegedly to remove the sites of potential infection.[85] For Russian Harbin, the plague had a critical symbolic dimension: it undermined the cultivated image of the young city as modern and European.

Seven years earlier, the *Harbin Herald* had ironically dismissed articles from the Siberian press that criticized the living standards in the recently founded railway town in China. Readers of such articles, the Harbin paper argued, might think that Manchuria was a region where

plague and cholera raged unimpeded; that the entire Russian population scattered along the railway line ... was fleeing the country, considering itself unsafe even in such a location in China as Harbin, inasmuch as the latter was no city, but something like a camping site bereft of any amenities and safety – a place, where Chinese died off like flies and uncollected Chinese bodies lay on the streets, impeding the movement of carriages and pedestrians.

The paper then described Harbin's modern buildings and institutions, concluding that urban development continued apace, "taking no heed of rumours about plague, cholera and other horrors, which, God knows, may exist anywhere else but not in a place with a Russian population, i.e. not along the line of the Chinese Eastern Railway."[86]

When plague did come to Harbin, Budberg felt that the Harbin Russian society was determined to fence itself off from the Chinese and be saved at their expense. He viewed himself as the spokesman for Chinese suffering and anxiety. He would later reiterate his criticism of the Russian administration in the book he published in Germany on the plague epidemics he had witnessed. There were also deeply personal grounds for his anger and resentment. To lead the struggle against plague in Harbin, the government in Saint Petersburg delegated a team of doctors and medical students led by the famous Ukrainian bacteriologist Professor Danylo Zabolotny (1866–1929). Harbin physicians interpreted this as an expression of doubt as to their ability to deal with the epidemic on their own. Tensions between the two groups came to a head at a meeting in which Zabolotny dismissed protests by the local doctors in terms some of them found offensive. Budberg enjoined

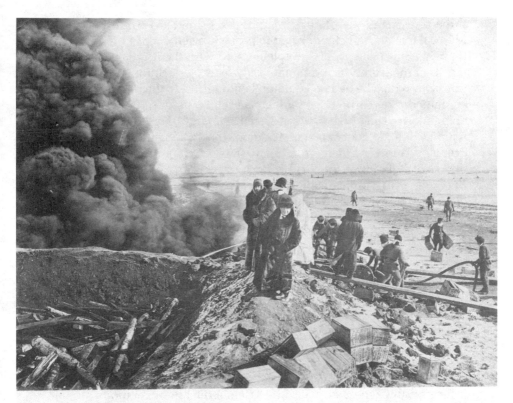

Массовое сжиганіе труповъ обливаемыхъ керосиномъ около г. Фудзядяни.

4.3. The mass cremation of plague corpses, doused with kerosene, near
Fujiadian. Photograph in the album *Chuma v Man'chzhurii v* 1910–11 g.g.
(Plague in Manchuria in 1910–11) (Moscow: Fototip. Sherer,
Nabgol'ts i Ko., 1911).

Zabolotny to apologize for his words, and when he declined to do so,
promptly challenged him to a duel for an insult to his honour. Rather
than accept this challenge, Zabolotny hastily left Harbin.[87]

Harbin and Fujiadian also had Chinese physicians, whose training in
traditional medicine kept them a world apart from the European doctors. They refused to recognize the disease as plague, offering various
methods by which it could be cured and often perishing along with
their patients. The Qing government in Peking hired and dispatched a
specialist of its own to Harbin, the young Malaya-born and Cambridge-
educated bacteriologist Wu Lien-teh (1879–1960). He was assisted by

three physicians (two Englishmen and a Canadian) from the Union Medical College in Peking. Eager to prove himself equal to, if not better than, his European peers, Wu collaborated with the Russians in enforcing strict measures, including intensely feared cremation, on a population with which he had no common language and which he considered benighted. This earned him Budberg's utter contempt. At the end of the epidemic, in April 1911, Wu was placed in charge of organizing an international plague conference in Mukden, the first such event in China. Scientists and physicians from many nations were invited, but on the orders of Zabolotny, the Harbin doctors were barred from attending. Budberg, who had made minute observations of patients and collected quantities of materials during the epidemic, saw himself robbed of an opportunity to present his research to the scientific world.[88]

Instead, Budberg addressed the Chinese population in a pamphlet titled *Baohu wenyi* (Protection from the Plague), which he had printed in Harbin at the Yuandong bao press in 1911.[89] Back in Tartu, he had addressed young Estonian mothers in a similar manner in 1902. Then too he had emphasized hygiene, but he spoke in the name of medical science; this time, in Harbin, he did not claim to possess superior scientific knowledge but was at pains to make his advice compatible with indigenous ideas. Although the Chinese text of the pamphlet is lost, its substance may be reconstructed from two articles he wrote for the German medical press in the same year. One of them, "Some Hygienic Principles in Chinese Popular Life," detailed Chinese methods of sanitation, stressing their use of the natural forces of light and wind. Spread out in the open air, rather than buried in the earth, human waste dried and was then productively used as fertilizer. Budberg drew on his experience as a prison physician to describe the clever way in which waste was channelled out of the prison quarters. Writing on the use of steam for both cooking and sterilization in Chinese cuisine, he conveyed his enjoyment of Chinese food and festivals by evoking a dish of pork, which "arrives at the table on New Year" so well steamed that it can be eaten only with chopsticks, with no need for a knife. He reported that his recommendation to the Chinese that they use steaming for disinfection during the plague met with "success and great understanding"; and prison inmates were grateful to him for introducing a steam iron to rid their clothes of lice.[90]

In the second article, Budberg began interpreting the epidemic he had just lived through, announcing conclusions that concur with medical knowledge today: pneumonic plague did not distinguish between gender, age, and physical constitution, and infection was passed strictly through breathing. He summarized the main precautionary measures contained in the pamphlet he had "disseminated among the Chinese people": when in the presence of infected persons, never expose yourself directly to their breath, protect clothes and hands from contact with suspect objects, and do not touch your face. Instead of the masks worn by medical staff in Harbin during the epidemic, which hardly allowed them to communicate with the patients, he recommended the head bandages he had seen used by Chinese physicians in Fujiadian.[91]

He had been interested in disinfection methods, as well as ready to take folk medicine seriously, from the early days of his medical and scholarly career.[92] In 1911, in an article he sent from Harbin to *Zentralblatt für Gynäkologie*, the leading Leipzig journal, in which he had last published as a Dorpat University physician before the Russo-Japanese War, Budberg wanted to share some of the professional knowledge he had gained in China with colleagues in Europe. This did not mean learning Chinese medicine; he was too staunch a believer in European science for that much acculturation. However, he told his readers that after observing the Chinese use of camphor oil for the treatment of wounds, he had now employed it successfully for several years in his own gynaecological practice.[93]

5
Daily Life in a Mixed City

The Russian and Chinese residents of Harbin, who had settled there for disparate reasons, interacted with one another regularly, though in a limited set of situations. When they left their homes and went out into the street, how did they interpret what they saw? What conceptual frameworks did they apply to their impressions?

Dress and Hair

In Harbin of the early twentieth century, European haute couture and gilt-buttoned Russian uniforms mixed and clashed with the long flowing gowns of Chinese officials and the nondescript grey of coolies' dress. To the Chinese eye, the foreigners' stiff clothing was strange and inconvenient. Objectively, it was ill-suited to the local climate with its harsh winters (–30 Celsius and piercing winds) and stifling summer heat. Outside the metropolis, the Cossacks who settled in villages on both sides of the Manchurian border had no difficulty wearing Chinese or native dress. They also adopted Chinese skills and borrowed household utensils from their indigenous and Han Chinese neighbours. Soldiers caught up in the Manchurian winter in 1904 welcomed the Chinese blankets, socks, gloves, and similar items, which the tsarist army found itself obliged to purchase in huge amounts from shops in Mukden.[1] In Harbin, however, use of Chinese clothing was almost unheard of among the Europeans. Instead, making few concessions to local conditions, Russian men and women continued to dress in East Asia much as they would have in Europe.[2] After the Revolution and during the Civil War, the sight of tsarist uniforms on the streets of Harbin nourished self-justifying "military myths"[3] while also rallying Russian youth to the struggle ahead, for many continued to believe that Harbin would contribute to toppling the Bolshevik regime.

The Chinese noticed the Russians' strong resistance to Chinese dress and resented it. Mao Hong, the rare local author to comment in print on aspects of shared Russian-Chinese life in 1929, wrote that fewer than a hundred Harbin Russians could speak Chinese "although they have been in Harbin for over thirty years"; even fewer, he claimed, dressed and ate like the Chinese.[4] Such comments combined modern nationalist feeling with the venerable belief that the self-evident superiority of Han Chinese culture transformed all aliens and minority peoples who came into contact with it – for hadn't even the Manchus become fully sinicized? Westerners in China, by this logic, should have wished to become Chinese, or at least imitated Chinese ways, whereas the opposite scenario of foreigners influencing the Chinese was unacceptable. Lamenting that the Chinese in Harbin had adopted Russian units of measurement, another local author paraphrased the ancient philosopher Mencius: "Alas, China did not transform the barbarians, but the barbarians have transformed China!"[5]

The insistence of Westerners in Harbin on wearing their winter coats with the fur on the outside was ridiculed in a local rhymed joke about the "old hairies" (*lao maozi*), which non-Chinese were of course not meant to understand. A Harbinite of mixed Chinese and Polish parentage who had made the mistake of putting on his coat the way his Chinese compatriots considered utterly wrong overheard that joke and remembered it decades later.[6] The weight attached to such seemingly trivial differences calls to mind the criteria attributed to Confucius himself for telling Chinese apart from barbarians: the *Analects* (Book 14:17) distinguished the latter as having loose hair and as fastening their robes on the left side instead of the right.

In the Republican era, however, "barbarian" fashions were readily absorbed by young Chinese, who discarded gowns and robes and who considered buttoned shirts and suits, leather shoes, wristwatches and glasses for men, high heels, short sleeves, and bobbed hair for women, and scarves and wedding rings for both sexes, the marks of a modern lifestyle. These novelties rapidly conquered Shanghai and more slowly but surely spread to cities throughout China. In Chinese Harbin, too, young people domesticated foreign clothing with an enthusiasm much deplored by nationalist and conservative commentators.[7] In a famous photograph of the couple Xiao Hong and Xiao Jun, reproduced whenever the two writers are mentioned, she wears her hair in bangs (with two braids and a pressed flower); he sports a fancy Ukrainian shirt (a *vyshivanka*) tied by a cord sash.[8] Self-consciously modern Chinese couples at the time wanted to get married in a "modern" ceremony and looked to Russian wedding customs as a model; they also took dancing classes.[9] Today, Chinese newlyweds in Harbin pose for pictures in front of St Sophia Cathedral, and every winter Russian-style fur coats are paraded on Harbin streets.

Clothing and hairstyle came as part of a larger package that included national identity and class distinctions.[10] Hair represented state allegiance: thus, Korean settlers in the Amur and Maritime provinces were naturalized in Russia on the condition of giving up their topknots; the Qing authorities, for their part, demanded that Korean settlers in Jiandao (Kando) shave their hair and adopt the Manchu queue.[11] To voluntarily change these elements of one's outer appearance was to transgress basic if not always articulated taboos. The elaborate hairstyle of well-born Manchu women, a chignon formed by rolling the hair around a bar placed on top of the head, made them instantly recognizable. Photographs of women with this impressive hairdo, wearing the characteristic high-platform shoes, added colour to travel reports from Manchuria.[12] Occasionally, though, confidence in recognizing a Manchu woman by her distinctive hair was illusory, as the Manchu hairdo was popular among Han women, too.[13] By contrast, there was no ambiguity about the duty of men to wear their hair in a queue and shave their forehead: this was a sign of submission to the ruling Manchu dynasty, and offenders risked the gravest punishment. By the eighteenth century, the male queue had acquired religious significance among Han Chinese and was perceived as inseparable from the body.[14] Tifontai's hesitation to part with his queue prevented him from becoming a Russian subject when he first wished to do so.

Russians, though, found the men's queue effeminate, and some made it an object of derision. Chinese men in Manchuria might be dragged by the queue to a Russian prison or police station.[15] A travelling Russian writer, incensed at the sight of a Chinese person being mistreated in this way in Port Arthur in 1898, drew a parallel between the queue and the Russian beard, the traditional mark of male dignity.[16]

It may have been more than fashion or personal predilection that inspired a number of senior Russian officials in China to let their beards grow. Already Jesuit missionaries in the seventeenth century noticed that the Chinese associated the beard with maturity and wisdom: accordingly, the bearded foreigner could expect a measure of the reverence accorded to a Confucian sage. The most outstanding Russian example in this regard was the railway manager Khorvat; and the Orientalist Shkurkin was even nicknamed "Boroda," The Beard, by his Russian students. After 1920, when Russians in Manchuria lost their extraterritorial status and became subject to Chinese jurisdiction, cases were reported of Russian men being seized by their beards.[17] A Chinese policeman who did so invented nothing new in terms of achieving the twin purposes of apprehension and humiliation, but rather modified a familiar method. Grabbing a suspect by the queue, or tying men together that way, was a common practice of the Chinese state's punitive apparatus until the end of the Qing dynasty.[18]

Sexuality

For the writer Nikolai Baikov, arriving in Manchuria in 1902, the Chinese women hobbling on their bound feet were simply ridiculous and nothing to look at.[19] The example set by Manchu and other banner families, for whom footbinding was strictly prohibited, made this custom far less common among the Han Chinese in the northeast than in metropolitan China.[20] Still, Russians in Manchuria came across women with bound feet, and like most Westerners in China they were uncomfortable with the sight. There were still few Chinese women in Harbin in those early years, because migration from Shandong was overwhelmingly male. This demographic pattern only changed when a steady proportion of migrants settled in Manchuria instead of returning to their villages, and men brought their families to join them. Baikov himself wrote more about animals, hunters, and trappers than about women of any nation. But some fiction by Russian writers in China, which focused largely on Russians, described Chinese women and used them to represent a romantic and exotic Orient rather akin to the Japan of French novelist Pierre Loti (1850–1923).

Harbin offered few models for stories about Oriental femmes fatales. The prolific writer Pavel Severnyi (1900–1981) published his first book in Harbin in 1924 when he was in CER employ and continued his literary career in Shanghai after 1932. He populated his pages with a cast of similar-looking Chinese characters. Most of them were fabulously rich men of noble birth educated in the mysteries of the Oriental tradition as well as the ways of the Occident (which allowed them to converse with Russians). The women were slender and bewitching daughters of nature or sophisticated heiresses. Members of both sexes resided in palatial villas and smoked opium, and the adventures involving their contact with Westerners were set against the background of Chinese legends and gory religious rituals "somewhere in China." Severnyi relied on personal experience in describing the Chinese hunters and bandits of "the Manchurian taiga": according to his son, during his time in Harbin his father was once kidnapped by *hong huzi*, and he got to know the people of the taiga when (apparently being unable to afford the fare) he walked from Harbin to Shanghai.[21] In his stories, Russian loners who came to live in the taiga of Manchuria always emerged fortified in spirit

from that primeval encounter. Severnyi's Chinese characters were creatures of a fairytale world that had very little to do with the reality of
twentieth-century China, and the "Chinese tradition" his stories constantly invoked was largely invented by him, but then being true to life
was hardly the point of these fictions, which meant to stimulate readers' fantasies. At the same time, Severnyi was never disrespectful of the
Chinese (he did seem fascinated by "the fairytale country," as he called
China), and his Russian characters were just as stereotyped.

It is notable that Severnyi's mildly titillating prose repeatedly turned
to the theme of interracial marriage or romance – again, something few
of his Russian readers in China would have tried though they could
experience it vicariously with his help. The novella lending its title
to the collection *A Porcelain Chinaman Nods His Head* (1937) is about a
Chinese widower, the last offspring of an illustrious clan. He was married to a Russian woman he had met in Moscow, and he still keeps her
dead body (embalmed by a Nepalese sage), as well as a gift she gave
him, a Russian-made porcelain figure of a "Chinaman." When Mr Lin's
jealous Chinese concubine attempts to smash the statuette, a pet tiger
he has raised on his estate breaks into the room and kills the young
woman. In the closing novella of the collection, "The Mists of a Damp
Moon," a Russian engineer must choose between the love of Lianhua,
"a luxuriant flower of Asia nurtured in the greenhouses of America,"
whom he first met in Germany, and that of Tamara, with whom he had
a relationship in Paris before the First World War; but instead of choosing, he dies in an accident on a mountain. And in the title novella of
Blue Heron Lake (1938), a Russian woman married to a perfect Chinese
gentleman she had met in Europe is torn between him and her pre-
revolutionary Russian flame, who suddenly arrives in China wanting
to take her to America (she eventually stays with the noble Chinese
husband, with whom she has a son).[22] It is hardly a coincidence that in
all three stories, the author makes his Chinese and Russian characters
fall in love outside China – as if to avoid having to imagine the circumstances in which such couples might have formed in China itself.

One marginal author of Russian fiction who dealt intensely with China
in his work, albeit for only a few years before repatriating around 1925,
was the Jewish writer Eliazar E. Magaram (Elie Maharam, 1899–1962).[23]
His collection of ten stories, published in Berlin in 1922 as *The Yellow
Visage*, had Shanghai rather than Harbin as its setting and appeared
determined to shock readers by portraying that city as the alien and
dangerous "Capital of the Yellow Devil." Magaram offered sketches
of the passive and servile Asian masses living in filth and stench. His
main theme was prostitution, and he offered graphic descriptions of

brothels, whores, and taxi-dancers of all nations, Russians and Jews not exempted. However sensationalist his tone, he clearly was well familiar with that environment. With none of Severnyi's attempted elegance, two of the stories dealt with interracial relationships, or rather their impossibility; in these, male Chinese sexual envy was frustrated by the unbridgeable gulf between white and yellow.[24] Magaram first used the title *The Yellow Visage* for "a miscellany of literature and arts devoted to China," which he edited in Shanghai in 1921.[25] Contrary to the impression this author created, however, sexual desire went both ways. Russian poets in Harbin and Shanghai professed their love to Chinese women – on paper, but probably also in real life, although the latter is more difficult to ascertain. An example is a poem by Kirill V. Baturin (1903–1971), "Nio-en" (1930), signed in Shanghai by a poet who had lived in Harbin: its enigmatic title transcribed the Chinese word *niang* (young woman), while the poem's last words did the same with *wo ai ni* (I love you).[26]

Chinese tradition forbade respectable women in the late Qing from conversing with men outside the family circle, and they did not venture outdoors on their own. In the first decade of the republic this situation underwent rapid change, with young women receiving education in the new schools and appearing in public. Yet for most Chinese women in provincial Harbin, the strictures of traditional conduct still held. The visibility and unrestrained behaviour of the city's Western women therefore presented a stark contrast. And their physique was obviously different as well.

Some Chinese visitors to Harbin – often travellers bound for Europe on the railway, who spent some time in the city – left comments on the Russian "babushkas," whose generous proportions were unusual to the Chinese eye.[27] While this type of remark let off some steam, a young Russian woman could be an attractive *and* disturbing presence for Chinese men. Sexual envy clearly figured in Chinese perceptions, and the bathing resort on Sun Island in the Sungari became an arena for tense encounters. The Russians had imported a modern Western practice, sunbathing, to Harbin as part of their construction of a European way of life in Asia. In the absence of a seashore, the Sungari River became a favoured haunt (for some, the fondest memory) for Harbin's Russian residents, as well as a principal motif for painters and poets.[28] For their part, Chinese were both shocked and excited by the sight of scantily dressed women. Mixed bathing had never been acceptable in China, and sunbathing was incomprehensible: propriety aside, northern Chinese women were reluctant to expose their skin to the sun, not wanting to turn "brown like peasants." Few Chinese of either sex would have been able to swim.[29] A 1929 publication in classical Chinese, titled by the formal name of Fujiadian, *Binjiang chenxiao lu* (A Record of Binjiang Hubbub), and advertised as "the only guide to life and travel in Harbin," contained the following description of Sun Island:

> At the height of the summer heat, the emigrant Russian men and women are vying to get into the water. All of them are accomplished in the art of swimming and some remain in [under?] the water for two to three minutes. It is a custom for men and women to splash water at each other, which they consider amusing. Looking from afar, one can observe hundreds of heads popping in and out, as if ducks, swans or some other water fowl were diving in for food. Every bath lasts many minutes, after which they come back ashore to stretch on the sand and receive the rays of the sun. Even though they wear slight bathing suits, the twin peaks of their bosoms bulge all the same [like] the wonderland of Peach Blossom; at times the spring scenery is offensive. Many Chinese onlookers go away hanging their head and covering their face, but those lying on their back go on just as before, barking as dogs and braying as donkeys, not paying the slightest attention, happy and self-contented; this is what one might call the strange habits of other races. Alas, though our people have a spot at the heart of the river, a place just perfect for refined strolling to escape the heat, it has become the pleasure ground of others![30]

The author, Liu Jingyan, who styled himself Liaozuo sanren (Traveller from East of the Liao), stated that he had lived in Harbin for ten years. Chinese descriptions of allegedly licentious mixing among foreigners are also known from Shanghai; one historian, citing a much older example, from 1863, comments that it stemmed "from envy and humiliation."[31] By the late 1920s, however, Chinese women in mainland China could be seen in swimming suits.[32] While the above passage makes palpable the sexual charge of the colonial city, the Sungari was a meeting place more than a place of conflict.

The CER manager Ostroumov promoted mixed bathing on the other side of the Sungari opposite Harbin, probably in the interest of saving space along the riverbank. A Russian memoirist wrote that this was unsettling at first for Russian and Chinese prudes but soon caught on among members of both populations.[33] A foreign observer of Manchukuo noted that during the summer heat, everyone, "White Russians" and "Bolsheviks," Chinese and Japanese, was bathing in the river "in sportsmanlike unity."[34] In winter, he would have seen people of all nationalities ice-skating. By the 1930s, the Russians and Chinese shared disquiet about the entirely uninhibited attitude toward nudity displayed by Harbin's Japanese residents.[35]

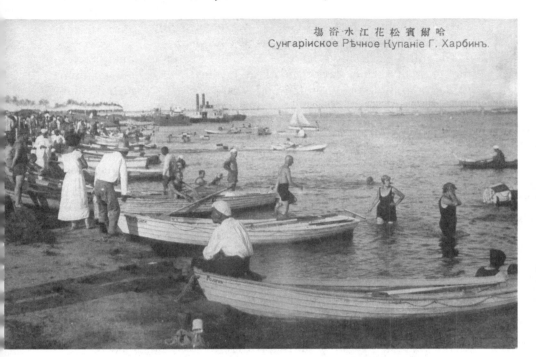

場浴水江花松賓爾哈
Сунгарiйское Рѣчное Купанiе Г. Харбинъ.

5.1. Sungari River bathing and boats. Undated postcard, author's collection.

The surplus of men created by the mass migration of single male workers to Manchuria was a stimulant to prostitution in Harbin. Chinese prostitutes were bought or abducted from families as far off as Jiangsu and Zhejiang provinces; others were Japanese.[36] Owen Lattimore, however, wrote that most prostitutes in Manchuria were local. They were "frequently 'redeemed' by men who take them either as wives or concubines. To be thus redeemed by a rich man is their commonest ambition."[37] In the popular Harbin daily *Kopeika*, in 1923, under the title "The Yellow Slaves," the poet and writer Venedikt Mart (Venedikt N. Matveev, 1896–1937), Magaram's match in Harbin as an explorer of the city's lowlife, published a sensational account of his tour of the brothels of Fujiadian. He presented the all-Chinese satellite town as a world apart from that of Harbin's Europeans.[38] While there is no direct indication that the Chinese sex industry in Fujiadian also catered to a Russian clientele, Russian brothels operated there, too. In daily life the boundaries between Harbin and Fujiadian – separated by an industrial buffer zone called Mostovoi poselok, Bridge settlement, in Russian, and

Bazhan, Eighth Section, in Chinese – were constantly crossed by Chinese people, although much less often by Russians.

The influx of destitute refugees after the Revolution made Harbin the centre of a white slave trade as well. When the League of Nations looked into the problem in the mid-1930s, it cited a French missionary's estimate of 3,000 prostitutes in Fujiadian, of whom 10 per cent were Russian, and another 1,800, 80 per cent of them Russian, in Harbin itself.[39] Moreover, Russian women were found to have "formed a source of supply for almost the entire occidental prostitution in ... China," among other ways by being trafficked from Harbin via Changchun to Qingdao, a port where the US Navy called every summer.[40] Some of Harbin's Russian brothels were available to Chinese men: the *Record of Binjiang Hubbub* listed addresses and prices, assuring readers that they would get along with the prostitutes in Chinese.[41]

Food, Drink, and Entertainment

"The first thing that amazed us was the absence of bread, either white or black," wrote one of Harbin's Russian pioneers about his arrival in southern Manchuria by ship in April 1898. The Russians needed their bread and took urgent measures "in order to have here, in distant Manchuria, everything we have been used to," said the same pioneer, who also claimed to have personally introduced potatoes into the region in the summer of 1899.[42] During the Russo-Japanese War, Russian troops in Manchuria had to make do with the small buns sold to them by Chinese villagers (which the soldiers found insipid and called "Manza bread").[43] Before long, Chinese farmers started growing more wheat to meet the Russian demand for flour in both Manchuria and the Russian Far East.[44] However, Chinese peasants did not change their usual diet of millet and corn in favour of Russian bread; nor did they begin to consume dairy products.[45] As Russians also missed milk, butter, and cheese, they opened their own dairy farms and creameries.[46]

Russian authors have often contended that Russian dietary requirements resulted in the long-term introduction of new crops and farming techniques in the region. One Harbin Russian publication argued, in this spirit, that "Russians introduced into Manchurian agriculture Russian cabbage, swede (rutabaga), turnip, beetroot, black radish, parsley, carrots, horseradish, parsnip, dill, Russian short cucumbers, peas, horse beans, Russian watermelons, melons, gourds, zucchini, tomatoes, asparagus, sweet peppers, and knob celery," and that these new vegetables were widely adopted by Chinese farmers.[47] Verifying or disputing such claims, which have also been made about flax, hops, oats, rye, lettuce, and strawberries, would require precise knowledge about the plant life and agriculture of northeastern China.[48] More solid documentation is presently available on the efforts of the Soviet government in the 1920s to persuade peasants in the Amur and Maritime provinces to begin growing rice and soybeans by learning from Korean and Chinese experience.[49]

The Chinese migrants from Shandong and Hebei brought their maize-flour cakes (*yumi bing*) with them to Manchuria. These were originally the staple food of the poor; Sun Yunxuan, raised in Shandong in the 1910s, remembered eating them because there was never rice in the house.[50] Rice, cultivated and consumed in southern China much more than in the north, did not grow near Harbin and had to be delivered to Jilin and Heilongjiang from southern Manchuria.[51] Harbin cuisine grew out of both sides' craving for the familiar, but once that basic need was satisfied, the city's inhabitants could begin to acquaint themselves with a mutually exotic gastronomy. The administrative elites had opportunities to sample each other's cuisine at its glittering best. So in August 1903, Russian officials were invited to celebrate the birthday of the Qing emperor at a banquet hosted by Chinese military and civil officials. At the end of the same month, this invitation was reciprocated by a festive Russian breakfast to mark the opening of the Russo-Chinese Bank. Only four days later, Chinese administrators treated the chief engineer of the CER, Alexander O. Iugovich (1842–1925), who was about to leave Harbin, to a farewell luncheon; and the Russian press relished describing the menu of swallows' nests, shark fins, Peking-style chicken, water lilies, sea cucumbers, and bamboo sprouts with lobster caviar.[52]

One aspect of the Russian heritage in Harbin manifest to this day is the food the city's people eat: the obvious examples are bread, red sausage, and ice cream. The famous Harbin *guobaorou* is a pork delicacy more subtly attributed to a chef by the name Zheng Xingwen, who created the recipe in 1907 as a Chinese dish that Russians would like. He had hit on the idea while preparing banquets for Russian officials.[53] The name of another local delicacy, *lidaosi chang*, originally referred to Lithuanian sausage. The Qiulin department store sells a canned drink called *gewasi*, advertised by the English words "since 1900" and, in Cyrillic letters, as "Harbin kvass." Even the store's name, Qiulin ("autumn forest"), is a transcription from the Russian "Churin."[54]

The heirs of Ivan Ya. Churin (1833–1895), a Siberian merchant, founder of the Churin chain of stores in the Russian Far East, opened a department store in Harbin in 1900. The firm had its own sausage and vodka factories as well as a cigarette brand, with additional enterprises and branches in other Manchurian cities. It sold everything: the Harbin

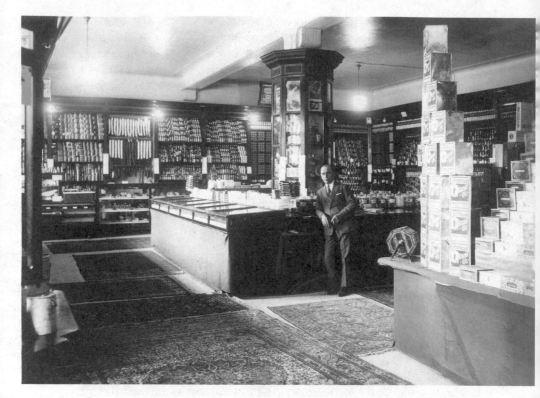

5.2. The interior of Churin's department store. Photograph from the archive
of Vladimir Ablamskii, courtesy of the A.M. Sibiriakov Museum
of Irkutsk City History.

photographer Vladmir P. Ablamskii (1911–1994), some of whose work is
reproduced in this book, documented each of Churin's many sections,
including women's and men's clothing, shoes, hats, home appliances,
watches, sports equipment, toys, records, and books.[55] As advertisements in the press attested, luxury products were imported to Harbin
from all over the world. In 1910 another large department store, the
Japanese Matsuura, with six floors, opened on Kitaiskaia Street; in the
1930s, these pioneering businesses were joined by two other Japanese
stores of comparable size. The Churin firm itself became the property of
the Hongkong and Shanghai Banking Corporation in 1931. It was then
taken over by the Japanese, sold to the Soviet Union in 1945, and finally
transferred to Chinese management in 1950. Its original building at the

corner of Novotorgovaia and Bol'shoi prospekt (New Trade Street and Grand Avenue) in New Town (now Guogeli dajie and Dong Dazhi jie in Nangang), enlarged to four floors, is still in operation.[56] A guidebook for Chinese tourists in Heilongjiang recommends tasting such Harbin specialities as *lieba* (from the Russian *khleb*; bread) and *shaike* (Russian *saika*, a small round bun), both freshly baked at Qiulin.[57]

Shopping for food made up a fair share of the contact between Russians and Chinese in Harbin, and the Chinese were typically the providers. Memoirs by Harbin Russians often evoke the strings of "sugared frozen apples," which peddlers offered on the streets of the city: *hulu*, or *tanhulu*, short for *bingtang hulu*, a northeast speciality that became a favourite especially with Russian children.[58] Street peddlers also sold "eggs, tomatoes, potatoes, live chicken and dressed poultry, salad, apples, pears and sundry eatables" so listed a press report in 1911.[59] Russians shopped not only in Russian stores such as Churin's but also in Chinese businesses, though they were served in Russian everywhere they went – for example, in the aforementioned grocery store, Shuanghesheng, and in the Harbin branch of a tea company based in Hankou and Shanghai.[60] And Chinese shops offered much more than groceries and tea. In 1934, or perhaps in 1935, the young musician Oleg N. Lundstrem (1916–2005) bought a Duke Ellington record in the Tongfalong department store, founded in 1929, and the rest is history, or so Lundstrem liked to recall it.[61] Lundstrem successively introduced jazz to Harbin, Shanghai, and (after 1947) the Soviet Union.

In the 1900s, Harbin had two main bazaars, a large one known as the Green Bazaar (the name Zelenyi referred to greenery), facing the southern side of Bol'shoi prospekt in New Town, and another in Pristan'. By 1903, the Chinese were already selling kvass at the bazaar, though the Russian authorities vainly struggled to ban it by arguing that Chinese-made kvass presented a danger to health.[62] By the 1920s the number of bazaars had reached five, not counting Fujiadian. These were sites of cross-ethnic contact between vendors and customers, and also between Chinese and Russian vendors, who worked and lived there next to each other.[63] A frequent theme in Russian memoirs is gratitude for the trust shown to them by Chinese peddlers, market vendors, and shopkeepers in Harbin, all of whom were ready to defer payments for their merchandise. To an extent, that Russians were now being trusted in financial relations meant they were being integrated into the web of Chinese society. They were not seen as liable to disappear tomorrow, with their debts unsettled. However, the use of credit to create debt and dependence was a common practice of Chinese trade. The same memoirs hint at the financial straits of émigrés, which made buying food on credit necessary.[64]

In wealthy private households and in Harbin's Russian restaurants, Chinese cooks prepared Russian dishes. Restaurants, which might advertise French or Georgian cuisine besides the Russian, did not, however, offer Chinese dishes. Nor did these regularly appear on the table in Russian households, nor were they listed in the recipe column of the popular entertainment journal *Rubezh* (published between 1926 and 1945).[65] Even so, Russians used rice and tofu (Russianized as *tufa*) as substitute ingredients when preparing their own dishes.[66] The child of a non-observant Jewish family in Harbin remembered Chinese food as "something we don't eat"; secretly, however, she would sometimes try "a very interesting, forbidden snack, bought from a street vendor."[67] Students and youth had their favourite cheap Chinese kitchens, which they frequented when not supervised by parents. Russians in Manchuria found it easiest to adopt *jiaozi* (Chinese dumplings) as the next best thing after *pelmeni*, the dumplings closely associated with Siberian life – so much so that a Russian remembering his times as a gymnasium student in Harbin about 1920 could say that after summer swims in the Sungari, he "would drop in a Chinese restaurant and eat pelmeni [*sic*]" with his friends.[68] An Italian would have used *ravioli* in the same sentence.

A strong sense of adventure attaches to Russian descriptions of gastronomic excursions to Harbin's "native quarter." Russians used the older name Fujiadian, not the current term Daowai (literally, "beyond the way"), but that area, outside the railway zone, evoked for them associations much like the English expression "the other side of the tracks": the poor and dangerous part of town. An outing to a restaurant in the all-Chinese suburb, where the streets had only Chinese names, was often recorded in language such as this: "Everything here seemed different, even the air, even the sky, even the sun. Another planet: this was the only way to call it."[69] Beyond the occasional dinner outings, disappearing into Fujiadian was a Harbin Russian fantasy. One person who was believed to ignore the borders between the two "planets" – Russian and Chinese, Daoli and Daowai – was the former White Army officer and poet Leonid Eshchin (1897–1930). Rumour had it that he led a double life among the Chinese in Fujiadian and had learned to speak their language. He had thus crossed the lines of decent Russian society before drinking himself to death in Harbin.[70]

Venturing into Fujiadian exposed Russians to smells they found offensive; more than one memoirist associated the place with the smell of garlic.[71] Sitting down for a meal there meant being prepared to join

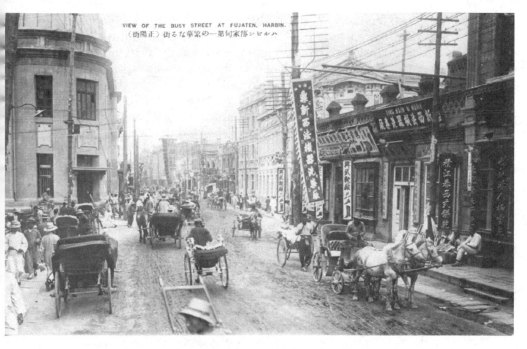

5.3. Former Zhengyang jie (now Jingyu jie), the main street of Fujiadian.
Undated postcard, courtesy of Olga Bakich.

in Chinese company and to be stared at – much as a Chinese customer
would attract curious glances at the Café Plage, a popular city institution on the riverbank. Russians were also kept away from Chinese eating places by the fairly accurate perception that these establishments
had lower standards of hygiene and that some of them were meant
more for smoking than for eating. Song Xiaolian compared Russian
alcoholism with Chinese opium addiction,[72] thereby linking two vices
for which each side could feel justified in despising the other. But alcohol was not solely a Russian problem, just as the opium dens did not
serve only Chinese customers. Vodka did not become popular with
the Chinese, though beer did. The favoured beverage of the Chinese
remained gaoliang wine (*shaojiu*), made from the sorghum plant closely
identified with northern China.[73] Russians drank it too, calling it *khanshin* (a pidgin word of mysterious origin) or "Chinese vodka."[74]

   In 1914, a CER committee acknowledged that Harbin Russians had
taken up opium. Networks for the smuggling of alcohol and drugs
(including heroin and morphine) into the city involved all nationalities.[75]

At least since the 1880s, Russian settlers in the Maritime province had been leasing their lands to Chinese for growing the opium poppy, which was marketed for consumption in China. By 1910, many Russians in the Maritime province had become opium smokers too. Cheap "Chinese vodka" was smuggled across the Manchurian border into the Russian Far East. In 1916, a Russian-Chinese package agreement was signed to outlaw the "liquor and opium" business, but it was soon rendered ineffective by the Revolution.[76] In Harbin, Eshchin was not the only Russian poet to describe smoking an opium pipe and sipping *khanshin* while lying on a *kang* in a *fanza*.[77] Obviously, many more did so without recording this activity in poetry.

If drinking needed an occasion, festivals and public celebrations supplied them. The tsarist administration loved jubilees and anniversaries – still a distinguishing feature of Russian public life – which of course were put to political use. In 1913, a year especially busy with such celebrations, the city marked the tenth anniversary of the CER, commemorated (with more than the usual pomp) the repelling by Russian troops of the first Boxer assault on Harbin, and joined the whole Russian empire in saluting the three hundred years of the Romanov dynasty.[78] Meanwhile in Peking, the Russian Orthodox Mission marked its two hundredth anniversary in China. Such organized activities bolstered the sense of shared identity among Russians.

The last great anniversary of Russian Harbin was the celebration of twenty-five years of the railway, in June 1923: a documentary history of the CER reaching back to 1896 was commissioned (although only the first of two projected volumes came out), while a large exhibition demonstrated the CER's achievements, and officials from both sides tried to outdo one another in mouthing slogans of peaceful Russian-Chinese collaboration. Two vodka companies showcased their products, incidentally attesting to actual acculturation and cross-ethnic business cooperation: a Chinese company offered a vodka-spouting fountain for all to enjoy, while another, the Russo-Japanese partnership of Borodin and Takata, built a model of the Eiffel Tower from its vodka bottles. A lavish costume party was remembered as the *bal poudré*, since the ladies of Harbin's high society dressed for it "in the perruques and panniers of French marquises."[79]

However, the following year, China officially recognized the Soviet Union and the two countries wrested control of the CER from the Russian émigrés. Only Soviet and Chinese citizens could now work for the railway; all other employees had to take the citizenship of one country or the other by 31 May 1925 in order to keep their jobs. As of 1 January 1924, the CER had 16,750 employees, divided into two main categories:

staff (9,000) and temporary workers or day labourers (7,600). Of the staff, 6,107 counted as "Russian" and 1,106 as "Chinese" in the official data; the temporary workers were almost equally divided between Russians and Chinese.[80] In the transition period to a new Soviet-Chinese administration, pre-revolutionary Russian settlers registered as "Soviets" independently of what they thought of the regime in Moscow. Other Russians took Chinese passports and registered as "Chinese" (and so helped populate the "Chinese half" of the railway staff); the rest were sacked on 1 June 1925. The Chinese police arrested the émigré manager of the CER, Ostroumov, who was then replaced by a Soviet appointee.

As hopes for the political restoration of old Russia faded, religion assumed an increasingly important place in the life of Russian Harbin. Most memoirs describe observing the Orthodox Christmas and Easter; some mention the annual church services in memory of the martyred Romanov family. They also evoke, however, such secular festivities as Tat'iana Day (25 January N.S., the occasion for student balls), Russian Culture Day (celebrated on Alexander Pushkin's birthday, on 6 June O.S., by Russian émigré communities worldwide since 1924), and Russian Child's Day (25 March O.S.; first marked in Harbin in 1930). Harbin Bolsheviks celebrated May Day and Revolution Day, the latter on 7 November N.S.[81] The intensifying Soviet presence in Harbin after 1924 manifested itself in an array of new Communist celebrations, which émigrés ignored, just as the school established for children of Soviet citizens (the "pink-coloured school," as everybody called it) studiously ignored the Orthodox holidays.

Chinese Harbin was more than a passive spectator at Russian festivals. Peddlers and grocers knew exactly what to supply for each Russian festival: buckwheat flour to make *bliny* for Maslenitsa on the last week before Lent in February or March; bouquets of willow branches (*verba*) for Palm Sunday before Easter and paper lanterns in which to carry home a lit candle from church on Maundy Thursday; bath brooms (*veniki*) and freshly cut grass for the Orthodox Pentecost in May or June. They had Manchurian fir trees ready for Christmas in lieu of the Russian *elka*, and they even offered boutonnieres for Tat'iana Day balls.[82] These services were in keeping with the established pattern of economic relations in the city, but Russian festivals and their accompanying distractions also influenced Harbin's Chinese society. The young people described in Xiao Hong's *Market Street* celebrated New Year twice, according to the Western custom on 31 December, which was welcomed as "modern" in the Republic of China, as well as by the lunar Chinese calendar.[83] Some Russians went even better, celebrating everything from European Christmas and New Year by the Gregorian calendar to Russian Christmas and New Year by the Julian calendar and through to the Chinese New Year, a string of festivals lasting from December to February.[84]

Coming to Harbin in the winter today, one will see local people and tourists enjoying rides on wooden sleighs across the ice-covered river. Until this mode of transport disappeared in the late 1950s, it was known in pidgin as *tolkai-tolkai*, literally, push-push.[85] It was originally devised as a practical solution for the winter season, to move goods as well as people. Carriages, pulled by horses or mules, also ran on the ice.[86] River sleighs have been revived as a leisure activity since the 1980s; both passengers and drivers are now Chinese and hardly anyone in Harbin understands pidgin any more.[87] But the most important winter recreation in Harbin, the one that has become the city's symbol, is the Harbin Ice Sculpture and Snow Festival. This festival began in 1963 and, after being interrupted by the Cultural Revolution, has been staged every January since 1984. The enormous ice sculptures and tall, brightly lit ice towers and Russian churches make for a great show, attracting domestic tourists and also visitors from across the border in the Russian Far East. The festival is officially presented as having evolved from the custom of northeastern fishermen of placing a candle inside an ice block to provide light in the dark winter months.[88]

Any mention of a Russian connection to the present-day Ice Festival is avoided. However, another popular activity, one that takes place during it and has become another iconic image of the Harbin winter, ice-hole swimming, is easily traced back to Russian influence. Harbin Russians of both sexes could be seen bathing in an ice hole on the day of the Baptism of Christ. This was the culmination of a mass procession, held annually on 6 January (19 January N.S.) after 1921. Russian Orthodox priests led the faithful toward a huge ice cross, erected on the frozen Sungari. The sight of thousands marching to the sound of tolling church bells attracted the attention of all city inhabitants irrespective of ethnicity and creed, and some non-Russian spectators joined the marchers. The towering cross was cut out of blocks of ice by "Chinese and Russian artisans" (according to a Harbin-born Russian scholar), and the water beneath the ice of the Sungari was transformed for the day into a baptismal font called a *iordan'* after the holy River Jordan. Religious vessels carved out of ice and illuminated from within were displayed in churches, which believers visited.[89] Photographs and postcards of the original ice sculptures strongly suggest that they were the origin of the Winter Festival, for which Harbin is internationally famous today. That festival has transformed religious Russian content into secular Chinese.

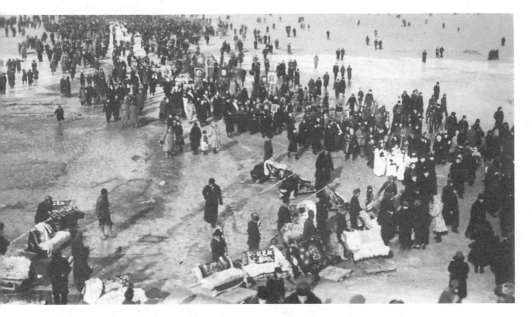

5.4. Ice procession on the Sungari River (note the sled taxis, *tolkai-tolkai*, in attendance). Undated postcard, author's collection.

Ascribing the making of ice lanterns and sculptures in Harbin to indigenous tradition rather than to the needs of the Orthodox religion, contemporary Harbin writer Ah Cheng (Wang Acheng, b. 1948) enumerates what he considers Russian influences on the shaping of "the Harbin person" (*Ha'erbin ren*), in a book so titled. According to Ah Cheng, the Russians brought beer-drinking to Harbin, along with their beer mugs, which however were later smashed by kvass-promoting Red Guards. Russians also introduced winter swimming in the Sungari, and Soviet songs are still being sung in karaoke. The Russian culinary heritage lives on in the ingredients of the Harbin breakfast and the large loaves of Harbin "Russian" bread.[90]

Just as there was a range of attitudes toward Chinese food, so also the extent of Russian awareness of Chinese festivals was a function of individual curiosity. All Russian Harbinites remember the Chinese New Year: the colourful celebrations that seemed magically to transform their hard-working neighbours into carefree holiday-makers. On the first day of the New Year, it was customary to pay visits to family and friends. This Chinese tradition (called *bainian*) closely resembled the customs of Russian Easter, but unlike the street processions, and the noise and clutter of the fireworks and paper dragons, it was invisible to Russian spectators because it took place indoors.[91] Shortly after Easter, which according to the lunar calendar was observed between April and May, Radonitsa (Russian All Souls' Day) was the occasion when "all of [Russian] Harbin" went to the cemeteries.[92] At the gates of the cemetery, Chinese were again in attendance, selling the flowers and eggs required by Orthodox custom. The future writer Ah Cheng was not the only child to climb over the fence of the Russian cemetery, collect the eggs left for the Russian ancestors, and eat them.[93] Only a few weeks later, the egg vendors went to sweep their own family graves on Qingming jie, Remembrance Day, celebrated on the third day of the third lunar month as the most important Chinese festival after the New Year. On these occasions as well as during funerals, they too left food for their dead, which at least one Russian has confessed to stealing with his friends as a child once the ceremonies were over.[94]

Harbin Russians enjoyed another Chinese holiday, which a writer in 1936 described as "almost as important as our Radonitsa": the midsummer or spirit festival, Zhongyuan jie. Numerous small boats, decorated with paper cut-outs symbolizing the dead, were set afloat on the river at night with burning lanterns placed inside them.[95] The sinologist Pavel Shkurkin, who playfully styled himself Master Shi, wrote an article to introduce the Russian public to "the Buddha's birthday," a festival observed on the eighth day of the fourth lunar month and accompanied by performances of Chinese theatre.[96]

Leisure was not, of course, limited to official festivals, and one thing people did in their spare time was play mah-jong. Chinese and Russians both enjoyed this tile game, even if they played it among themselves rather than with each other. Some Russian women took to mah-jong in Harbin or Shanghai and made a lifelong habit of it in whatever country they moved to after leaving China.[97] Other leisure activities, especially those that did not require understanding of the other language, did bring Chinese and Russians together. One was sports: here, Russian-Chinese contacts developed during the 1920s and reached a peak during the period of political friendship between Soviet Russia and Communist China in the 1950s.[98] In the early years, the presence of members of the Chinese elite at a performance of the circus of Nikolai K. Borovskii in Pristan' merited a notice in the *Harbin Herald* (Borovskii named his troupe The First Courland Circus, probably in reference to his place of origin).[99] Also in 1904, during the Russo-Japanese War, the *Herald*'s reporter attended a show, presumably a Chinese opera, in Tifontai's theatre. In "the huge building … packed full of spectators," he spotted "several Russians: military physicians and civilians, and two or three Russian ladies," who shared the best places on the balcony with Chinese women (members of "the Chinese beau monde," as the reporter called them).[100]

More evidence of such social mixing appeared in the railway's Chinese-language newspaper, *Yuandong bao*. Although this CER organ had a stake in promoting the image of Chinese-Russian cooperation, its reports on Russian cultural activities in Harbin seldom mentioned the participation of Chinese in them, or vice versa – which lends greater credibility to the short newspaper articles that did point this out. For example, in May 1911 it was reported that Chinese had bought cheap tickets to watch an airplane rise in the sky above the racecourse in Majiagou as part of a Harbin "aviation week."[101] In November, Chinese and Russian spectators filled up a hall near Danilov's theatre to see a display of wax figures of famous personalities from Bismarck to Li Hongzhang.[102] By the 1920s, attending the races at Harbin's two racecourses, betting on races, and horse breeding were passions shared across ethnic lines. The Chinese governors of Jilin and Heilongjiang and the mayor of Harbin kept their own stables, as did wealthy Russians.[103] The circus became all the more attractive when entrepreneurs combined the performances of Russian and Chinese acrobats: the Izako family circus, originally from Siberia, offered an elaborate mixed program along with wrestling, advertising it in *Yuandong bao* so as to draw a Chinese audience.[104]

The same newspaper printed ads for performances at Harbin's teahouses, but there is no evidence that the storytellers and theatre troupes, who entertained the Chinese public in these locales beginning from 1908, aroused more than the passing curiosity of the city's Russians.[105] Chinese theatre, also called Chinese opera in English, flourished in Fujiadian, where the popular genres were *bangzi* (the "clapper opera" of northern China) and, increasingly by the 1930s, Peking opera and a modern Hebei variant known as *pingju*. Like the operettas, which enjoyed great popularity in Russian Harbin, Chinese theatre had an enthusiastic fan culture and brought guest performers to the city, delighting their respective audiences.[106] To attend a *pingju* or an operetta was to enter a protected cultural space, presumed to be incomprehensible to outsiders and thus safe from their intrusion.

One evening in 1934, two young Chinese Communists – a student of Russian from Jiangsu, who was to become well-known as a translator of Russian drama, and a Manchu painter and poet raised in Fujiadian – went to watch a classic play by Alexander Ostrovsky (1823–1886) at the Commercial Assembly theatre in Daoli, and realized they were being observed by the all-Russian audience around them. These audience members would have been surprised to learn that Jiang and Jin had both read *The Thunder-storm* in the original.[107] More Chinese spectators may have frequented the cinema theatres, introduced to Harbin by the Russians in 1905, especially when the films were silent.[108] Once voice (often the English of American movies) was added in the early 1930s, Harbin moviegoers could choose between Russian, Chinese, and Japanese cinemas.

Religion, Myth, and Rumour

The Russian education system in Harbin, which was sketched out in chapter 3, was oriented inward, to meet the perceived needs of the Russian community. The railway administration constructed some of the social apparatus that ordinarily served to bring the local population into the orbit of Russian civic life within the empire, but contrary to policy followed within Russian borders, in Manchuria it did not take the next step toward making these new attributes meaningful to the Chinese.[109] It is important to bear in mind that in terms of international law, Harbin and Manchuria always lay beyond the Russian border with China as last fixed in 1860. Parts of Manchuria were occupied for almost four years between the Boxer Uprising and the Russo-Japanese War, but they were not annexed by Russia, nor did the Chinese in Manchuria become subjects of the tsar. Quite the contrary, some of Harbin's former Russian subjects (including Mordechai Olmert in 1928) temporarily adopted Chinese citizenship. By 1932 the number of "naturalized Chinese citizens" in Harbin stood at 6,793, compared to 27,633 holders of Soviet passports and 30,044 stateless émigrés.[110]

Russia refrained from promoting Russification through schooling in Manchuria. Indeed, after the late nineteenth century, missionary activity did not form part of the Russian strategy toward Asian peoples even within Russia's borders.[111] The official purpose of the Russian Orthodox Mission, which had operated in Peking since 1713, was to attend to the needs of the "Albazinians": descendants of Russian soldiers who had been taken to Peking after the Qing army sacked Albazin fortress on the Amur River in 1685. The mission evolved into an extension of Russian diplomacy, a nest for spies, and a cradle of Russian sinology. Although Chinese conversions to the Orthodox faith were viewed as desirable, they were undertaken with caution so as not to undermine the mission's more vital activities. About 6,000 Chinese (two or three hundred annually in the earlier period, rising to five or six hundred in the last seven years) were baptized at the mission in Peking between 1902 and 1917, at which time the centre of Russian religious life in China passed to Harbin.[112]

The conquest of Chinese souls was even less of a goal for the Russian clergy in Harbin. As late as October 1945, a bishop sent by the Soviet-controlled church in Moscow to oversee the unification of the émigré eparchies of Harbin and Manchuria with the Moscow Patriarchate, noted the complete absence of Russian missionary work among the Harbin Chinese; rather naively for the time, he outlined a plan for launching such work forthwith "in China, Manchuria and Korea."[113] There were Chinese Christians in town, such as the educator Deng Jiemin and, later, the businessman Wu Baixiang (1879–1966), but their faith did not necessarily make them better disposed toward the Russian Orthodox Church.[114] The visual presence of the Russian religion, which remained alien to the vast majority of the Chinese population, accompanied the city from its inception in 1898. Panoramic photographs and postcards of Harbin featured the "onion domes" of its churches until the mid-twentieth century. Nine Russian churches were built from 1898 to 1921, and another twelve between 1921 and 1928. By 1941, Harbin had fifty churches with parishes and three monasteries.[115] Like the Russian schools, the churches in Harbin and along the CER line served as havens of "Russianness" for their adherents at a time when China was tightening its embrace. A former resident wrote that "the Church together with the Russian school helped our generation of Harbinites ... to conserve to some extent our 'Russian soul,' the best characteristics and traditions of Russian culture."[116]

The towering churches that reminded Russians of their native country became a curiosity for the Chinese, for no other city in China featured them in comparable profusion. For the nationalist author of *Record of Binjiang Hubbub* it must have been a deliberate choice not to include any pictures of them in his guide, which instead offered readers views of Chinese sites.[117] Some believers in the Chinese popular religion found the churches disturbing. The principles of geomancy and respect for nature's "veins and arteries," as well as concerns not to block the path of benevolent spirits, limited the built landscape in Manchuria as elsewhere in northern China to one-storey dwellings.[118] Taller temples, pagodas, and shrines to local deities were scattered across the Manchurian countryside, but the locations of these were chosen in consultation with experts in *feng shui* (literally "wind and water"). Some Chinese in Harbin perceived the first and most important Harbin church, St Nicholas Cathedral, constructed in the centre of a square named after it in New Town between 1899 and 1900, as a disruption of *feng shui* and an omen of ill luck.[119]

However, Russian sources nowhere indicate negative Chinese attitudes toward the symbols of Orthodox religion. Instead, they insist on positive ones. Placed prominently at the Harbin railway station was the icon of St Nicholas of Myra, whom Russians called St Nicholas the Miracle Worker. It has been claimed that he was the object of Chinese veneration.[120] The Chinese called the figure in the icon *vokzala stalika*,[121] or even, affectionately, *kholoshaia stalika* (pidgin for "old man of the railway station" and "the good old man"), and some, so Russian memoirists maintained, believed in its miracle-working powers. According to a tale oft repeated with slight variations, a Chinese boatman (or a merchant) was once about to drown in the Sungari. In despair, he summoned all his idols, yet none came forward to save him. But when he shouted in pidgin: "Russian God Nikola of the railway station, come and help me!" St Nicholas, the patron of all seafarers, walked on the water and carried the man safely to the shore – and then vanished. The grateful Chinese rushed to the railway station, where bowing and crying before the icon he told the crowd of his miraculous salvation.[122]

Obviously, "the type of story which predominates at any one time can tell one much about the community in which it is popular."[123] The story of Chinese reverence for a Russian saint closely associated with his namesake the tsar and believed to be the protector of Harbin was popular among Russians and served the purpose of confirming the influence of Russian religion. After the agreement under which the railway passed into joint Chinese-Soviet control in 1924, the Soviets began taking possession of the property of the Russian Orthodox Church, but a Chinese court, mindful of Zhang Zuolin's anti-Soviet positions, prevented complete confiscation.[124] Harbin Russians explained such Chinese resistance to Soviet demands as a consequence of the affection for St Nicholas among the Chinese people. A Soviet agent in China, Oskar Erdberg (1901–1938), heard this version of the events after noticing an icon of St Nicholas in a CER train in 1925; he quipped that the Lycian saint must have accepted Chinese citizenship along with some of Harbin's émigrés.[125] The icon only left the railway station in 1947, when it was moved to the Chapel of Our Lady of Iviron (the Harbin analogue, constructed in 1933, of Iverskaia Chapel in Moscow, which the Bolsheviks had demolished), in the courtyard of St Nicholas Cathedral. It was destroyed along with the chapel and the cathedral in August 1966. The story was told that when the Red Guards set the cathedral on fire, a Chinese priest flung himself into the flames in a vain attempt to save the icon of St Nicholas.[126]

The Chinese were accustomed to worshipping local gods, protectors of the villages or towns where their temples stood. However flattering this was to Russians, it is conceivable that some Chinese in Harbin accepted the notion of St Nicholas as the divine patron of the

Russian-built city.[127] There are comparable examples of Russians show-ing respect, and even adopting, manifestations of native faith they encountered in Siberia.[128] Chinese informants told Owen Lattimore that Russian ship captains on the Sungari respected the local custom of burning incense on the bridge and letting off firecrackers so as to appease the spirits of the rocks just above Sanxing, where the river is difficult to navigate. " 'When they come as far as this,' they say, 'their Russian gods are no good. They have to respect our spirits.' "[129]

Some ordinary folk in Manchuria took to making the sign of the cross when speaking with Russians as a way of demonstrating their sincerity. One physician, who observed the Chinese with unusual interest and sympathy during the Russo-Japanese War, noticed that beggars who approached the Russians in Qiqihar made the sign "correctly" (mean-ing the Russian Orthodox way of tracing three fingers from right to left, as distinct from the motions of Chinese Christian converts).[130] At a station on the western section of the railway, around 1920, a Russian memoirist "met a Chinaman who was passing by and was predicting fortunes for our friends living there"; he had his own fortune told and years later marvelled at the accuracy of that prognostication, delivered in Russian-Chinese pidgin.[131] Religious syncretism and the develop-ment of cults require time; whatever homage was paid by the Chinese in Harbin to St Nicholas and by Russians in the periphery of Manchu-ria to Chinese and native traditions may have been early steps in that direction, steps that were later cut off by the Russians' departure and the imposition of Communist atheism.[132]

Deeply ingrained religious perceptions became determining factors in interethnic relations as, for those who lived by them, they justified cultural and racial insularity. Some Cossacks and other Russian Ortho-dox settlers in the Far East believed that "the Chinese had no soul." This idea helped justify "hunting" Chinese and Koreans in the Ussuri taiga and in the Manchurian borderlands. To shoot and rob an Asian was no more of a sin than killing any "beast" (Russian: *tvar'*).[133] Besides reflecting the perception that Asians were not fully human, that prac-tice was the manifestation of a violent frontier society: Russians also "hunted" for Russian gold miners and rovers (*brodiagi*).[134] Cossacks in eastern Siberia who accused the Chinese of killing a Russian child in order to eat him mirrored a Chinese tradition of suspecting Europeans of cannibalism and of the abduction of Chinese children.[135] A number of Russian sources blamed the eruption of Boxer violence in Manchuria to rumours that spread among coolies after the bones (in another ver-sion, the paw) of a bear were discovered near the railway tracks and suspected as being those of a Chinese person.[136]

Such sinister rumours about the Russians reached far and wide outside Manchuria, or so one Harbin sinologist claimed, telling his local readers that people in southern China believed "that Russians could not come across a foreign woman without violating her and were constantly waging war in order to exterminate all children in the occupied lands." The children would be eaten, their inner organs used for preparing European medicine, their eyes for camera lenses.[137] These rumours, however, were part of a Chinese discourse that developed in the second half of the nineteenth century and was directed mostly at the Protestant missionaries rather than at Russians.[138] The medical context was key to it; in times of emergency, such as epidemics, involuntary contact with Russian physicians rekindled similar suspicions in Harbin. The spread of rumours indicated absence of knowledge about the other side and an effort to compensate for that lack of information, and it reflected popular fear.[139] Finally, one cannot fully trust the attribution of beliefs to other people. If more Chinese records of religious perceptions and fantasies about the Russians were available, they would offer more reliable indications of popular Chinese thinking than descriptions of the same in Russian writing.

6

Trials and Endings

In July 1912, Roger Budberg published an essay in the *German Medical Weekly* (the vehicle he had previously chosen for his piece on Chinese principles of hygiene), which soon enough was reported back to China and embroiled him in a new controversy. The subject was the Chinese queue, or braid, and the recent drive by modernizers in China to eradicate the practice. Budberg described in detail how Chinese parents arranged their little boys' hair. He enumerated the advantages of the queue and the shaved forehead, which, he believed, ranged from improving blood circulation, and therefore intelligence, to helping unify the empire, for the queue made men of different ethnicities all feel Chinese. In addition, it prevented wrinkles, protected one from the elements of nature, and could be used for a pillow. He foresaw that Chinese men who changed their hairstyle would suffer from lice and skin diseases – in fact, he had already heard such complaints from his patients. Medical advantages apart, he added that a shaved forehead hid the natural ugliness of the male Chinese physiognomy. Old Chinese men looked handsome thanks to wearing the queue from childhood. Budberg also praised traditional Chinese clothing for its perfect elasticity and contribution to hygiene. Published in the year marked by the collapse of the empire and the rapid crumbling of its symbols, the article indulged in mockery of the young Chinese reformers, who by wishing to imitate the West were leading their nation to "an ugly suicide."[1]

The Berlin journal ran this diatribe from Harbin in a section separated by the heading "Feuilleton" from a preceding report by the former chief physician of the German naval quarantine station in Tsingtao, eastern Shandong. In 1898, the year Harbin was founded, the German navy acquired a colony at Kiaochow (now spelled Jiaozhou) Bay. Tsingtao

(Qingdao), the colony's capital, where Dr Erich Martini was stationed, was one of three foreign-built cities in northern China, along with Harbin and Dalian. As the German delegate to the recent international plague conference in Mukden, Martini described this conference as a success indebted to two Chinese men who had "entered modern times": Wu Lien-teh and Alfred Sze. German plague prevention in Shandong had succeeded because of the dissemination of Western medical ideas and the willing acceptance of these by the Chinese populace. In sum, China had suffered a plague but learned about modern medicine, and the Mukden conference had been "a friendly revolution" compared to the violent one that was still in process.[2] The contrast with Budberg's message was stark indeed.

In an ironic footnote at the end of Budberg's article, the editors made it known that they were "ready and willing to give the word to a completely modern Chinese to express himself *against* the queue." Presumably, the journal did have some Chinese readers, who would have been outraged by Budberg's piece. No riposte to it was sent to Berlin, however, whereas a sceptical review in *The British Medical Journal* called the author "more Chinese than John Chinaman himself."[3] The ensuing debate played out in China, but among Europeans rather than Chinese. In September, Budberg's article appeared in Russian in a Harbin newspaper.[4] At the same time it was reprinted (minus the concluding sentence on the "ugly suicide") in *Der Ostasiatische Lloyd* in Shanghai.[5] And in October this German newspaper, the oldest in China, published a response by a physician in Guangdong province who had worked in China since 1907. Like Budberg, Hermann Vortisch-van Vloten (1874–1944), previously of the Swiss Basel Mission on the Gold Coast in Africa, spoke Chinese and was familiar with Chinese life, yet he disproved Budberg's defence of the queue point by point. He too described the daily uses of the queue, adding some playful ones, but, having encountered "thousands of patients," he argued that the queue stood for no "hygienic principles"; it was actually conducive to skin disease and bad for sanitation. For all the reasons he listed, he welcomed the queue's end and reminded his Harbin colleague that, far from a unique attribute of the Chinese, queues were also worn by Africans, while in China they had not been imposed until the Manchu dynasty.[6]

This article was written in a humorous vein, but in January 1913 Budberg reacted to it in the pages of the *Ostasiatische Lloyd* in a tone of haughty indignation. He declared China infinitely superior to Western "culture bearers," contending that the prospect of China losing its culture would put the entire world in peril. Quite blind to his own faults in this respect, Budberg accused his opponent of cultural insensitivity for making light of the queue and daring to compare Chinese and African customs. Presenting himself as a scholar who for many years had taught "at the German University of Dorpat," he maintained that "we Germans" stood near to the Chinese in character. But only very few Europeans – such as himself, he implied in a transparent hint to his marriage – were privy to the mysteries of Chinese family life. Before other Europeans could even be introduced to these, they "first had to learn much, very much, from the Chinese."[7]

After the victorious 1911 revolution, queue cutting was forced on a reluctant population. Many educated Chinese perceived the campaign against the queue as a betrayal of tradition and a symbol of Western cultural invasion. One prominent conservative opponent of the movement was the Governor General of Manchuria, the Han bannerman Zhao Erxun, who in late 1912 moved to Peking and became the official historian of the defunct Qing dynasty.[8] Phantom pains were a common complaint among men who had lost their queues. In the northeast, many refused to cut them off even in the 1920s. However, it is not the section of Budberg's article on the changing Chinese hairstyle that causes astonishment, coming as it did from someone who professed to love China. On the personal level, his strident opposition to the reformers of China ran into a contradiction since one such modernizer was Alfred Sze, the American-educated high official in Harbin, whom he was pleased to call a friend. His outburst had much deeper causes than the queue, since for him, the people and ideas at which he lashed out represented the dangers posed by modernity itself. He seems to have perceived the Chinese Revolution of 1911 as an assault on his way of life – that of an aristocrat and an admirer of Chinese tradition. This challenge to the basic premises of his existence, the fall of the monarchy in his adopted country, was, as he was soon to discover, only the opening salvo.

Arrests and Trials

In what Baron Budberg persistently called his "struggle for truth and justice," he conspicuously failed to live up to the second part of his heraldic motto, *Fortiter in re, suaviter in modo* (Steadfast in action, gentle in manner). His manner was not gentle, and when he finished fighting one battle, he looked for the next. In 1913, his target was morphine dealers in Harbin; in an article for *St. Petersburger Zeitung*, he described his battle against them and the attacks he had to endure as a result, while vowing to remain steadfast in his anti-drug campaign.[9]

The hostility he had incurred from Russians loomed behind Budberg's arrest, a year into the First World War. Harbin was then boiling over with anti-German sentiment. After Germany's nationals were ordered to leave the CER zone within a month (many of them moved to Hulan), popular suspicion turned to Russian subjects of German extraction.[10] In Russia itself, Saint Petersburg was renamed Petrograd in an attempt to erase its German legacy, and a patriotic mob destroyed the German embassy as well as the offices of *St. Petersburger Zeitung* over the course of a day in August 1914. In 1915, all the German-language press in Russia was shut down (the newspaper to which Budberg had contributed from Harbin would not be published again until the 1990s). In even more distant Madrid, the tsar's ambassador, Baron Theodor Budberg, was discharged from his duties, for his German name as much as for ill health.[11] Of out sheer terror, ethnic Germans in Russia were soon changing their surnames to Russian-sounding ones. Jews, meanwhile, were suspected of collaborating with the enemy, one reason being that Yiddish speakers understood German.

Half a million of the inhabitants of Budberg's native Courland, including almost all the Jews, had been expelled by the summer of 1915, or fled on their own into the interior of Russia amid spiralling violence; many would remain there after the war. Prominent Baltic Germans were deported to Siberia before they could welcome the German occupation, and in Siberia itself and in the Russian Far East, German businesses collapsed. The manager of the Kunst & Albers trading firm (founded in Vladivostok in 1864), the competitors of Churin, was charged with espionage and arrested.[12] A pseudonymous Russian journalist in Petrograd published a series of maliciously sarcastic reports that portrayed Baltic Germans as agents of Germany. One of his many allegations was that they had devised a system for signalling to enemy planes and receiving coded messages from German pilots; in this context, the author mentioned a suspicious airplane passing "above the dacha of the aristocrat Budberg" near Riga, apparently an allusion to Magnushof.[13] Even on the front lines, the loyalty of senior commanders of German ethnicity, such as generals Aleksei Budberg and Pavel Rennenkampf, was questioned after the Russian army's defeats.[14] Arrests in Harbin included the pharmacist Leonhardt Tomson, whose sister-in-law was a German subject, Budberg's good friend the physician Friedrich Raupach, and the city's chief rabbi, Aaron Kiselev (1866–1949).[15] Even the Russian Consul in Harbin, Vil'gelm Vil'gel'movich (alternatively, Vasilii Vasil'evich) Trautschold, was later suspected of helping Germany.[16]

The *North China Herald* in Shanghai reported: "Baron Budberg, the official doctor in Harbin, who was recently arrested, has been charged with high treason. Incriminating documents have been found which show that he has been actively helping German prisoners to escape.

The police also found in his residence sixty pounds of opium."[17] Because of the crime imputed to him, although Budberg was a civilian, on 28 October 1915 he was incarcerated in the military guardhouse of the Trans-Amur District Border Guard, the special force in charge of security along the CER. In November, the railway manager Khorvat, in secret telegrams to Petrograd, referred to Budberg as the latest victim of the "shameful" witch-hunt of persons with German surnames in Russia and Harbin.[18] The arrests in Harbin had been ordered by the Russian counter-intelligence service, whose agents collected rumours about alleged supporters of Germany in the railway zone and staged provocations to unmask them. Half a year later, while Budberg was still imprisoned, the Harbin Chief of Police, Roman von Arnold (1871–1930), who owed his own safety to being of Swedish rather than German descent, was questioned on his case. He and Budberg were friends, and, hoping to shield the baron from the grave charges against him, he told the special investigator sent by the court in Irkutsk that Budberg was a naive and gullible person, nicknamed "a German-turned-Chink" for his adoration of China. Having become more Chinese than German, he posed no danger. A dreamer who lived in a fantasy world, he was nevertheless an upright man dedicated to his medical work and no traitor to the tsar.[19]

During the thirteen months he spent in harsh conditions in the guardhouse, on the southern outskirts of Harbin, Budberg was mocked and humiliated both as "the German spy" and on account of his Chinese marriage. He later wrote that the officers and personnel had tried to persuade him that his wife was unfaithful to him and that she was the ringleader of a *hong huzi* band in German pay.[20] The shock to his dignity was evidently severe. In April 1916 he attempted suicide in his cell.[21] By the time of his unexpected release in November of that year, he was shattered both physically and mentally.

The war between Germany and Russia tested the loyalties of many who had been rooted in different respects in both countries, forcing them to choose sides. A fellow member of the old Baltic German aristocracy, who cultivated the legacy of his Teutonic ancestors, Baron Roman Ungern-Sternberg (1886–1921) from Estland, signed up eagerly to fight the Germans under the command of General Rennenkampf, his great-uncle. Later on he achieved notoriety as a maverick warlord in the White Army, pursuing the utopian goal of restoring the Romanovs and the Qing as well as the spiritual leaders of Mongolia and Tibet.[22] Born to a Russified German family in the Urals, Baron Pavel Olbrich volunteered for the First World War as a youth of sixteen, "not simply as an expression of patriotism [but] wanting to prove that, being a German,

[he] was prepared to fight the enemies of Russia for the Faith, the Tsar and the Fatherland." After becoming a popular writer of the Russian emigration in China under the pen name Pavel Severnyi ("Northern"), he was approvingly called "the German with the Russian soul" by one critic.[23] The Harbin journalist Iustina V. Krusenstern-Peterets (1903–1983), whose father, a Baltic German officer from Estland, travelled to the front with the Trans-Amur Guards and was killed in battle in 1916, resented the baseless accusations of disloyalty that were made against Russian Germans in Petrograd at that time. Yet as a patriot of tsarist Russia, she maintained that the physician Budberg was a spy and a Russian-hater.[24]

Not all suspicions levelled at ethnic Germans in Russia and Manchuria during the war were figments of nationalists' imagination. Budberg had often declared his close affiliation with Germany and its interests, while constantly criticizing Russia; his wartime sympathies must have been with Germany. And Germany did operate agents and spies in China and Manchuria, who invested particular efforts in sabotaging the CER. In December 1914, the German military attaché in Peking, Baron Werner Rabe von Pappenheim (1877–1915), personally led a mission to blow up either the CER bridge over the River Nenjiang or the CER tunnel in the Greater Khingan Range, allegedly taking with him "eight hundred Hunghutzen [*hong huzi*]." Soon after arriving in Hailar, the attaché and six other Germans under his command were killed by local Mongols on Russian orders. Efforts to mobilize Manchurian bandits to blow up the Sungari bridge in Harbin, and the bridge across the Ussuri, likewise came to naught in early 1917.[25]

A secret agent familiar to Russian counter-intelligence was Roger Budberg's close friend, a German from Alsace named August Stöffler (1874–1946).[26] Stöffler came to Manchuria as a member of the Société des Missions Étrangères de Paris in 1902. He spent a decade as a missionary there, including two years at the Catholic mission in Fujiadian. He resigned in 1912, after claiming to have been mistreated by his French superior because of his German origins, but remained in Manchuria. In 1919, Stöffler was deported from China along with most German residents in the country. Decorated for his wartime service for the German empire, but denied a chance to continue his intelligence work, Stöffler, now a French citizen, married and settled with his German wife in Borneo, resuming correspondence with Budberg from that island. He eventually repatriated to French Alsace.[27]

It is easy – too easy, at this distance – to see what perhaps brought Budberg and Stöffler together. Although they belonged to different social classes, both were by birth people of border regions with complex connections to Germany. Both admired China and had tried on alternative identities. While the archival files listing Germany's wartime agents in China do not name Budberg in this capacity, it becomes clear that Stöffler, who collaborated with the German legations in Mukden and Peking, used his friendship with Budberg to promote his intelligence career.

A long letter by Stöffler to the German Foreign Office, which he wrote after being deported, shows him echoing Budberg's opinion on the absurdity of the Christian mission's work among the Chinese, "whose civilization is much older and who have a religion as good, if not better, than ours." He presented himself as a German patriot and a speaker of accent-free Chinese, who had travelled through the whole of Manchuria as an expert on trade and an adviser to German firms. During the war, he had spread German propaganda and assisted German prisoners of war who had escaped to Manchuria from captivity in the Russian Far East.[28] Stöffler claimed special credit for helping Lieutenant Baron Paul Wolff von Todenwarth (1876–1965) reach the consulate in Mukden. With some assistance from Budberg as well, this officer was able to return to Germany. He was sent out again in 1916 to foment a pro-German rebellion in Libya and later described his escape from Russia and adventures in China in a colourful memoir.[29] According to Russian military reports, only about one hundred of the 200,000 German and Austro-Hungarian military prisoners who were held in camps in Siberia and the Russian Far East managed to escape into China between 1914 and 1916.[30] Many more did so in 1917 and 1918, but instead of being conducted to safety by German agents, most of these refugee soldiers ended up in Chinese internment camps in Jilin town, Hailun (central Heilongjiang), and Qiqihar.[31] In August 1917, China joined the Allies' side against the Central Powers and interned German subjects on its territory as enemy aliens.

In an article published by the organ of the Harbin Russian Orientalists in the autumn of 1916, sinologist Pavel Shkurkin still urged the unmasking of German spies wherever they were.[32] The political upheavals of the following year overtook Russian concerns about treasonous Germans in the railway zone, although these were not forgotten, while Budberg's legal troubles continued. In September 1917 the charge was levelled at him that, as chief physician of the hospital for prostitutes in Pristan' from 1907 until his arrest in 1915, he had taken bribes from Japanese brothel owners. Sophia E. Antonova (1871–1934), a midwife and nurse who had worked with Budberg since the beginning of his medical career in Harbin, and the physician Władysław Wyrzykowski (Vyrzhikovskii, 1877–1942), a Polish graduate of Dorpat

University, who had replaced Budberg during his imprisonment, were also accused. Defence statements by Budberg survive in the archives, handwritten in almost faultless Russian: he denied improper conduct and announced that he was ready to resume work at the hospital for prostitutes free of charge, out of a sense of medical duty. Citing the involvement of Japanese nationals, he requested that he be tried by the foreign consular court.[33]

Instead, the Russian Border Circuit Court in Harbin forwarded the case to the Judicial Chamber in Irkutsk, to which it had been subordinated until 1917: that chamber had been abolished by the Bolsheviks in January 1918 but had been reconstituted six months later by the Kolchak government. A ruling in the case against Budberg and the others was made in June 1919.[34] Between the opening of these juridical proceedings and their conclusion, the pendulum of power had swung in Harbin, too, though not nearly as violently as it had in Russia. While Budberg was incarcerated in the military guardhouse, the only junior officer there, whom he later remembered with gratitude for treating him with respect and even spending whole nights talking to him in his prison cell, was the young Martem'ian N. Riutin (1890–1937). After Budberg's release, these conversations led to a friendship despite the age gap and Riutin's political convictions.[35] In December 1917, Riutin, a Bolshevik, who had cabled Lenin for guidance on the situation in Harbin and received orders from him to seize control of the city, attempted a coup against the CER manager Khorvat. The result was a swift takeover of Harbin by Chinese troops.[36] They protected Khorvat with the support of the foreign consuls, who were anxious to maintain order and prevent the spread of the Bolshevik revolution into Manchuria; but thereafter Chinese power would rise quickly at the expense of the Russians, and Khorvat was soon compelled to leave Harbin.

For several years, Budberg had supplemented his income as a physician by operating a steamer called the *Harbin* and three barges (one of which he had named *Zhong-De-Hua*) on the Sungari. His experience with shipping and barges went back to the Russo-Japanese War. River conditions permitting, the *Harbin* transported grain to the southwest as far as Bodune (also Boduna; now Songyuan), an inland port at the confluence of the Sungari and the Nenjiang. In June 1918, Budberg sold the steamer and an iron-hulled barge, the *Podruga* (female friend, in Russian), to a Chinese company.[37] Many Russian firms participated in shipping on the Sungari, and most of them sold out to the Chinese after 1917.[38] The charges made against Budberg in his first trial included that he had allowed two escaped German POWs to sail on the *Harbin* to Bodune, Stöffler's base at the time.

Budberg's relative and good friend Paul Lieven, who had strolled with him through Mukden during the Russo-Japanese War and was in Khabarovsk in 1918 as representative of the Red Cross, came over to Harbin to see him. This was the only visit he ever received from a member of his extended family in Europe.[39] The correspondence with Antoinette had broken off after his first arrest, and in wartime, he could not write to Germany. In August 1919, however, Budberg was arrested for the second time. Harbin was then a vital transportation node for the White resistance in Siberia and the Far East, and a pro-Bolshevik strike on the railway had cut off supplies to the Kolchak regime in Omsk. Kolchak's counter-intelligence service responded by issuing telegraph orders for arrests and deportations, and persons who were summoned to Omsk often did not return.

From his cell in the prison where he had been employed as a physician, Budberg wrote appeals against his deportation to Omsk in the effort to forestall his arbitrary execution. No one in Harbin could tell him (nor did they know at the time) what the charge against him was, and he was not put on trial. His ten-year-old daughter urged her mother to commit joint suicide, while well-wishers pressured the young woman to leave her husband and renounce any rights to the girl, so that Zhong-De-Hua could become eligible to inherit from her father. Far from being a mere victim, however, Li actively involved herself in efforts to get Budberg out of prison, conferring with his friends and approaching Russian officials. In September, Budberg gave his blessing for his child to be admitted into the Lutheran faith. In addition to her Chinese name, she was christened with a double European name: Antoinette Cecilia, in honour of her father's favourite sister, who now became the child's godmother, and of his grandmother, whose memory he cherished.[40]

According to Budberg, the Chinese Chambers of Commerce in Harbin and Fujiadian expressed their concern for him to the Russian CER authorities.[41] More decisive was the support of General Khorvat and especially his trusted assistant, General Mikhail E. Afanas'ev (1857–1936). They repeatedly wired Omsk about Budberg's case and eventually secured his release. Two friends then paid Budberg's bail, which was set at 100,000 rubles. These were the tobacco factory owner, Il'ia A. Lopato (1874–1934), a well-known figure in Harbin and leader of its small Karaite community (a sect within Judaism), whom Budberg praised in glowing terms, and the prominent Jewish physician Iulii E. Eliason (?–after 1936), a veteran of the Russo-Japanese War.[42]

Budberg was released in November 1919 after three and a half months in prison and was immediately reinstated as the same prison's physician. Only in 1922 did he learn that he had been arrested after being named as a German agent working for the Bolsheviks in a series of letters purportedly from the German high command to the leaders of the Russian Revolution. In 1918 the US Committee on Public Information had endorsed those letters as evidence of a "German-Bolshevik conspiracy." Only in the 1950s were the "Sisson documents" definitively proven to have been audacious forgeries produced by the Polish adventurer Ferdynand Ossendowski (1878–1945), formerly resident in Harbin.[43]

Writing to his "dear old friend" Stöffler from his cell in October, Budberg had called the conditions of his second imprisonment "paradise" compared to the first. Since he was infinitely curious about human nature, being behind bars offered him a great opportunity for studying criminal psychology.[44] Completely unlike the situation at the military guardhouse in 1915 and 1916, the prison director treated him as a colleague and did all he could to offer him help and encouragement. The Harbin city prison, which Budberg got to know intimately both as a long-time physician and as a prisoner in 1919, was a large compound at the corner of Kitaiskaia and Politseiskaia Streets. Established by the Russians in 1901, it was used by all successive administrations in Harbin until 1967.[45]

In March 1920, Budberg was again able to write to his sister. He told her about being robbed by a gang of masked marauders, who invaded his house – an experience he described as one of the most interesting in his life since it, too, was a lesson in criminal psychology. He and his wife were held at gunpoint and were nearly shot amid the sobbing of their daughter, while Li showed remarkable courage – and, incidentally, her fluent Russian – by mocking the bandits and offering to sacrifice herself to protect her husband and child.[46] Crime was rampant in Harbin: the perpetrators of this particular robbery were a band of Russian outlaws, who had escaped from the city prison and were later killed in a joint action by the Russian police and the Chinese military in February 1921.[47]

Amid all that, Budberg was as busy as always, treating patients at his hospital, at the city prison, and at home. On the eve of his arrest, he had also been employed in the CER Ninth Section Hospital and Infirmary, on Kazach'ia Street in Pristan' (Cossack Street, now Gaoyijie, in Daoli), alongside the midwife Antonova, five nurses, and his old friend Stepan G. Migdisov (Migdisiants, 1867–1933), chairman of the Armenian National Society in Harbin, who had studied medicine in Dorpat, served in the Russo-Japanese War, and worked with Budberg in times of plague.[48] In addition, he was engaged as a specialist in the private hospital of Dr Nikolai S. Kirchev (1866–1945), an ethnic Bulgarian, born in Romania and trained in Russia, on Novogorodniaia Street, corner of Polevaia (New Town Street and Field Street, now Shangzhi dajie and Tiandi jie).[49] A free man once again, he wrote in the spring of 1920 that he allowed himself the luxury of keeping three horses and greatly enjoyed riding out of the city in the mornings.[50]

But even as he was writing to his sister, rejoicing at being recently informed that their mother was still alive, she was no longer. Having left Riga to stay with Antoinette, she died in January 1920, aged eighty-three, in Augustusburg Castle, which by then had been transferred from German jurisdiction to the newly reconstituted Poland. When the news of his mother's death reached him through a letter from Stöffler in Borneo, Budberg wrote to his sister that she had bequeathed to them "tradition": "Being conscious of mother's still living made it easier for me to live on in the light of tradition, especially now that the suffocating democratic winds are raging through the world, levelling everything."[51] Together with the loss of his mother he mourned bitterly the disappearance, during his arrest the previous year, of his most valued possessions: a box containing the letters of his ancestors, dating back to the eighteenth century, and his own entire correspondence with his grandmother. The utmost importance he attached to the history of his family demonstrates how he combined loyalty to the culture in which he was raised, and his adoption of China with its ancestor worship. He would never stop demanding the restitution of these precious effects, which, after confiscation, were apparently lost while being transported from Harbin to Omsk. Writing about them to the still acting tsarist consul in Harbin, Budberg reminded him of his duty to protect Russian subjects abroad.[52]

Roger Budberg was arrested and imprisoned twice as a Russian subject. However, after the tumult of the First World War and the Russian Revolution, the map of Europe was being redrawn, with some states erased and others created. Under the wartime German occupation, the Baltic German nobility supported the re-creation of the Duchy of Courland and Semigallia, extinct since 1795. Acknowledged by the Kaiser in March 1918, it was included in a United Baltic Duchy, incorporating Estland and Livland, in September.[53] But after Germany's defeat and the Kaiser's abdication in November, the regions to which the Budberg family traced the Baltic component of its identity became part of the new Republic of Latvia. In December 1919 a Latvian Consulate opened in Harbin, one of only two in China (the other being in Shanghai), and one of more than twenty foreign consulates in the city.[54] In 1920 the Harbin press informed all persons born in the territory now incorporated

by the Latvian state, irrespective of their ethnicity, that they were enti-
tled to apply for Latvian citizenship, with a deadline of 5 September.[55]

Budberg did not take up this opportunity to shed his last links to
tsarist Russia, the now defunct country he had so much to blame for,
in favour of the Latvian republic. Since the confiscation of all his documents upon his arrest in 1919, he had been living without any identity
papers.[56] In his correspondence with his sister and his published writings, one finds no reference to the founding of a new state in his place
of birth: the one exception is a late letter to the family lawyer in Riga
in which he condemned Latvia for its land policy.[57] He hardly noticed
ethnic Latvians and Estonians in Harbin, although he had spent most
of his life among these people before coming to China (he did seek out
and establish contacts with Germans, and with graduates of the multinational medical faculty of Dorpat University, a surprising number of
whom were present in Harbin).[58] Similarly, Latvian diplomats in Manchuria showed no interest in Budberg – their focus was on Latvians, not
German barons. And even had Budberg applied for Latvian citizenship
in 1920, he probably would have been turned down, since, as of that
year, Poniemon still belonged to Lithuania (which briefly established
a Budberga parish at that location). In March 1921, after long negotiations, the boundary between Latvia and Lithuania was drawn through
the former Budberg family estate, leaving two thirds of it on the Latvian side.[59]

In May 1920 the recently appointed first honorary Consul of Latvia in Harbin estimated the total number of Latvians in Manchuria at
between 500 and 600. About 240 of them (presumably, ethnic Latvians)
were members of patriotic organizations.[60] The consul rightly antici-
pated that the numbers would increase with the arrival of émigrés from
Siberia and the Russian Far East: in January 1924, the Harbin consulate
reported to the Foreign Office in Riga on 835 registered Latvian citizens.
Because of re-emigration, only 350 such persons were still in Harbin as
of 1926 (there were only another 204 in all the rest of China).[61] China
recognized Latvia in 1923 but established diplomatic relations with it
only in 1936, four years before Latvia lost its independence to a Soviet
invasion.

Endings

Five days after the death of Alexandrine Budberg, her second son Gotthard died in Tobolsk, western Siberia, at the age of fifty-six. From
1907 to 1909 Gotthard Budberg ran a printing house in Riga's Old
Town.[62] He could have earned a modest place in history for publishing,

alongside a number of books in Latvian and Russian and a liberal paper in German, the first-ever Yiddish newspaper in the Baltic region – the *Nazional-Zeitung*, which appeared between August and November 1907. However, his Jewish collaborators were too baffled by the notion of a German baron promoting the Jewish press to properly record his name.[63] By 1915, Gotthard was living near Tobolsk with Joseph,[64] who combined a career as a judge with a life dedicated to hunting. An expert marksman, Gotthard shared his older brother's passion.[65] After appointments to Ufa and Omsk, Joseph Budberg served on the circuit court of Tobolsk beginning in 1900. When his request to be reassigned to the Baltic after the death of his father in 1906 was rejected, he remained in Tobolsk, where he held a respectable position.[66] He informed Roger that their brother Gotthard made ends meet by hunting and fishing – the former gentleman's sport having become a means of subsistence – while his wife kept a small shop. But in the winter of 1916, Gotthard was arrested in Tobolsk. He was later released in the distant village of Berezovka and only returned after about a year, a broken man who soon lost his sanity.[67]

In August 1917, Nicholas II, who had abdicated as tsar in Petrograd, was escorted to Tobolsk with his family by order of the Provisional Government. The Romanovs were kept there until the following April, when the Bolsheviks transported them to Ekaterinburg in the Urals, where they were soon executed. The few members of the nobility in Tobolsk must have feared for their own lives. Joseph resigned from his post as a judge in March 1917, retiring to a nearby Tatar village, where he had a small house. He and his wife supported themselves by gardening. In August 1919, just prior to his own arrest, Roger telegraphed his brothers urging them to find safety with him in Harbin.[68] He learned of Gotthard's death from the last letter he ever received from Joseph, in April 1921.[69] Between 21 February and 8 April, Tobolsk was the main city controlled by forces of the Western Siberian Uprising: a large revolt by peasants against the Communist dictatorship and the confiscation of grain. During that period, on 11 March, the Peasant City Council in Tobolsk reinstated the circuit court and reappointed Joseph Budberg as one of its judges.[70] Five days after the Red Army reconquered Tobolsk, on 13 April 1921, Budberg was shot and robbed outside the city. His corpse lay on the street for two days before his wife found him.[71]

Aged fifty-eight at his death, he had married in his fiftieth year, the only one of the eight Budberg siblings with a Baltic German spouse, and he died childless. Joseph's wife, Elfriede (Frida), was a widowed commoner from Riga. Left destitute in Tobolsk, she managed to return to Latvia, later to end her days in a nursing home next to the Raczynski family in occupied Poland in 1944.

In Harbin, a mysterious infection had meanwhile carried away Roger Budberg's wife. She died in late November 1920, having just turned twenty-seven. The image of this unforeseen tragedy is the first photograph in the book Budberg published in Germany in 1923 with a dedication to his "beloved wife Li-jü-dsehön." It shows Li on her deathbed, flanked by Buddhist figurines: the bodhisattva of compassion Guanyin holding a child, a Buddha on a lotus throne, and incense sticks in a Chinese bowl. Budberg wrote how terribly he missed her, reproaching himself for not spending enough time with her while she lived. He often visited her tomb in the Chinese cemetery.[72] Baroness Budberg, or woman Li of the Bu family, was buried in Taiping qiao (Taiping Bridge). At the time, that area belonged to Binjiang County, northeast of Harbin; today it is part of Harbin's Daowai district, although its old cemetery is long gone.[73] In February 1921, the same cemetery at Taiping qiao became the site of a mass burning of corpses during Harbin's second epidemic of pneumonic plague.

In the spring of 1921, by which time Latvia and Lithuania had divided Poniemon between them, and Joseph's death had removed the eldest heir, Roger Budberg's remaining siblings were forced to deal with the Latvian state. The sisters Marie Belloni, who had married an Italian in 1900 and lived with three sons in Rome; Cecile Diestelhorst, who had lived in Dresden as the wife of a German physician since 1897 and had a son and a daughter; and Alexandra (formerly Alexandrine, known as Lelly in the family) Paine, who had been widowed in 1904 from her first marriage to an Englishman, and in 1911 emigrated to the United States, where by 1918 she had remarried and divorced, now with five children, attempted to recover what remained of their parents' property. Antoinette, in Poland, was less involved; she was in the best circumstances financially, although she was also beset by family problems and a mother of five, whereas Roger in China declared himself in correspondence utterly uninterested in money and depressed by the pecuniary disagreements between his sisters. As he put it to Antoinette, "the letters, now, that deal with the inheritance business, are bad enough to make me morally disgusted. It even seems to me as if I have become more of an aristocrat through contact with the lowest strata of the Chinese population, than this should have been inculcated in us through blood and education."[74]

Writing this, he would have remembered the earlier family dispute, which saw their mother pitted against all her children with the exception of Marie and Wilhelm over ownership rights to the Magnushof estate after the death of her husband in 1906.[75] Their brother Wilhelm had since gone missing: during his Harbin trial in 1915, Roger Budberg testified that he had no information of his whereabouts.[76] In early June 1921, within weeks of hearing of the death of Gotthard and on the same day he had received Elfriede's letter about the murder of Joseph, Budberg met Luis Karlovich Bubnik. A German-speaking widower with two children, who introduced himself as a former timber merchant, Bubnik had taken refuge from Ufa in Harbin, where he opened a bakery. He said he had known Wilhelm, an alcoholic, in Ufa and had nursed him and taken care of his burial around 1911.[77] This earned Bubnik Baron Budberg's lasting gratitude: at least from early 1924, but probably sooner after that first meeting, the Bubnik family moved into an apartment in Budberg's hospital.[78] After learning of Wilhelm's death, Roger Budberg regarded himself as the last male offspring of his line.

None of the surviving siblings and claimants to the Budberg inheritance lived in Latvia; indeed, all five resided in different countries. Thus, in 1922 Marie and Cecile travelled together to Riga to sort out furniture, artworks, and all other objects that remained behind in the country that would never again be their home. The logistics proved difficult, and rather than await everybody's answers on what they wished to do with these belongings, Marie – the favourite daughter and main beneficiary of their mother's will – sold many items locally and shipped the rest to Rome.[79] Responding to this news in a letter to Antoinette, Roger was furious, recalling an ancient feud with Marie back in 1893, which had made him never want to set foot in Poniemon again.[80] But the situation, in which the siblings had to communicate again over legal matters, briefly brought them together across the great geographical distances. Marie soon started to write to Roger not only about their parents' furniture, but also to fill him in on her life; he found one long letter from her "not lacking in warmth." Lelly wrote, too, proposing to translate his essays on China into English for publication in America.[81] But little came of their endeavours to be recognized as the rightful owners of Poniemon, or Magnushof.

This was because a radical agrarian reform in Latvia in 1920 had expropriated the land of the Baltic Germans for redistribution among peasants and war veterans (similar measures were enacted in Estonia, where the Budbergs had relatives). The owners received inadequate compensation or none at all, and they were usually left with only small parcels of land on their former estates. In Poniemon, this amounted to a mortgaged outlying farm of 57 hectares, which was not worth taking, whereas Magnushof had been expropriated in its entirety. By the spring of 1924, Joseph's widow Elfriede was nursing the scheme of applying for Lithuanian citizenship, so as to become eligible to inherit the part of Poniemon that had passed to that country.[82] The restitution claims brought forward by the lawyers retained by Roger's sisters were not resolved by the Latvian judiciary until as late as 1938, when Marie's money was finally collected on her behalf by the Italian ambassador in Riga. Alexandra Paine, an American citizen, had to wait until 1932 to be informed that her claim had been rejected.[83] Her daughter Tamara, who had married a Latvian officer, was the last family member remaining in Poniemon until she too, by then a widow with a small child, left for the United States in 1930.

Between October 1920 and May 1921, pneumonic plague returned to Manchuria after a decade's absence and under much changed political circumstances. As in 1910, when tsarist Russia had weighed in to take control of the measures to contain the epidemic, Roger Budberg was closely involved in the medical work in Harbin. Once more he did every-thing to make himself unpopular with his Russian superiors and col-leagues by accusing them of profiteering from the plague and of gross insensitivity toward the Chinese poor. More than 3,000 lives were lost among the Chinese population of Harbin and Fujiadian. However, when it came to isolating those who had contracted the plague, so as to prevent them from infecting others, Budberg was uncompromising in his medi-cal standards and made proof of his impartiality. In the numerous press reports on the epidemic, which were reprinted in the weekly organ of the CER, Budberg's name comes up in connection not with the protests he lodged against the Russian administration but rather with his demand that the medical police find and apprehend the Chinese secretary of the Binjiang District Court, who, a few days after his wife got infected and died, fled Harbin by a private car together with his daughter.[84]

Apparently, Boris Ostroumov, who had replaced General Khorvat as the head of the Railway in April 1921, thought of Budberg as a potential bridge builder with the Chinese and intended to make him director of the CER Central Hospital, for which Budberg had worked since 1906.[85] However, according to Budberg himself, the planned appointment encountered strong opposition within the Russian community and was never made. Ostroumov had indeed launched a thorough reorganiza-tion of the Central Hospital at that time, and he appointed a new direc-tor in June.[86] As for Budberg, when the Chinese authorities took over the Harbin prison hospital in July, his long-time wish to enter Chinese service was fulfilled.[87] Not only did he keep his job as the prison phy-sician, but in August he was also appointed medical inspector of the Harbin police, which had been under Chinese control since the previ-ous year.[88]

He did not stay long at that new post, the peak of his official career: by early November he had been dismissed for what was vaguely described as insubordination.[89] Budberg saw things differently, telling the Russian press he had left of his own free will because he refused to receive his salary out of a budget that the city reserved for the treatment of prostitutes: being "a follower of Confucius," he declared that "he would rather work for free."[90] In fact, the Chinese police department had stopped funding Budberg's hospital for prostitutes, the only institution in Harbin that treated venereal diseases. In October, this crisis had prompted an unusual petition by the prostitutes themselves, so Budberg may have been caught between loyalty to his patients and to his new bosses.[91] Over the next two years, he approached the CER administration, which was still in Russian hands, contesting a decision from 1920 to have his dilapidated hospital torn down. Notably, he succeeded in mobilizing leading representatives of the Chinese community, including the Chamber of Commerce and the Association of Chinese Employees of the CER, to support his motion for prolonging his lease of the land so that he could build a new hospital on it.[92] In 1924, however, the Harbin City Council decided to construct its own venereological hospital rather than continue subsidizing Budberg's private one.[93]

A strikingly original book Budberg published in Hamburg in 1923, *Bilder aus der Zeit der Lungenpest-Epidemien in der Mandschurei, 1910/11 und 1921* (Pictures from the Time of the Epidemics of Pneumonic Plague in Manchuria), conveyed the anxiety and suspicion that permeated Harbin when it was struck by "the Black Death."[94] Alongside a detailed memoir of the two epidemics, the book included 140 photographs, beginning with a frontispiece portrait of the author in his white medical gown. He had gone to the Chinese cemetery at Taiping qiao, where his wife was buried, and had himself photographed in front of the temple built for the spirits of the unburied dead (who according to popular belief would become hungry ghosts), and with the naked corpses and skulls of the victims, who had been burnt and thrown into mass graves.[95] He took most of the other photographs himself, while others were contributed by August Stöffler and the Harbin old-timer Richard Kegel (1864–1922), a former German subject, who had also been questioned and detained during the spy scare of 1915.[96]

One photograph, taken in 1921, shows a dead infant lying in a field, barely covered by a bundle of reeds; a pig in the distance is described as "on the lookout for a good bite." For Budberg, this was just the occasion to warn Westerners who witnessed such scenes in Manchuria against concluding that the Chinese did not love their children. The opposite was true, but only immersion in "the soul life [*Seelenleben*] of the Chinese" could reveal the reason for the practice of feeding dead children to animals. His own detailed explanation had Buddhist overtones: people believed it was necessary for a child's soul to join the soul of an animal in order to reach the cycle of transmigration.[97]

Budberg had to rewrite both *Bilder aus der Zeit der Lungenpest-Epidemien* and his *Memoirs*, published in Russian, after all his papers were confiscated in 1919. He updated both manuscripts by including his second arrest and the second plague epidemic. A review of the German work in *The China Medical Journal* (published in English in Shanghai) called it "a very interesting book with a very personal note," containing "vivid descriptions of the two great Manchurian plague epidemics, seen with a keen eye, a kind heart and a very sensitive mind," by an author who "is a friend of the Chinese people, and ... describes them as having been despised, bullied and ill-treated by the Russians." Yet the reviewer also noted that "accusations, many of a personal character, fill a great part of the book."[98] The Harbin paper *Zaria* (The Dawn) commented that for Budberg, "the epidemic of 1910 was a war with Prof. Zabolotny."[99] There were at least four reviews in the German medical press, and all of them were appreciative of the book, both as a contribution to medical science and as an addition to the genre of plague literature.[100] Though one-sided and opinionated, this remains the only work by a Harbin author to place Russian-Chinese relations squarely at its centre. Hardly any copies of the book reached libraries beyond Germany. Along with the rest of Budberg's writings in both German and Russian, and his singular life story, it was quickly forgotten.

In a glowing review of the Russian *Memoirs* for the newspaper he edited in Riga, the prominent Baltic German author Oskar Grosberg (1862–1941) called Budberg a forerunner of Eurasianism.[101] Budberg himself never made the connection to this stream of Russian geopolitical thought. His second book was a vigorous polemic against the Russian administration of Harbin, the protest of a deeply wronged man who was fighting to restore his good name. To this end, he reproduced the interrogation protocols and official correspondence related to his trial from 1915 and 1916 (copies of which he had obtained), along with his diary and numerous petitions to the Russian and Chinese authorities from 1919 and 1920.[102] Besides the litany of complaints and accusations, the book contained descriptions of Harbin's criminal world – of thieves and murderers the author had met both as a prisoner and as a police physician. It was interspersed with Budberg's religious ruminations on the forces of good and evil, as well as passages on the love and sacrifice of his wife, the suffering that she and their daughter endured, and their shared love of nature. The final sentence expressed his longing to be soon reunited in soul with his wife, whom he called his heroine.

The book's red cover made a richly symbolic display of the two languages and cultures that mattered to him most: above the Russian title,
Memuary, a coiled yellow dragon (the Chinese imperial colour, thus
joining the auspicious colour red) divided in two an inscription in Chinese, reading, from right to left, *tiandi liangxin*. This adage translates as
"[May] Heaven and Earth be your conscience" – an injunction to speak
the truth. The author's formal signature, "Dr med Baron Boenningshau-
sen Budberg," in his cursive German script, appeared beneath the Russian title. The frontispiece carried his portrait in profile, now inscribed
with the shorter version of his name and title of nobility. A dedication to
his mother was followed by the arresting juxtaposition of the Budberg
coat of arms and Latin motto, *Fortiter in re, suaviter in modo*, with the
four Chinese characters, *tian di liang xin*, encircling the coiled dragon.
By these visual means he affirmed the equivalence of the German and
Chinese traditions and again proclaimed his loyalty to both.[103]

Budberg expected a scandal to erupt in Harbin when this book came
out; and he intended to have his book on the plague epidemics translated into Russian as well.[104] But in the only local response to the *Memoirs*
that has come to light, a reviewer referred to the author as a mystic and
a dreamer, a lover of China who had combined Christianity with Con-
fucianism, and a person of rare integrity, whose name shone brightly in
petty-minded and greed-ridden Harbin.[105] Budberg told his sister that
Harbin writers and journalists phoned and visited him.[106] Some of the
intrigues and conspiracies he attributed in the *Memoirs* to his enemies
within the Russian administration were obviously the products of his
imagination. Others, like the Sisson documents, were strikingly real
(and serious people believed them). And there was indeed a dangerous
plot to take advantage of him, which he entirely missed.

The experience of having been arrested twice had shaken his grip on
reality. More and more, he began to view coincidences as omens and the
shadows around him multiplied. He believed in the continuous communication between the worlds of the dead and the living and often felt
himself in the presence of benevolent ghosts. Sharing these visions in
letters to his sister, on one occasion he admitted that his intense mental
life and flights of the spirit may have taken him beyond the bounds of
"normality" as most people understood it.[107]

He knew he was in poor health and was worried about his daughter's future. On 3 June 1924 he signed a will in which he left her all his
property. He appointed Luis Bubnik, the German merchant from Ufa
who had buried Wilhelm, as his executor.[108] The notary and three witnesses were all Russians, among them Vladimir V. Ponosov (1899–1975).
Also originally from Ufa, soon after coming to Harbin in 1922, Ponosov

joined the new Society for the Study of the Manchurian Region. He was
to become one of the most prominent scholars of Manchuria, leading
several ethnographic and archaeological expeditions and working in
Harbin museums for many years.[109]

Budberg considered himself a sinologist, yet he ignored the Harbin
Orientalists in his writings, much as he did Western studies on China
in general. Being entirely self-taught, he did not join their organizations
(until a late stage, the Society of Russian Orientalists only accepted people with formal sinological education, so this might not even have been
possible); it seems that he did not read their publications. Yet in 1925, the
archaeologist and keeper of the OIMK Museum in Harbin, Vladimir Ia.
Tolmachev (1876–1942), a senior collaborator of Ponosov, included photographs of artefacts from Baron Budberg's private collection in an essay
on the antiquities of Baicheng, the Jin dynasty capital in the thirteenth
century, also known as Huiningfu. He wrote that as of 1924, those artefacts were being exhibited on temporary loan at the museum.[110] In the
years that proved the last in Budberg's life, there were indications such
as these of guarded rapprochement with the Harbin Russians, especially
those among them who shared his deep engagement with China. Perhaps he had softened his antagonism toward the Russians once they
were no longer the masters of the city, backed by the tsarist empire, but
émigrés, who now needed to behave differently toward the Chinese.

The artefacts Budberg allowed to be exhibited at the museum of the
Society for the Study of the Manchurian Region were part of a sizeable
collection of Chinese art he had built since settling in Harbin and that
he described as his own "rich museum." Apparently, it had been of
no interest to the Russian robber gang that had broken into his house;
even so, he moved the collection to the museum as a precaution against
future robberies, or fires.[111] Most unusual among these objects were
anthropomorphic figurines made of bronze, which Budberg told Tolmachev he had purchased on his trips to Ashihe. They dated back to the
Jurchens and must have been found locally.[112]

Ashihe, the town near Harbin where his wife may have been from,
was easy to visit, being a stop on the CER. (It was renamed Acheng
in 1909 and became a district of Harbin in 2006.) It was a place where
foreigners from Harbin – those who dared venture beyond Fujiadian, including Russian students of Chinese – journeyed to see "the
real China." Budberg also took photographs of people and temples
in Ashihe and sent some of these to his sister Cecile in Germany.[113]
A leading Harbin sinologist who often went there, Ippolit G. Baranov
(1886–1972), opened a long essay on the temples of Ashihe in 1926 by

describing it as "an ancient Chinese town, closest to Harbin, which has preserved the type of Chinese towns of former times."[114]

Collecting Chinese art connected Budberg with a more knowledgeable and affluent collector, who lived in Peking rather than Harbin. Johan W.N. Munthe (1864–1935), a Norwegian, came to China in 1887 to work for the Imperial Chinese Maritime Customs, an organization run for the Chinese government under a British inspector general. It had an international staff dominated by Westerners but including Japanese and Chinese employees. After serving in Shanghai, Chefoo, and Ningbo, Munthe took leave between 1895 and 1897 to work in Tientsin for the "model army" founded by General Yuan Shikai, and in this capacity he is credited with reorganizing the Chinese cavalry. In 1900, the Russian General Staff engaged Munthe as an interpreter during the suppression of the Boxers. He rejoined the Customs Service in Tientsin in 1902, then in 1911 resumed work for Yuan Shikai, who had appointed him an aide-de-camp with the rank of major-general, in charge of the security of the Legations Quarter in Peking. Yuan, who became president in 1912, died in 1916. That same year, Munthe left the Customs Service, though he remained in Peking. At the time of his correspondence with Budberg, he still commanded his security guard in the capital. Munthe died in Peking in 1935, having spent forty-nine years in China.[115] He is best known for having donated Chinese art to the museum in Bergen, his home town, where the Munthe collection is prominently displayed and the general, with his phenomenal military moustache, is an iconic figure.[116]

It is unclear how Budberg and Munthe met. Budberg mentions him as a friend in the final pages of his *Memoirs*, but the immense emotional burden of the relationship is revealed in his letters to Antoinette from 1922 to 1925. As Roger explained to his sister, he had always depended on soul-to-soul contact, the possibility of sharing his innermost thoughts with another person. The first such person was their maternal grandmother, and the second was his wife. After her sudden death, the role of intimate confidant fell on Munthe.[117] Budberg admired the general for living in China far longer than him, for speaking better Chinese, and for having made the kind of career in Chinese service to which he himself aspired, although he also criticized Munthe for remaining distant from the Chinese in spirit.[118] Yet their friendship would evolve into a nightmarish obsession on Budberg's part that consumed all his mental energy. In letter after letter to his sister, he complained bitterly about Munthe's coldness and his determined silence with regard to his own entreaties for clear answers.

The answers Budberg implored the general to give him concerned two issues. One was matrimony: according to Budberg, soon after his wife died, Munthe had promised to find him a new wife in Peking. He even said that the Manchu General Yin Chang (1859–1928), a former ambassador in Berlin and the Qing Minister of War, would look for a suitably high-born candidate; later another matchmaker was discussed, a former lady-in-waiting at the Peking court.[119] The other issue was publishing: since his wife's death, Budberg had taken to writing Munthe daily, and sometimes more than once a day. This correspondence has been lost along with Munthe's Peking archive, but several of Budberg's letters survive because he appended them to those he sent his sister. They are of intense lyrical expression in an elevated register of literary German, presenting a vision of cosmic harmony in which the natural and human worlds are merged. Budberg expected Munthe and his wife to publish his letters and then demanded that they do so. He was sorely disappointed by the couple's indifference to his requests.[120]

Another permanent theme of contention with Munthe as well as with Antoinette was the adherence of both to Christian Science, which Budberg resolutely rejected along with theosophy and anthroposophy.[121] The relationship with Munthe seems to have ended after the general wrote to Budberg that he and his wife "were sorry to find out that you have become mentally ill."[122] Quoting these words to his sister, Budberg blamed Munthe for ruining his life; he was now convinced that Munthe had been tormenting him with false expectations "for six years" on instructions from the leaders of Christian Science in the United States.[123]

Frustrated by Munthe's responses, or his silences, in 1924 Budberg began writing long letters on his cosmological thought to Aunt Lonny, his childhood caretaker, now bedridden in Estonia. He asked her to forward these letters to Antoinette so that she could edit a collection of them.[124] While he seemed to consider his correspondence with Antoinette of lesser value, when writing to her, too, he may have imagined that one day his letters would become public. The collapse of his friendship with Munthe left Budberg in a state of emotional depletion, and he was driven to search for another solution to his urgent need for spiritual exchange as well as, quite simply, company.[125] His large house on Kavkazskaia was empty now: he had lodged Zhong-De-Hua "with good people" in his hospital for prostitutes, where he passed by in the evenings to wish her good night. Budberg wrote to his sister that he felt unable to take care of the child without a woman beside him; considering the violent robbery he had lived through, he may also have feared for her safety.[126]

Way to the Great Light

In a letter to Munthe in May 1922, Budberg described a desperate visit he made to a woman fortune teller, confessing to his friend that he had been "so ill in [his] soul."[127] And so he found his way to the Rosicrucian movement. Only the "beautiful" and "ancient" Rosicrucian Order could restore his peace of mind when he felt alone and abandoned. Now a teacher started coming to his house to instruct him in the secret teachings, "the way to the great light."[128] By late 1922 he had decided to turn his cellar into a Rosicrucian temple and residence of the order's Young Master, whose name he did not reveal.[129] There is no more information about this person in the letters to his sister. In January 1925 he regretted the temporary departure of his "Chinese master," who had gone to visit his native place and was only expected back in Harbin after the Chinese New Year.[130]

The Rosicrucian Order appealed to Budberg because it revealed the deep mysteries of life and the conspiracies that abounded in the world, and because it was German.[131] However, although someone may have stressed to him the German origins of this esoteric movement, the variety practised in Harbin drew on the tradition of Russian Rosicrucianism, originally a branch of Russian freemasonry. The émigré Rosicrucians in China emphasized the Russian sources of their teaching, expressing "no sympathy for oriental mysticism."[132] In Harbin in the 1920s, Budberg seems to have been alone in trying to combine European occultism with the Chinese world view as he understood it.

A vision that did blend the Russian occult with the Orient, although it was inspired by India and Tibet rather than by China, was yet to manifest itself in Harbin in the 1930s. A rare copy of *Lectures in Occultism*, "read in the esoteric circle of the Rose Cross in 1923 and 1924," by Viacheslav P'iankovich (1881–1935), a blind Harbin occultist and former tsarist colonel from the Ufa gentry, was bound by its first owner together with two publications by followers of the émigré painter and mysticist Nicholas Roerich (1874–1947), who stayed in Harbin in 1934.[133] P'iankovich, who lived in Harbin after 1919, founded his small occult circle in 1922. In the other Rosicrucian circle, which began meeting in Budberg's cellar slightly later (but may well have been inspired by P'iankovich's example), he was derided.

We know this from letters to Roerich and his wife Helena (1879–1955) by Petr A. Chistiakov (1879–1965), a department head at the CER, who was a colleague and friend of Roerich's Harbin-based brother Vladimir (1882–1951). Before switching to Roerich's teaching, Chistiakov had joined Budberg's Rosicrucians. He described going through a ritual ceremony of initiation "in some underground space hastily turned into 'the temple' of the order." According to Chistiakov, as of April 1923, the Rosicrucian circle in Budberg's house had about ten members. Presenting itself as "the Philomatic circle" to the uninitiated, it venerated Master (or Mahatma) Morya, a sage it shared with Roerich's theosophical system of Living Ethics, also known as Agni Yoga. The circle was dominated by "a German from Ufa" known for his talents of magnetism and ability to determine "the character, past and present of any person." Chistiakov also reported that the financial crisis and loss of security of the Russians, in a city rapidly falling under the sway of Chinese power and inundated by new refugees from beyond the Soviet border, have encouraged the recent turn to mysticism: "never before has Harbin had such a number of fortune tellers, palm readers, astrologists and plain charlatans."[134]

The spiritual and the supernatural attracted Budberg even in their manifestations among Orthodox Russians. In the first half of the 1920s, as the Bolsheviks intensified their assault on religion, demolishing churches and executing priests, Russia was swept by a wave of popular revival marked by the "reawakening of icons." This form of religious fervour did not skip Harbin. Budberg's midwife Sophia Antonova, one of the people closest to him and to his wife, as many references in Budberg's *Memoirs* attest, believed in these miracles and discussed them with him. As Antonova told Harbin's Archbishop Mefodii (1856–1931), the doctor, a Lutheran who had become an enthusiast of occult practices, did not deny that icons could glow again. However, in conversations with her he "explained this phenomenon by the concentration of magnetism and electricity in the atmosphere after the earthquake in Japan [in September 1923] and the tension of magnetic energy in humans due to a special condition of the sun." She asked Budberg whether he would believe in the reawakening of icons if this happened with her own. And indeed, on 14 December, an icon that Antonova had inherited from her great-grandfather began to glow. After three days, all of the saints' faces on it had brightened. Regarding this as an act of providence, Antonova offered a *moleben* (prayer of thanksgiving) in front of the icon in her apartment. According to her account, as quoted by Mefodii in a short book he published in Harbin in 1925, *On the Omen of the Reawakening of Holy Icons*, Budberg participated in this rite, "praying as if he were a Russian Orthodox."[135]

For years, he lunched daily at Antonova's apartment, on 65 Politseiskaia Street, which was near both the Harbin prison and his hospital. In a letter he wrote in 1923, he acknowledged that he was now in close contact with "Orthodox spirituality."[136] His own influence over his Russian nurse was significant. Antonova's daughter Nadezhda, who was born in Nagasaki in 1902, graduated from the Harbin Commercial School with a gold medal in 1920 and, with Budberg's help, went to study in Germany, receiving her physician's diploma from the University of Munich in 1928.[137] Back in China in 1930, she followed in her mother's and Baron Budberg's footsteps by opening a maternity clinic in Shanghai. Her mother also moved to Shanghai; when she died there in 1934, the *North China Herald* wrote that Antonova had worked for Baron Budberg ever since being decorated for her medical service in Manchuria in the Russo-Japanese War.[138] In Shanghai in 1946, Nadezhda M. Antonoff married an Australian and changed her name to Nadine Beal. A worldly medical professional, soon after immigrating to the United States in 1950 she nonetheless reported, just as her mother had done in Harbin in the 1920s, that an old Russian icon she had brought with her suddenly shone again.[139]

By 1924, Budberg was a firm believer in magnetism. In 1910 he had written that the Chinese recognized such forces in the natural world as "electricity, magnetism, somnambulism and many others," so his espousal of these beliefs was a synthesis of the China he imagined and the tenets of his occult movement.[140] After his daughter had suffered for weeks from headaches and an eye disease (for which she was examined by Dr Göldner, the colleague from Dorpat), he was afraid to apply his magnetic powers to her, for he considered them too strong. Instead, Luis Bubnik cured the girl with his powers, which derived from his standing as Old Master in the Rosicrucian Order. As Budberg wrote to his sister, his best friend could heal the most difficult cases of epilepsy in only five minutes.[141] In an earlier letter, Budberg had told Antoinette that Bubnik, "the old occultist," was completely devoted to him and lived for his sake.[142] Bubnik was also financially savvy; he had promised Budberg to improve his situation, which had become rather strained, by renting out a plot Budberg owned on Kommercheskaia (Commercial) Street (now Xi erdao jie), which ran parallel to Kavkazskaia. Lacking a passport, Budberg was refused a bank loan, but he was far from destitute: his other properties included a house he had bought in Harbin's New Town, as well as land and houses at the CER's Yimianpo station southeast of the city (now part of Shangzhi, a town under the Harbin city jurisdiction).[143]

He was still receiving patients and was proud that women of many nationalities came to the morning consultation hours at his clinic. He told his sister that since opening his first practice in Harbin, he had never charged his Asian patients, so as to increase trust in Western medicine. In 1925, Budberg wrote that "out of eight to nine hundred

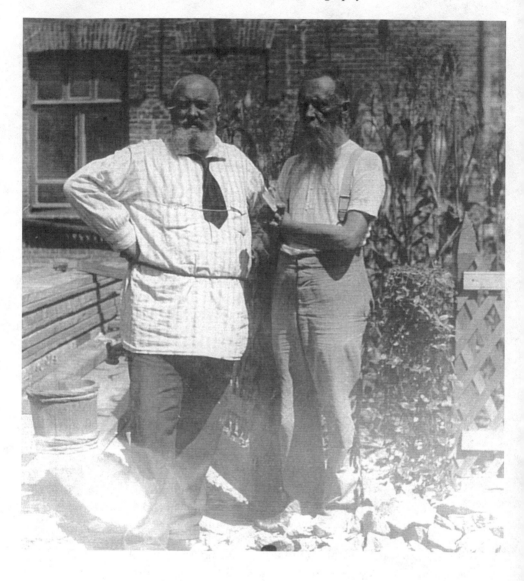

6.1. Roger Budberg (right) and Luis Bubnik. Courtyard of the Budberg house
on Kavkazskaia Street. Photograph in Popoff family album.

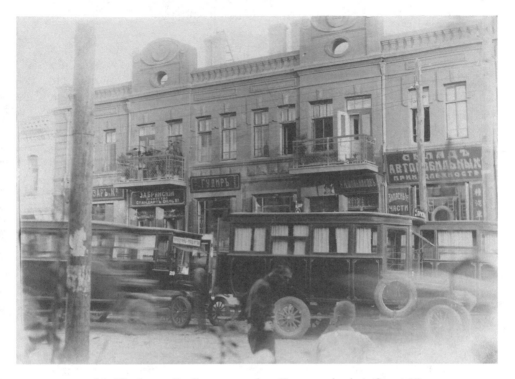

6.2. The house Budberg owned on Kommercheskaia Street 15,
Harbin. Photograph (1925) in Köhler family album, Germany.

Budberg rented out this house, located on a parallel street to the one where he lived.
In August 1925 he sent this photograph, signed and inscribed on the back, to his sister
Cecile (or perhaps Cecile received it via their sister Antoinette). It affords a glimpse into
Harbin of that time and its manifold international connections. The signboards may be
identified with the help of Harbin's Yellow Pages (*Ves' Kharbin na 1926 god*, 153–4): from
left to right, these are E.V. Frezar and Co., which represented the Ford Motor Company
in Harbin; E.A. Brianskii, which represented Standard Oil (Frezar, on the left, and Gudir,
on the right, were both Brianskii's agents); next door, there was A.A. Shil'nikov's "Depot
of Automobile Parts." The bus from Pristan' to Modiagou (in Chinese: Daoli to Majiagou)
is just passing by on this busy street (the bus schedules are also listed in *Ves' Kharbin*,
64); through the bus window, a child can be seen seated on a bench, perhaps waiting for
another bus to arrive. Two men at the front of the picture are engaged in conversation, not
noticing the photographer behind them.

Another photograph of this building in 1933 (in the Popoff family album) showed it
topped by the huge sign of Dunlop Rubber Co.; Standard Oil was still there, now flanked
by International Harvester and by an agent Sakamoto, who represented the recently
founded Japanese manufacturer of auto parts, Bridgestone; Shil'nikov's depot advertised
parts for Cadillac, Chandler, Dodge and other automobiles. Like Budberg's home on
Kavkazskaia Street, this house has been demolished.

European physicians in Harbin" (an exaggeration, since Harbin had around two hundred Russian physicians at that time), he was "the only one with such a large clientele of Japanese and Chinese patients." He also mentioned treating Manchus, Russians, and Tatars.[144] One Jewish patient's young son still remembered him eighty years later.[145]

In January 1925, Budberg submitted to the Chinese court his medical opinion on the life-threatening condition of Harbin's best-known political prisoner. The previous October the Chinese police had arrested the deposed manager of the railway, Ostroumov, along with other prominent figures in the Russian administration, including the last tsarist governor of Amur province and most recently the head of the CER Land Department, Nikolai L. Gondatti (1860–1946). All were charged with corruption. Declining further responsibility for Ostroumov's health if he remained in prison, in February Budberg obtained the court's permission to gather a medical concilium in order to examine Ostroumov in his cell. The Russian press by then described the engineer as dying.[146] Budberg may have overstated the case to get Ostroumov released. (His daughter Olga had visited Budberg, and he recorded her exclamation at seeing his house: "How different everything is, here at your place, so unlike other people's!")[147] Once Ostroumov was free, Budberg looked upon his release as a personal achievement, and his references to this Russian official show surprising admiration.[148] He also went on issuing public challenges and protests, for which he had become famous among some and notorious among others. In July, he denounced the appalling conditions in the prison hospital, arguing that the best wards there had been taken over by the employees for their apartments.[149]

In August, the press reported on "Doctor Budberg's adventure": having gone out boating on the Sungari with some friends, he was ambushed by armed Chinese bandits. But as soon as the *khunkhuzy* were addressed in Chinese and realized Doctor Bu ("Bu daifu") was in the boat, they let the party continue unharmed on its way.[150] Ten days after that river excursion, Budberg warned readers of the daily *Rupor* (The Mouthpiece) about the quality of water in the Sungari, claiming under the heading "What Are We Drinking?" that it was radioactive and dangerous even for bathing.[151]

On 26 August, Ostroumov, Gondatti, and other former high officials of the railway during its now bygone "White Russian" era were finally released from the Chinese prison. In celebration, some members of the distressed Russian community staged a ceremonial presentation of icons. At that very moment, before being presented to Gondatti, a time-worn icon of St Vladimir Mother of God suddenly began to glow in the hands of *hegumenia* Rufina (1872–1937), a recent refugee from

Vladivostok. Archbishop Mefodii personally served the *moleben* in front of the restored icon and made this manifestation of divine agency the climax of the book he was then writing on holy omens. Rufina, in turn, founded the Convent of St Vladimir – the first Russian Orthodox convent in Harbin – to commemorate the event.[152]

Meanwhile, on 25 July an ill-famed criminal by the name Ivan Kornilov was executed by garrotting after spending five years (interrupted by a daring escape) in the Harbin prison.[153] The *North China Herald* described Kornilov as a bandit "found guilty of several murders" and "a ruthless robber who made free use of his revolver." The newspaper also called him the first foreigner executed in China "since the Canton factory days in the early eighteenth century." It reported that "the priest and the prison doctor, Dr. Baron Budberg, only arrived after the execution was over. Korniloff's body was examined by Dr Budberg who wrote out a death certificate."[154] Amid the growing frustration of Harbin Russians over the treatment of their prisoners, Budberg must have been unhappy with the way his Chinese superiors had used him as rubber stamp. Nevertheless, in September he examined the medical condition of two Russians, arrested at the Suifenhe railway station in possession of "infernal-machines and a large quantity of pyroxylin." The Chinese authorities suspected them of being Soviet agents, sent to blow up Zhang Zuolin's arsenal in Mukden.[155]

On 1 November 1925, however, Budberg was fired from his position as prison doctor after fifteen years of work, the last four of which had been in Chinese service.[156] The Harbin reporter of the *North China Herald* now wrote that Budberg, "most popular among the Chinese," was being held responsible for letting another condemned foreigner, a Turk, commit suicide before his scheduled execution. He commented that "Dr. Budberg does a great deal of good to the poor and needy, whom he treats free of charge, his hospital receiving no outside support. He also has a lucrative private practice, thanks to his long residence here, where his name is equally known to foreigners and Chinese."[157] Budberg himself told the Russian press that he had been surprised by his discharge, which had come with no explanation. He emphasized how dangerous his job was; a few years previously, he had narrowly avoided death during the escape of some prisoners. He pointed out to Harbin's *Zaria* that he was the "only European here decorated by the high order of the Double Dragon."[158]

The Chinese chief prosecutor, speaking to *Zaria* via an interpreter, justified Budberg's dismissal by his habit of issuing medicine to prisoners without consulting the prison administration.[159] The following day, Budberg rejected the accusation that he had provided the Turk with the poison that allowed him to escape Chinese justice. He wished to make clear that studying both law and medicine in Dorpat qualified him as a legal medical expert notwithstanding his other specialization in midwifery. There appeared to be no bitterness this time: he thanked the Harbin court and his colleagues for their past confidence and friendly attitude.[160]

He did not give up on the idea of marrying again until his final rupture with General Munthe in autumn 1925. After becoming a widower he had imagined that his union of souls with his deceased wife was strong enough to sustain "a bond of three" with a new spouse; he also felt that his daughter needed to be raised by a woman.[161] In June 1925 he was still musing that, although "his dear wife had been Chinese," he would like Munthe to find him now a Manchu woman.[162] In January 1926, however, a newspaper carried a riposte to an unidentified interview Budberg had given on mixed Russian-Chinese marriages. He had rejected them completely, since he believed that no European could attain the advanced culture and "spiritual beauty" of the Chinese and that "no European woman could ever measure up to the elevated and beauteous image of the Chinese woman." He presented his own case as an exception, describing himself as "a learned biologist, who has devoted [his] entire life to science and has never cut off [his] ties to nature." The reaction in Harbin's Communist daily *Molva* (Common Talk) was milder than might be expected: the pseudonymous author caustically reiterated the epithets "respected doctor" and "respected Baron" but pointed out that by claiming that European women were inferior to the Chinese, Budberg had offended his own mother. The author avowed that all his female kin were European, yet this gave him no right to deprecate women of other nations. In a curious example of what a Harbin Russian might say on these charged issues in 1926, he concluded that "every race presents both positive and negative exemplars of humanity." It was common knowledge, he added, that the baron's daughter from his Chinese marriage was being given a European (German) education, rather than being educated "at some pension in Fujiadian."[163]

Soon after turning fifty, he began calling himself an old man; the *Memoirs* contained many references to his "old age," and he had felt near death both in prison and after his release in 1919. By early February 1926, Budberg's health had deteriorated so sharply that the Russian press informed readers about this. He suffered from bronchial asthma and was being treated by five Harbin doctors; Boris Ostroumov visited him at home.[164] Budberg's last short book, *On Life* (O zhizni), appeared in June. Once he realized that the Munthes were not going to publish his writings, he decided to do so on his own. *On Life* contained many ideas originally expressed in his letters to Munthe and to Antoinette (and surely in other correspondence no longer extant). Its tone was very different from that of the *Memoirs*: Budberg finally seemed ready to address not the Russian courts but Russian readers in Harbin, the public he had so often criticized in his writings, but with whom he had never conducted a dialogue. Now he wanted to convey his admiration for China and explain it to them.

He spoke in the manner of a wise old man, a doctor of medicine who in the book's subtitle called himself an *akusher*, a male midwife. This was no mere modesty, as he wished to be seen as a person who by his profession stood near the mysteries of birth and life. He called on readers to abandon Western individualism and the illusion of the independent self. As an alternative, he presented a harmonious merging with Life, Nature, and the whole of Creation, ideals that he found in the Eastern traditions but considered consonant with Christianity.[165] *On Life*, supported by evidence from physics, biology, and psychology, also hinted at the turn of his thought toward the occult. *Molva* reviewed this book favourably in a brief notice despite running a violent attack against Budberg's anti-Soviet publisher on the same page.[166] It was the first of several issues of "conversations" with readers, which he was preparing: two other titles, announced as forthcoming on the back cover of *On Life*, were never to appear after the author's death and his publisher's relocation to Shanghai.[167]

Baron Budberg died in Harbin in the early morning hours of 25 August 1926. Though he had hardly left the city for some years, on the previous day he had returned from a two-month journey to Halun-Arshan (Chinese: A'ershan), a hot spring in Inner Mongolia about 700 kilometres northwest of Harbin; he must have gone by rail to Hailar and then spent four days travelling south on horseback to reach it. In accordance with the Mongol belief in the curative powers of snakes, reptiles shared the waters of the resort with humans. Despite the difficulties presented by the journey, by the 1920s Halun-Arshan had become popular with Russians, as several Harbin-published guides attest.[168] The day before he died, so the *Russkoe slovo* (The Russian Word) reported, Budberg said that bathing in the springs had done him good. As was his usual custom, on the last day of his life he went for a boat ride on the Sungari. "He collapsed at home; Dr Raupach, who was called to his bed, stayed until midnight. In the morning, the house manager Mr Buznik [*sic*; misprint for Bubnik], who spent the night in the neighbouring room, heard coughing; the baron was already dead of cardiac arrest."[169] He was fifty-nine years old. The newspaper referred to his "great popularity among the Chinese population."

The next letter that Antoinette Raczynski received from Harbin was from Luis Bubnik. Writing in German on her brother's stationery, he informed her of the baron's death and his own appointment as guardian of the orphaned child in accordance with Budberg's will.[170] Once the news from Harbin had reached the Baltic, standard death notices with summaries of Budberg's biography appeared in Estonian and German in Tartu (formerly Dorpat), and thereafter in the German-language press in Latvia.[171] Then in November, the main German newspapers in Riga and Tallinn published a lengthy eulogy by Oskar Grosberg, the writer who had reviewed Budberg's *Memoirs* the previous year. Grosberg drew on Russian press reports from Harbin to focus on the rare cross-cultural nature of the funeral in that city. According to him, members of all of Harbin's communities expressed their love and gratitude at Baron Budberg's grave. They acknowledged Budberg as a righteous and upright person known to "half of East Asia," and as a protector of the Chinese in Harbin, who had saved "tens of thousands" through his battle with the Black Death and had been decorated by the Empress of China; a man, so the Baltic obituarist concluded, "in whom the old Baltic tradition blended harmoniously with the views of Confucius."[172]

Between Harbin and Riga some confusion and embellishment had taken place, and even the opportunity to berate the Russians was not missed. Yet this eulogy reflected the way Roger Budberg saw himself, the role he believed he performed in Harbin, and the persona he had fashioned through his writings – probably just how he wanted to be remembered. The description of the funeral is confirmed by other sources. The *Russkoe slovo* too reported that both Orthodox and Buddhist clergymen took part in the funeral procession, which stretched for nearly two city blocks. Wreaths had been sent from the German and Danish consuls, the German club, and personally from Luis Bubnik and Boris Ostroumov. A brass band performed Chopin's funeral march as the cortège made its way to the Lutheran church, where a service was held. From there, the cortège continued to the baron's final resting place at the New Cemetery.[173]

Next to this report, *Russkoe slovo* placed four private statements of grief, offering condolences to Budberg's daughter: by Luis Bubnik, who was "devastated by the loss of his best friend"; by Bubnik's partner, Aleksandra G. Zamesova; by Dr Stepan Migdisov (who had succeeded Budberg as medical inspector of the police in the Special Region of the Eastern Provinces) jointly with nurse Sophia Antonova and feldsher Mikhail Popov (who had worked with Budberg for many years in the emergency room of the Harbin police station); and by doctors and nurses of the First Settlement Hospital (Pervaia poselkovaia bol'nitsa), formerly the Hospital of the Harbin Congregation of Sister of Mercy of the Red Cross.[174]

The reports on Budberg's death and funeral in *Molva* presented him as an important scholar of Manchuria (*kraeved*) and as a "biologist" who had published widely both in Harbin and abroad. The paper also called him a veteran of Harbin (*starozhil*), a term that by this time differentiated between recent émigrés and pre-revolutionary settlers; Budberg "had lived here for twenty years, spoke fluent Chinese and studied Buddhist philosophy." Unlike *Russkoe slovo*, *Molva* commented that "the doctor had many friends among both the Russian and the Chinese populations." It mentioned a memorial service (the word *panikhida* is suggestive of the Russian Orthodox ritual), for which numerous friends had gathered in the Budberg apartment on the day of his death. On the following day, the funeral procession was so long that it caused traffic on Kitaiskaia Street to halt for the duration:

> The deceased was buried by the Russian Orthodox, Chinese and Lutheran clergy. Chinese Buddhist monks [*bonzy*] walked in front of the coffin with all the paraphernalia of the Chinese funerary ritual, followed by three Chinese and Russian music orchestras. Behind the hearse walked the Lutheran and Orthodox clergymen and a large crowd of mourners. The latter included representatives of the medical and legal circles, as well as important Russian and Chinese public officials.[175]

We do not know whether Budberg left instructions regarding his funeral. With priests of three religions officiating, it was an apt final statement to the divided city of Harbin, which he had made his own. Budberg's death may have elicited grief among the Russians in Harbin as well as the Chinese, although only Russian- and German-language descriptions of his funeral are available. An article in *Zaria* on the previous day called Baron Budberg a uniquely gifted yet profoundly lonely person and a romantic mystic, whose eccentricity almost brought about his ruin when the spy scare spread in Harbin during the World War. The writer predicted that "a great multitude of simple Chinese folk from Harbin and Fujiadian would surely accompany their 'Doctor Bu' to his grave with the warmest feelings of love and gratitude."[176]

For many Russians in Harbin in 1926, Budberg's name and title evoked a disappearing tradition (the old imperial aristocracy, the beginnings of the Russian colonization in Manchuria) that was already being missed. Previously, his "going native" had earned him the image of an eccentric German-turned-Chink. Budberg rarely acknowledged that, however peculiar his convictions appeared to most people in Russian society, they were not uniformly rejected or ridiculed: beginning with the generals, who allowed him to immerse himself in the study of China instead of serving with the army before the Russo-Japanese War was over, he had always been able to earn respect and friends among Russians. That his wholehearted adoption of China also won him the trust and affection of Harbin's ordinary Chinese population is a claim for which we have largely had to rely on his own words. He had written about having "lost in [his] heart almost any touch with European society" and having formed instead, together with his Chinese wife, a "natural and warm bond with the Chinese people ... whose nicknames for us, 'sister' and 'elder brother', never left our consciousness."[177] Visiting temples during the plague in 1921, he felt that they were holy places for him, too, for he had long been united with the Chinese people in his soul.[178]

One of the letters to his sister in 1922 included a remarkable account of spending his evenings in the company of humble Chinese fishermen and boatmen, who lived on the left bank of the Sungari opposite the city. He helped them build a small temple in memory of the cholera epidemic, which had raged there while he was in prison in 1919. He wrote that he was learning much from these simple people, whom he called his friends.[179] Did any of them cross the river to walk in Doctor Bu's funeral procession? Did his Chinese "boy," a domestic often mentioned in his last letters (unnamed, but described as an amateur photographer) join it? And what had happened to Sjödro, who may have been his "adopted son"? How many people of Harbin, all gone now, remembered the German-Russian baron, who loved China, and passed on his story by word of mouth?[180] This memory would have lasted for another generation among Budberg's patients, their children, and the descendants of many other people who knew him, including his Chinese teachers and domestics and, possibly, his wife's relatives.

At the last station of his journey, it was the Lutheran minority in Harbin, consisting of Germans, Latvians, and Estonians, that embraced him as their own.[181] It would have been impossible for Budberg to be interred at the Chinese cemetery, beside the tomb of his wife, if he had wanted it, but we don't know that he did. As the place of the dead is more often determined by their ethnicity and the religion they were born into than by the more complex identities they may have developed while alive, his body was committed to China's soil in the Lutheran section of Harbin's New Cemetery. On 15 September 1926, a notice by Baroness Antoinette Cecilia Budberg-Boenninghausen in *The Russian Word* informed friends and acquaintances of her father that the Lutheran pastor would that day conduct a memorial service at Baron Budberg's grave.[182]

7

Russians and Chinese under Japanese Rule

On the first day of 1927, a seventeen-year-old bride of mixed Chinese and German extraction, who had grown up in Harbin, married her twenty-six-year-old Russian groom in Shenyang (the city then known as Mukden). Nikolai Popov had served in Kolchak's army and was presently a military instructor with the Fengtian Army of Zhang Zuolin. Young Antoinette was the daughter of the Harbin physician Baron Roger Budberg, who died in August 1926. She had a Chinese name as well, Zhong-De-Hua, meaning Chinese-German Flower. Her mother, Li, who had also married in her teens, died when the girl was eleven. In the wedding ceremony on 1 January, the role of father of the bride was filled by a Chinese officer remembered as chief of Zhang Zuolin's headquarters, a General Li, or perhaps Yi.[1] The father of the groom was alive and a former tsarist colonel,[2] but he was not present at the wedding of his son in Manchuria as he had immigrated to Bulgaria (the groom's mother died in Shanghai in 1923). Thus the role of father of the groom was assumed by General Georgii I. Klerzhe (Clerget; 1883–1938), who had also fought under Kolchak and was now chief consultant to Zhang Zuolin. A wedding reception was held in Klerzhe's house.

Russian Soldiers in Warlord Armies

Our only source about that day in Mukden also reports that the witnesses for the bride were Captain Kuroki of the Japanese Imperial Army and an unnamed adjutant to Zhang Zuolin. While the bride's side was represented by Chinese and Japanese military men, the groom's was composed strictly of Russians: the war pilot Colonel Dmitrii A. Kudlaenko (1893–1944), formerly of the Russian General Headquarters, now senior instructor to Zhang Zuolin's air force;[3] General Arkadii P. Slizhikov (1882–1940), formerly Assistant Director of the General

Headquarters Academy after its evacuation from Saint Petersburg to Siberia;[4] the cavalry master (*rotmistr*) Gavriil F. Kulebiakin (1892–1962), instructor of the Manchurian Army's armoured troops;[5] and the engineer Leon I. Korganov (1873–1932), who represented the Cossack *ataman* Grigorii M. Semenov.[6]

The connection to Semenov (1890–1946), who had lived in Dairen (Dalian) under Japanese protection since 1922, was shared by several of these men. "Captain" Kuroki, by his full name Kuroki Chikayochi (1883–1934), had been Semenov's close adviser and his representative in Harbin in 1918 and 1919. With the rank of major, he resigned from the Japanese Imperial Army in 1920 to protest Tokyo's decision to abandon Semenov.[7] General Slizhikov had served in Semenov's army from 1919; General Klerzhe was director of Semenov's headquarters in 1921. The groom himself, Lieutenant Nikolai Popov, or Popoff, would maintain his contacts with Semenov until the 1930s, as attested by correspondence that has survived in his son's archive. The list of wedding guests comes from a late communication from Popoff to Baron Nikolai Budberg (1894–1971), the last genealogist of the Baltic German noble family, into which Popoff had married.[8]

In the 1920s, Russian émigrés like Popoff entered the employ of Chinese warlords, a phenomenon that stunned and embarrassed Western observers in China. Since Russia and China were neighbours, however, beginning in the 1650s, and especially after the Albazin fortress on the Amur fell to a Qing attack in 1685, Cossacks had passed into service in the Qing "Russian Company," which was part of the Bordered Yellow Banner. The Manchu rulers settled the new recruits in Peking, where some people to this day identify themselves as descendants of the "Albazintsy."[9]

Russians served in other Asian states besides China. For a brief period in 1918, Georgii Klerzhe was commander of the Persian Cossack Brigade, which was established in 1878 and remained active until the early 1920s. Chinese and other Asian recruits from within and beyond Russia's borders, such as Buryats and Mongols, joined the Special Manchurian Detachment, which Semenov created to fight the Reds in early 1918. In an attempt to make the enlistment of Asians palatable to supporters of his cause in Europe, Semenov argued that the ethnic composition of his army was intended to shame Russian soldiers into realizing their patriotic duty, and he announced that he believed in healthy competition between nationalities. At the same time, he justified his reliance on Japanese funding by emphasizing his near-native fluency in Buryat, Kalmyk, and Mongolian and by popularizing the image of Japan as a friend of the Russian people despite the legacy of the Russo-Japanese

War.[10] Other White Russian military leaders recruited soldiers in China and its borderlands: most notably, *ataman* Ivan P. Kalmykov (1890–1920), who was arrested and shot by the Chinese authorities after escaping into China; and Baron Roman Ungern-Sternberg, a former deputy of Semenov's, and appointed a lieutenant-general by him, who was captured by the Bolsheviks after being betrayed by members of his Asiatic Division in Mongolia and executed in Novonikolaevsk (present-day Novosibirsk) in 1921. From 1918 to May 1920, China contributed about 4,000 troops to the Allied intervention in Siberia. The Bolsheviks, for their part, drafted Chinese migrants as "volunteers" in Siberia and the Far East and moved them across the enormous country. Their presence among the Red Army forces was remarked on as far west as in Latvia.[11] Shared military life, then, has been a largely neglected aspect of the Russian-Chinese encounter in the twentieth century; an early example was the "Chinese detachment" formed by Tifontai (Ji Fengtai) during the Russo-Japanese War.

Resistance to the Bolshevik Revolution, which had suffered repeated defeats in European Russia, continued longest in Siberia. In January 1920, however, Admiral Kolchak, who had declared himself Supreme Ruler of Russia in Omsk in November 1918, was arrested in Irkutsk and soon afterwards was shot nearby without trial. In March 1920, retreating White Army troops began crossing the border into China at Manzhouli; many more men, about 11,000 by a local Chinese account, escaped into China in November after Japan had withdrawn its support from Semenov, who had declared himself Kolchak's successor and commander of the Far Eastern Army. These troops were disarmed and their weapons added to the arsenals of Manchurian warlords.[12] The last detachments of the White Army that had resisted the Reds in the Russian Far East evacuated in October and November 1922. Most of these men, who were accompanied by their wives and children, would never again set foot on Russian soil except as prisoners of the Soviet Union.

Russian service in the northern arena of Chinese internal warfare began with the defeat of the Fengtian Army by the army of warlord Wu Peifu (1874–1939) in the first Zhili-Fengtian war in 1922. That was also the year that Zhang Zongchang (1881–1932), known as the Dogmeat General, began working with Zhang Zuolin, nicknamed the Old Marshal. As one of his first assignments, Zhang Zongchang took charge of the border-crossing of the remnants of the White armies into Manchuria at Suifenhe and Hunchun in the extreme east of Jilin province, in late October and early November 1922.[13] In 1923, Zhang Zuolin made a first attempt to form a Russian detachment under the command of the veteran cavalry general Mikhail M. Pleshkov (1856–1927). This initial venture was soon called off, but not before Zhang engaged more than three hundred "volunteers" from among former Russian soldiers, hitherto employed in logging.[14] Zhang famously had Russian bodyguards accompany him as he moved about in an armoured car. As is evident from the list of the Popoffs' wedding guests, he used more specialized Russian personnel as aviation experts. These pilots would have reported to the eldest of Zhang Zuolin's many sons, Zhang Xueliang (the Young Marshal), who, promoted to the rank of major-general at twenty-two, was in command of the Fengtian Army's air force two years later. Zhang Zongchang, too, had an air force, a more modest one, commanded by a Chinese pilot said to have been trained in Soviet Moscow.[15]

One should backtrack a few years from 1 January 1927, as well as widen the frame. In the 1920s, that Russian soldiers served Chinese warlords contradicted the hierarchy of races: Western nations maintained their concessions and extraterritorial rights in China, and the idea of white superiority in Asia still had strong defenders. A number of British "adventurers" enlisted in Chinese service, including that of Zhang Zuolin, but they did so as individuals rather than forming military units.[16] The half-Asian composition of the Russian empire did not make it easier for Russians to march to the orders of Chinese commanders. Racial thinking was embedded in the world view of these soldiers, and despite their resentment of other Europeans in the Far East, the educated men (largely, the officers) among them saw themselves as part of the European world.

Beyond the question of whether to serve under Asian commanders, there was a more basic one: why become a soldier in China? As soldiering was these men's profession, one answer was that being impecunious émigrés, they were doing what they knew best, regardless of who employed them or why, and would continue to do so as long as they were being paid. In other words, they were mercenaries, or in the definition some historians have adopted, "soldiers of misfortune."[17] At least one leading figure among the Russian officers is reported to have put it this way. No lesser man than Konstantin P. Nechaev (1883–1946) rejected any ideological motives and even the baggage of "White ideas," stating simply: "We are mercenaries, *Landsknechte*."[18] Nechaev, who had followed the classical trajectory from the First World War to the Civil War, was named a lieutenant-general by Semenov. In 1924, when summoned to head the Russian *otriad* (detachment) that Zhang Zongchang was forming in anticipation of a second Zhili-Fengtian war, he was a coachman in Harbin.[19] Thereafter, he commanded the Russian forces under Zhang until the summer of 1927, and he remains the

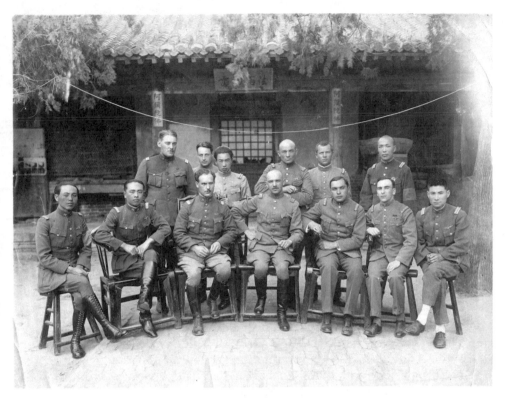

7.1. Russian and Chinese pilots in Mukden. Undated photograph,
courtesy of Olga Bakich.

figure most identified with them. However bluntly he stated his motive
in conversation, money (sporadically paid) was only part of it.

For Nechaev and many of his troops, enlisting with the northern warlords was a way of shifting the battleground of the Russian Civil War
to China and thereby continuing the resistance against the Bolsheviks,
which had ended in failure in Russia itself. Former soldiers of the White
Army were told by their commanders, and may have told themselves,
that the military forces they had joined in China were fighting the Reds.
Wu Peifu, head of the Zhili clique, collaborated with the Chinese Communist Party until early 1923, when he turned against the Communists,
suppressing the strikes they organized.[20] The perception that they were
helping the anti-Communist warlord Zhang Zuolin and his subordinate Zhang Zongchang fight against Wu gave some meaning to the
service of White émigrés. So did fighting against warlord Feng Yuxiang (1882–1948) and the Kuomintang Army of Chiang Kai-shek, which

initially received Soviet aid and military advisers. It became harder to explain operations against Chiang after he broke with the Communists in April 1927.

Nechaev also reportedly argued that participating in warfare in China was a means for Russians to earn the right to establish a permanent Russian detachment in Manchuria; once this detachment was created, it could be "enlarged and used to fight the Bolsheviks."[21] A variant of this reasoning was the expectation that after the Chinese got rid of their own Communists, with the assistance of Russian émigrés, they would help the Russians eradicate Communism in Russia.[22] When in December 1926 the army of Zhang Zongchang prepared for a battle against the Kuomintang, the rival army was identified (e.g., in an order issued by the Zhang headquarters to the Russian troops) with "Red Canton." Their Russian commander reminded the officers and men that "our victory over Bolshevism in China brings this country peace, statehood and culture."[23] Despite such echoes of tsarist imperialism, the only interest that members of the Russian emigration took in the Chinese wars of the 1920s lay in the possibility that they might curb the spread of Communism.

In the orders in Russian that were issued on behalf of the Chinese command, Zhang Zongchang was occasionally called the White Marshal.[24] The Soviets, too, associated the northern Chinese warlords with the White Army, using the term *belokitaitsy* (White Chinese) for the regimes of Zhang Zuolin and Zhang Xueliang. This analogy with *belogvardeitsy* (White Guards) operated on the semantic level to demonize opponents of the Soviet Union in bordering countries, while reflecting no political reality.[25] Curiously, a present-day Russian historian of White émigrés in Chinese service uses *belogvardeitsy* interchangeably with *naemniki* (mercenaries), as if the White Army's struggle had indeed been transferred to Chinese territory.[26]

In the recruitment of Russians to Chinese armies, leadership and personal ties loomed large. The men were attracted to these units by the names of their commanders and by the rank they carried from their past service in the tsarist and White armies. The Chinese command appointed the Russian officers at their former rank and subsequently promoted them. This helped maintain the illusion of continuity from the tsar's army, through the White Army's resistance, to the fighting between warlords in China. It was not insignificant that Zhang Zongchang himself, a native of Shandong who came to Harbin as a young man, could speak Russian and had collaborated with the Russian military during the Russo-Japanese War. Thus, he had worked for Russians before a change in the balance of power enabled him to hire them. As their commander-in-chief for four years, he knew how to earn their respect, for example, by rewarding their leaders and honouring the Russian dead at a cemetery set aside for them in Jinan.[27]

In addition, for young recruits, who may have come to Harbin as children and would have been aged twelve to fifteen in 1918 or 1920, joining an army in China five years later was a way of reliving the battlefield experiences of their fathers' generation in Russia, which had been presented to them in a heroic light. A stream of young "volunteers" flowed into Zhang Zongchang's Russian detachment from Harbin, Shanghai, and other cities. By the spring of 1926, that force had more than 1,500 members despite the heavy casualties it was sustaining at the time.[28] Paradoxically, even as service with the Chinese armies drew young Russians south into China rather than closer to the Russian border, it may have been a way for them to return to Russia in their imagination. Soviet Russia would have had no place for them except in camps and prisons; service under the Chinese amounted to a leap backward in time in that it was an attempt re-create a tsarist military unit. In the troops' daily lives, this imaginary construction was supported by the symbolic language of Russian battle orders, the religious services of Russian Orthodox priests and Muslim clerics (notably, a minority among the volunteers were of Russian Muslim background), and frequent rhetorical evocation of the White Army's ultimate cause, the restoration of the monarchy in Russia.

Yet the fantasy of a tsarist Russian army in 1920s China was often punctured by reality. During the first two months of fighting in 1924, Zhang Zongchang attached a Japanese military company to his Russian detachment. When his army reached Tientsin in November, and consuls in that treaty port protested against the presence of foreign troops in its ranks, Zhang denied having Japanese soldiers and apparently soon dispersed them, but he said that his "Russians" were Chinese of Russian origin.[29] Indeed, members of Zhang's Russian forces were required to take Chinese citizenship.[30] Incongruously for a force consisting mostly of ethnic Russians, an order by Nechaev in January 1926 phrased the New Year wishes as "the liberation of China from the Russian-Bolsheviks, whom we too hate."[31] In December 1926 the Russian commanders held a parade to honour those among their men who had received the Order of St George, the highest military decoration in tsarist Russia. But they also awarded the St George star to Zhang Zongchang and accepted Chinese decorations from him.[32]

There were always Chinese in the higher command of "the Russian detachment," and the enemy against whom the Russian forces were engaged was Chinese as well. In addition, the detachment itself always included Chinese troops, who became the majority in the forces as more

Russians resigned from service.[33] The armoured trains, the most vivid symbol of the Russian intervention in Chinese wars, did draw largely on Russian staff. Still, Chinese commanders were often in charge, which is probably why a Russian major recorded in his diary that he shouted out "Stoi, russkie, mamandi!" – "Hold on, Russians, hold on!" (the last word in Russian-Chinese pidgin) – when attempting to stop one of those trains and board it.[34] When the Chinese troops switched sides, as warlord soldiers frequently did, the Russians became targets for robbery or for extradition (for a reward) to the enemy. Russian soldiers captured by the opposite side after being wounded in battle were in danger of meeting a terrible death by torture and beheading.[35] Trust between the Russians and Chinese serving in the same units seems to have been minimal in these circumstances, and Russian complaints regarding Chinese desertions and poor fighting spirit are ubiquitous in the records, although there is also some evidence suggesting comradeship in battle.[36] Communications with the higher command and among the troops were channelled through interpreters and at a more basic level relied on pidgin. The day-to-day fighting in the Chinese wars constantly brought the Russian soldiers into contact with the Chinese population, both in the countryside and in the cities their armies reached. Entering a village presented an opportunity to rob the peasants (the usual practice of Chinese armies), which Russian soldiers called *fatsai*, "to get lucky," a pidgin calque of the Chinese *facai*.[37] Besides regular fighting, the Russians were sent out on missions against local bandits, the *hong huzi* (redbeards); they also became involved in conflicts and negotiations with members of the sectarian movement called *hong qiang hui*, the Red Spears Society, through which villagers defended themselves from marauding bandits and soldiers alike.[38] The "red" symbolism in these encounters was, however, too coincidental to provide additional motivation.

In the second Zhili-Fengtian war, between 15 September and 24 October 1924, the Russian detachment of Zhang Zongchang's army won a victory in its first battle against Zhili forces in northern Liaoning on 28 September. It then became known and feared for its armoured trains, devised by Colonel Innokentii Kostrov. In November the Russian "army group" was moved south and used in the occupation of Tientsin by the Fengtian Army. By the summer of 1925 the group was stationed in Tai'an and nearby Jinan.[39] It suffered a heavy blow in early November 1925 when Kostrov was killed along with half the staff of the armoured trains he commanded in a clash with the forces of warlord Sun Chuanfang (1885–1935) near Gucheng, a station on the Tientsin-Pukou Railway. In March 1926, Nechaev was severely wounded, losing a leg; he later recovered and resumed his role as commander. Led by an armoured train, the Russian forces entered Peking the same month and celebrated Orthodox Easter there. After the troops returned to the Jinan base in May, an incident demonstrated how easily their commanders could lose their authority: the Russian general who had replaced the convalescing Nechaev was thrown into prison along with another colonel for insubordination to his Chinese superiors. Stripped of their tsarist ranks, both were then sacked "without the right ever to return to Chinese state service." A General Zhao assumed "temporary" charge of the 65th Division, as it was then known.[40]

In July 1926, Chiang Kai-shek launched his Northern Expedition from Guangdong, setting out as a coalition of Nationalist and Communist forces for the unification of China under Kuomintang rule. As the Russian troops moved to the banks of the Yangtze to assist the army of Sun Chuanfang (this warlord, whose troops had killed Colonel Kostrov and many of his comrades the previous year, had meanwhile entered into a coalition with the other northern warlords against Chiang's expedition), they had an indirect encounter with Soviet Russia. The troops detained the Soviet steamship *Memory of Lenin*, which was bound for the port of Hankou. They threw the Communist propaganda materials they found into the river and arrested all on board, including the wife of Chiang's Soviet military adviser, Mikhail Borodin (1884–1951).[41]

Soon afterward, the Russians had to retreat from Nanking along with the army of Zhang Zongchang. As they did so, they sank the *Memory of Lenin* to the bottom of the Yangtze. One of the two Russian armoured trains was abandoned near Nanking, while in March 1927 the other became involved in dramatic fighting against the Kuomintang in the Zhabei quarter of Shanghai. At the end of that battle, the surviving Russians surrendered to the authorities of the International Settlement rather than to the army of Chiang Kai-shek, thereby shedding their provisional "Chinese" identity in favour of a European one.[42]

In September 1927 another detachment of the Russian forces participated in a failed assault by Zhang Zongchang's army on the base of Feng Yuxiang in Kaifeng. They remained behind after the rest of Zhang's army retreated and then surrendered to Feng, eventually spending fourteen months in humiliating captivity.[43] Meanwhile, Zhang was quickly losing ground even in Shandong. In the course of reorganizing his army in January 1928, Zhang disbanded the Russian infantry brigade, and most of the Russians in his service resigned; by April, up to 2,000 of them had left, with about 800 remaining.[44] The last Russian soldiers to serve under Zhang Zongchang switched sides in September 1928, either surrendering to Zhang Xueliang (the Young Marshal) when faced with the prospect of fighting against his Mukden Army, or using the same occasion to pass into Nationalist (Kuomintang) service.[45] The Young Marshal had inherited power in Manchuria after the assassination of his father by the Japanese in June. In late December he signed an alliance with the Nationalist government.

The service of Russian soldiers with Chinese warlords was not simply a story about men. The families of these soldiers often followed them. Thus, an entire Russian community had to be evacuated from Jinan when Zhang Zongchang lost his base there in April 1928.[46] Zhang not only had Russians fighting his battles, but also kept Russian women in what envious observers called his harem. Defeated by the Kuomintang army, Zhang moved to Japan. On a return visit to Jinan in September 1932, he was assassinated on the orders of another warlord.

General Klerzhe, the host of the wedding reception in Mukden in January 1927, had worked for Zhang Zuolin since 1922. He ended his service later in 1927 and moved to Shanghai in 1935. In January 1938 he was taken into Japanese custody in Tientsin, by then conquered territory, and shot as a suspected Soviet spy.[47] Colonel Kudlaenko, however, having been promoted to major-general by his Chinese commanders, made a smooth transition from Zhang Zuolin to Zhang Xueliang and died in China a year before the Soviet invasion. The last to survive was Semenov, whom the Soviets arrested in Dairen after the Japanese defeat in summer 1945 and hanged in Moscow a year later. In the mopping up of former White generals and collaborators with Japan in Manchuria, Nechaev too fell into Soviet hands; he was executed in Chita. Still in 1927, Nikolai Popoff quit his own much less illustrious military career in China and left for Belgium with his wife. He knew some French and had received a visa from the Belgian Consulate in Shanghai to study engineering at the Institut Gramme in Liège.

Little can be discovered today about Antoinette Popoff's short life outside of her father's writings. When she was eleven, she fell dangerously ill with pleurisy.[48] She lost her mother by the end of the same year and then stayed for a while with her Manchu nanny in Hulan.[49] She was often ill in adolescence, too. While her mother lived, "everybody at home spoke Chinese," but her father found a governess from Dorpat to teach her German, and he expressed his "heartfelt wish" that one day his Antoinette should visit her Aunt Antoinette in Poland.[50] Yet he also hoped she would continue the "cultural work" he had begun in China.[51] At thirteen, she had learned to play the piano well enough to give a recital in Harbin; a Russian newspaper published the photograph of the musical prodigy, Baroness Budberg, and her father was proud of her.[52] That same year he decided she would be better off living with the staff of his hospital. She reminded him too much of his deceased wife, and he claimed she was assailed by painful memories whenever she stayed at his house.[53]

Looking now at the photographs in the family album, which she managed to bring out of China, one is tempted to identify her opium-smoking Manchu nanny, and perhaps governess Neiper from Dorpat. Or was it her home tutor Fräulein Krantz, who returned "to her father in Reval" (the German name of Tallinn) in July 1924, travelling to Europe with Janja, Luis Bubnik's daughter, who was about to begin medical studies in Prague?[54] Or again, was it the "lady educator" her father hired after finally giving up the idea of a second marriage, when she was already sixteen?[55] There are also several photographs of Zhong-De-Hua as a young child with her parents, some taken in front of their house, which had a garden with peach and apricot trees that gave out beautiful blossoms in the spring.[56]

Her parents called her Zhong-De-Hua to symbolize the blossom of two cultures, the Chinese and the German, although their own identities were a richer blend than could have fitted into those neat categories. A single letter by her own hand survives: at her father's request, at age fifteen, she wrote to her cousin Joseph Alexander, who was then nine. Father inscribed the address on the envelope, as well as the sender's name, Dschung-dö-hua Antoinette Cécile v. Budberg. She produced two versions of the letter, one in German and the other in classical Chinese. Displaying an exemplary calligraphy, she tried to initiate the boy in Poland into the mysteries of Chinese characters; in the German version, she echoed one of her father's favourite terms by emphasizing the difference between Chinese and European "soul lives" (*Seelenleben*).[57] She signed the Chinese letter Bu Zhong De Hua; the German, Cousine Cäcilie.

While clearly proficient in Chinese, it cannot be known what contacts, if any, she had with Harbin Chinese society. She never attended school, having been educated at home, and she spent her adolescence in her father's venereological hospital in the company of the Bubnik children. She wanted to study medicine in Germany and might have done so had her father lived longer.[58] Sometimes she went bathing in the Sungari.[59] Some hints in Budberg's last letters suggest that by late 1925 he had liquidated his hospital and brought Antoinette back home. Marrying at seventeen, only four months after her father's death, she soon found herself in emigration in another country, speaking Russian with her husband, who called her Zhunda.

Nikolai Popoff (1900–1964) apparently married her by entering into collusion with her guardian Luis Bubnik, who initially planned to marry the baron's orphaned daughter to his own son.[60] Popoff lived off his wife's inheritance, buying a house in Liège in 1928 and making two trips back to Manchuria (in 1933 and again in 1937) in order to recover and sell the last Budberg properties in Harbin. In Liège, Antoinette often counted the beads of her rosary. Her father advocated the use of a rosary with precisely 116 beads in his book *On Life*, as he advised readers to combine this form of religious devotion, common to Buddhists and Catholics, with the autosuggestion method of the French psychotherapist Émile Coué (1857–1926).[61] Zhong-De-Hua's rosary, which she must have brought with her from China, would have offered her a measure of spiritual comfort in the midst of a disorienting relocation. Her aunt and godmother Antoinette Raczynski visited her in Belgium in 1930, bringing along her sons.[62] Antoinette Cecilia Popoff also had children, two boys and a girl. Her youngest child was only three years old when she died of tuberculosis on 6 March 1934, her twenty-fifth birthday.

A Manchukuo Minority

In the China that Zhong-De-Hua left, to spend her last seven years among the Russian émigrés in Belgium, rapid changes in the political situation affected the standing of the Russians who remained in Manchuria. After the loss of extraterritoriality and consular protection in 1920, Russians had become the first Westerners subject to Chinese law. Their sense of humiliation was exacerbated by multiple abuses perpetrated on them by the warlord administration of Manchuria. In the second half of the 1920s, Russians got used to working for the Chinese: even the former all-powerful manager of the CER, Boris Ostroumov, who remained in Harbin after his release from a Chinese prison, accepted an offer of employment from General Wu Junsheng to help build a new railway, between Hulan and Hailun, from 1925 to 1928.[63] Few Russians in Manchuria were prepared to take Chinese nationalism seriously, as its local representatives were the ex-*khunkhuz* Zhang Zuolin and (after he and Wu Junsheng were blown up in their train in 1928) his son Zhang Xueliang. The transformation from a colonizing elite to a defenceless minority was difficult to stomach.

Suddenly, in the first days of 1932, it seemed as if all the pent-up frustration broke loose. A Russian child was caught stealing a cookie from a Chinese pastry shop; the owner called the police, who gave the eight-year-old a beating and took him to prison. The uproar was such that it made the pages of the *New York Times*: "With five Russian civilians killed, twenty-two wounded and the Chinese casualties unknown,

Harbin's streets are barricaded and tension and clamor reign, recalling the wild days of the French Revolution." The newspaper's reporter noted with surprise that "the Russian mobs, mainly armed with sticks and stones" had won a victory "over the Chinese armed police and soldiers," and that, for the first time, Reds and Whites had joined forces against a common enemy. They then demanded an international commission to investigate "the frightful oppression under which the Russians have been existing under Chinese rule."[64] No such commission was created, and once the Russian crowd that had thronged Kitaiskaia Street dispersed, following an apology from the city governor, so did the coalition of "Reds and Whites." Clearly siding with the Russians and recounting recent kidnappings by bandits and the "squeeze" practised by the city police, the reporter told readers in New York that "Chinese pretensions to maintenance of law and order in Harbin are a mockery." The irony of the situation was that within a month the Chinese administration would have to relinquish its powers.

Many Russians (Whites rather than Reds) welcomed the change of political authority when Japan's army marched into Harbin on 5 February. They imagined that Japan might treat them better, and they saw Japan's takeover of Manchuria as deliverance from the threat of forced repatriation, which had hung in the air during the years when Soviet influence on the CER had grown. Some even fantasized that Japan, which had previously intervened in the Russian Civil War, might again support White plans to overthrow the Bolshevik regime.[65]

By the late summer, however, everyone's attention had been diverted to the forces of nature. A flood of the Sungari on 7 August left Fujiadian submerged. Two days later, the water covering the streets of Pristan' was 2 metres deep, turning the inhabitants into hobby photographers eager to capture the surreal sight of rowboats floating on Kitaiskaia as if along a Venetian canal.[66] Besides all the levity, thousands of Chinese, Russians, Koreans, and Japanese in Harbin, and in many towns and villages affected by the flood, had to leave their homes for refugee camps hastily created by the new Japanese regime, which invested heavily in relief operations as an opportunity to bolster its legitimacy. When the Japanese responded to cases of cholera from the polluted water by imposing inoculation of the entire population, the wife of the US Consul in Harbin, in an article she wrote for *National Geographic Magazine* (richly illustrated with her husband's photographs of flooded Harbin), mentioned that the Chinese "flocked to the Russian doctors," preferring to be vaccinated by them rather than by the Japanese police.[67] This vignette contrasts with Chinese fears of the Russian medical staff during the earlier plague epidemics but accords with available data on the steady increase in the number of visits by Chinese patients to the Russian-run Harbin Day Clinic in the 1920s.[68] It suggests that by 1932 some Harbin Chinese trusted their Russian neighbours more than the Japanese newcomers; we may recall Xiao Hong's turning to such a Russian clinic that year. There is evidence that Harbin Russians, too, occasionally turned for medical care to Chinese and Japanese physicians, who advertised in the Russian press; and that Russians adopted Chinese methods of medical self-help, such as "opium, ginseng, boiled water, massage and acupuncture."[69]

Notwithstanding any political developments, the religious narrative affirming Russian influence over the Chinese continued unabated. When Bishop Nestor (1885–1962), a leading figure of the Russian Orthodox Church in Harbin, visited Belgrade in 1933, he opened a series of lectures on Russian life in the Far East by reporting that "in the unanimous opinion of the natives," the previous year's flood had been retribution for the banning of the annual procession on the ice of the Sungari in January. He also retold the stories about how Chinese love for St Nicholas protected his icon from removal by the Soviets in 1924, and about the Chinese man who believed he had been rescued by St Nicholas after begging for his help during a storm on the river; even now, that person kept coming to the Harbin railway station to light candles in front of his saviour's icon. So great was the appeal of Russian religion that a small icon of St Nicholas was worshipped in a Daoist (formerly shamanist) monastery run by Manchu priests on the mountain Mao'ershan east of Ashihe, while at Yakeshi station of the CER in Inner Mongolia, the Chinese beseeched Harbin Russian clerics to pray for rain and were grateful for the miraculous effect of the Orthodox ritual. In Easter, Nestor added, the splendour of Harbin churches drew in "Jews, the heathen Japanese and Chinese, and others of non-Russian faith."[70]

In 1931, a remarkable educational map was published in Harbin – one of the most impressive maps of China produced in the twentieth century. Called "Pictographic map of the people and topography of the Chinese Republic," it easily covered a wall.[71] Each region of China was shown on it through drawings of the local landscape, the typical animals, and the representative nationality: so, for example, looking at Xinjiang one saw blue mountains, mosques, yaks, and Uighurs in their traditional clothing. The author of the map, identified as "John Diakoff," was Ivan A. D'iakov (1881–1969), a Russian Orientalist and traveller across Asia and the Pacific, who arrived in Harbin from Hong Kong in 1931. His map hinted to Chinese schoolchildren that there were still Russians in Manchuria: Harbin was represented by the figure of

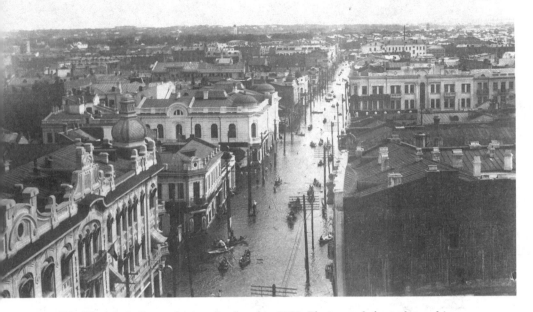

7.2. Kitaiskaia Street during the flood in 1932. Photograph from the archive of Vladimir Ablamskii, courtesy of the A.M. Sibiriakov Museum of Irkutsk City History.

a uniformed railway employee not evidently belonging to any ethnic group, but wearing a moustache and a peaked cap. He looked rather similar to another, bearded man, drawn along the CER track between Hailar and Manzhouli – surely a Cossack (see figure 7.3). The railway uniform and peaked cap seem to have remained symbols of "the Russians": a chart of the nationalities of Manchukuo, published in 1939, showed a similarly dressed miniscule Russian standing for the smallest national group in Manchukuo, with only 70,000 people. The following groups, all depicted as men in traditional clothing and headgear, were Japanese with 500,000, Koreans with 750,000, Manchus and Mongols estimated at 800,000 each, and the towering figure of a Han Chinese representing the absolute majority of 32 million.[72]

In 1942, D'iakov was appointed inspector of schools in Trekhrech'e, a sparsely settled part of Hulunbuir (Russian: Barga) in Inner Mongolia,

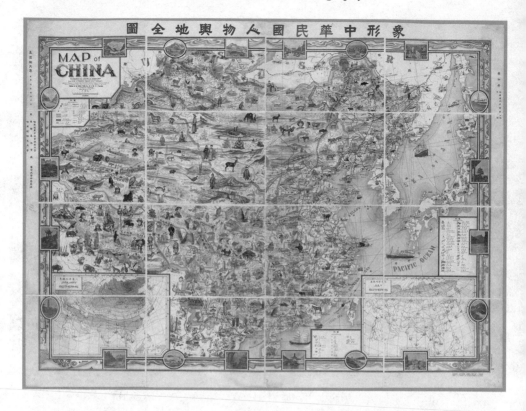

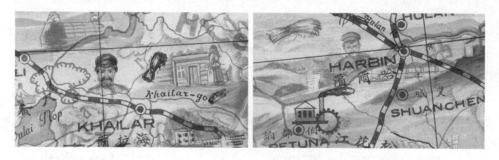

7.3. Map of China, compiled by John A. Diakoff (with excerpts
showing Harbin and Hailar). The David Rumsey Map Collection,
davidrumsey.com.

where Cossacks and Old Believers were still the largest group (around 9,000).[73] He barely survived his attempt to criticize Japanese education policy, and described his arrest and torture in a memoir ironically titled *Amaterasu* – after the founding goddess of Japan, whom Russian schoolchildren of Manchukuo were ordered to worship after 1940.[74] Being a denunciation of Japanese rule, this memoir is similar to a better-known book published in English in 1943 as *"Bushido": The Anatomy of Terror*, although D'iakov's is the more reliable of the two since the author of *"Bushido"* had never lived in China.[75]

The journal *Aziia*, only four issues of which appeared in Harbin, in April and May 1932, was subservient to the Japanese but also expressed the world view of its editor, the aforementioned Vsevolod N. Ivanov. In the inaugural issue, under the title "The Russian Colony in Manchuria," Ivanov wrote that Manchuria offered the perfect conditions for "preserving the Russian national face [while maintaining] the rights of a national minority." This was so, he explained, because the danger of assimilation, a major threat to Russian youth in exile, did not pertain in northeastern China. Ivanov did not notice the contradiction between fearing assimilation, on the one hand, and calling for Russians to acknowledge their "common destiny" with Japan, on the other.[76] Even more incongruous, considering that Ivanov had been a Soviet citizen since 1931, was his next long essay on "Europe, Asia and Eurasia." In it he criticized Europe for imposing its values on the rest of the world, and condemned the Soviet Union for appropriating European rationalism and materialism, while praising the Catholic and the Russian Orthodox churches, along with fascism and National Socialism, for being loyal to tradition. He expressed gushing admiration for Asia, which had given the world literature and philosophy of unsurpassed heights and had developed a splendid model of monarchy. Unlike new China, which was forgetting its tradition due to Western influence, Japan represented the harmonious fusion of Asian heritage and European know-how; under its leadership, a new Eurasian civilization was being created, which opened possibilities to forge a new Russia.[77]

The Russians of Manchukuo were pressed by the propaganda machine of the new puppet state to play a small part in a supposed paradise of nations. Determined to enhance the lie of inter-racial harmony among "five nations" in the new country, the Japanese invited Russian authors to write on the "natural place of Russia in Asia" and the special affinity of Russia to Japan – or rather to Nippon, as the Japanese censors insisted the Russian press now call it. Statements in this spirit could hardly be taken at face value when reiterated by the Cossack generals (all of them connected with the *ataman* Semenov), whom the Japanese authorities placed at the head of BREM, the Bureau for the Affairs of Russian Emigrants in the Manchurian Empire, created in 1934. The Cossacks underwent a transformation in status in the 1930s from a military caste at the margins of Russian society to its main public voice, self-styled protector and symbol of the continuing struggle against Red Russia.[78] A reflection of the prominence of military men among the émigrés who reached Harbin after the October Revolution, this development left liberal-minded Russians uneasy about having retrograde and often openly anti-Semitic *atamans* as the supposed leaders of their community along with the Russian fascists, whom the Japanese also promoted. Jews and the many other minorities of the former Russian empire, whom the Japanese counted together with the ethnic Russians and likewise aimed to bring under the leadership of BREM, made every effort to obtain recognition for their separate ethnic and religious organizations. When such recognition was granted, it came at the cost of collaboration with Manchukuo.

In 1934 the eccentric and charismatic painter and occultist Nicholas Roerich arrived in Harbin with his family in preparation for an American-funded expedition through Manchuria and Mongolia. A vocal supporter of Manchukuo,[79] Roerich imagined creating another new country. His Great Plan envisioned the coming of a Messiah, or a World Leader, to unite the Russians in Manchuria and the nations of Asia; together they would identify Him with Buddha Maitreya, the Buddha of the Future. A new Mongolian–Siberian nation, with a capital called Zvenigorod, would then be founded in the Altai Mountains.[80] Roerich had left Russia in 1918 and lived in the United States from 1920 to 1923 before embarking on a five-year expedition through India, Turkestan, Mongolia, and the Tibetan Plateau, where he searched for the kingdom of Shambala.[81] According to Roerich's cosmology, the white race had evolved as the fifth incarnation of beings formerly inhabiting the moon, Venus, and the lost continents of Lemuria and Atlantis.[82]

During his time in Harbin, Roerich, whose own Baltic German roots were in Courland, contributed an introduction to the first collection of stories by Al'fred Kheidok (Alfrēds Heidoks, 1892–1990), a Russian writer of Latvian origin.[83] Like so many who met Roerich, Kheidok accepted him as a lifelong spiritual teacher. In the stories in his collection, *The Stars of Manchuria*, Russian émigré protagonists left their Western enclave to roam in the unknown and threatening Chinese countryside, or the Mongol desert. There, in a dilapidated temple, they encountered a beautiful Manchu princess, or a Buddhist monk who bestowed upon them the gift of immortality. Kheidok's stories were regularly published in the Harbin press and must have responded to a need felt by his reading public.[84] Another admirer of Roerich was Vsevolod Ivanov.[85] People who found any of this convincing would have drawn some comfort from seeing a dethroned emperor reinstated as the nominal ruler of Manchukuo. Monarchism and mystical Orientalism were often part of the same ideological package – as they had been for Baron Budberg and in different ways also for Roerich and Baron Ungern.[86]

Yet few people could be made to believe in the prospect of living on under the Japanese occupation. Many Harbin Russians, those who could afford to leave, went elsewhere after 1932. The most popular destination came to be Shanghai, which succeeded Harbin as the centre of the Russian emigration in China during the 1930s. The nun Rufina transferred her entire convent of St Vladimir from Harbin to Shanghai; after her death there, it moved on to the United States. Many Chinese escaped from Manchukuo as well, among them young intellectuals such as the writers Xiao Hong and Xiao Jun, a couple who went to Qingdao in June 1934 and then to Shanghai. There, the following year, Xiao Jun published his anti-Japanese novel, *A Village in August*. Xiao Hong experienced the desecration of her native land by a brutal occupier with more pain than was felt by the Russians who departed for Shanghai at that time. She expressed these feelings at the end of her memoir, *Market Street*.[87] A popular song from 1936 about leaving Manchuria during the occupation, "My Home Is on the Songhua River in the Northeast," is still taught in Chinese schools.[88]

To an extent, what has since become known about the horrors of the Japanese occupation, and the brutality that mainly targeted the Chinese population, has coloured our view of the years between 1932 and 1945 in hues too uniformly black.[89] Russian life continued in Harbin under Japanese rule, although survival strategies became increasingly difficult to reconcile with personal integrity as far as contact with the state was concerned.[90] While some prospered, many fell into desperate hardship. In 1932 a newly arrived American resident claimed that Harbin had "the unsavory reputation of having more beggars than any other city of China, and most of them are Russians"; her lightweight report went on to describe these Russian beggars in some detail. The same author's insistence that "uncountable numbers of [Russian] girls ... work in cabarets" was, even if overblown, not completely far-fetched.[91]

The Soviet decision to sell the CER to Manchukuo in 1935 was no act of decolonization, for the railway passed to the Manchurian empire rather than to China. Rather, it marked the symbolic end of the tsarist colonial enterprise, launched in 1896. One Russian, born in Manchuria as the son of a railway stationmaster, was shocked to hear of the sale in

the United States, where he had moved already in 1922. In a late interview, he said: "My Russia was Manchuria. There was a predominance
of Russians in that particular area. Of course, we came in contact with
the Chinese, but anyway we considered it to be part of Russia, and
when the Russians sold the Chinese Eastern Railway to the Japanese,
I had actually angry tears in my eyes – they had sold my land, the land
where I was born."[92]

The plight of Soviet citizens who did not repatriate in 1935, instead
remaining in Manchuria, was especially difficult and became even more
so after Japan entered the Second World War by attacking the US Pacific
Fleet in Pearl Harbor on 7 December 1941. Most of them surrendered their
Soviet passports. With many Russian residents having left, whether for
Soviet Russia or for Shanghai, the demographic data for the early 1940s
yield an average of about 30,000 Russians in Harbin – slightly under half
the Russian presence in Manchuria as a whole. The total Harbin population, overwhelmingly Han Chinese, numbered around 700,000 and was
rapidly growing.[93] A tiny group of people who could not be easily classified as belonging to either "the Russians" or "the Chinese" were the
descendants of mixed couples. These people were categorized as "Eur-
asians," a now discarded English term, which, outside Manchuria, was
applied especially to the children of Western fathers and Chinese mothers; "half-castes" (the corresponding Russian word, *polukrovki*, literally
means half-blood); or "those of 'mixed' or 'confused' blood" (*hunxue'r*,
as they were referred to in Chinese then and still today). This was the
kind of person Zhong-De-Hua (Antoinette Budberg) was: one of the first
such children in Harbin, she surely had been called these names behind
her back or to her face before leaving China.

This group received special attention in the 1930s, and not simply
because its members were growing up. Once Manchuria fell under Japanese control, and when, after 1937, China also lost its sovereignty on
territory within the Great Wall, some Chinese began treating the émigré
Russians as the weaker side against which to assert their own national
superiority. Thus, in Chinese short fiction, Russians were often portrayed as beggars, prostitutes, and petty criminals. The dual identity of
those of "mixed blood" was perceived as most dangerous in wartime.
Seen from this perspective, being Chinese *and* Russian (or Chinese
and German, "Zhong-De," as Li and Budberg named their daughter)
was not an option; everyone needed to possess a specific racial and
national affiliation. Because the hybridity of the descendants of mixed
couples – living symbols of the cross-ethnic encounter – was physical
and unerasable, they could never satisfy these demands and become
purely Chinese, try as they might.[94]

Poverty did force Russians to work with or for the Chinese. It also made more Russian women in Harbin marry Chinese men beginning in the 1920s, even if this led to their being ostracized by other Russians. Chinese society was sceptical about these women, too: it was widely presumed that "a Western woman could not make a proper Chinese wife."[95] Mao Hong, telling readers in 1929 that not a few of his male friends had married Russians, was quick to comment that those wives never learned good Chinese, adapted to Chinese ways, or shed the habit of looking down on Chinese people.[96] Liu Jingyan confirmed that mixed marriages were common enough, although he had never heard of a Chinese woman marrying a Russian. He added that the Chinese husbands always learned Russian but not vice versa; the "mixed" children became proficient in both languages and interpreted for their parents, a spectacle amusing to behold.[97] Writing in 1931, Owen Lattimore accurately distinguished between perceptions of intermarriage on the two sides: while the two communities, in his opinion, despised each other, Russians viewed intermarriage with the Chinese as a mark of failure, whereas the Chinese considered marrying a Russian a mark of success and upward mobility.[98]

Marriages between Russian (most often Cossack) women and Chinese men in the border areas of Manchuria, the vicinity of Heihe and the villages of the former Trekhrech'e region in Inner Mongolia, have left a small community of descendants, which today makes up the officially recognized "Russian minority" in China. In Harbin and elsewhere in Manchukuo, Russian-Japanese couples also came together, usually to separate after the evacuation of the Japanese army and civilians in 1945.

In 1938, when the Harbin State Medical Institute opened its doors, aspiring Russian students found themselves in circumstances similar to those of the young Chinese who in the 1920s had taken Russian classes to enter the Polytechnic or the Faculty of Law. Japanese was by then being taught in Russian schools, but getting through medical school in that language was obviously a huge challenge. Four Russian students of the first intake graduated as physicians; among the second intake (which proved the last to complete their studies, as the institute closed down in 1945), only two Russians did so.[99] Others learned Japanese in order to survive: homeless in Harbin in 1939, a fourteen-year-old Changchun-born Russian youth, whose parents had been killed by Chinese bandits, enrolled in free Japanese courses offered by the South Manchuria Railway because it offered scholarships, the prospect of a translator's diploma, and a guaranteed job. He graduated and found work as a translator and interpreter, first for the railway and then for a large Russian firm. In 1945, the Soviet army, having initially used his language skills, sent him to the Gulag under allegations of spying for Japan.[100] Among the Russian military men who served Chinese warlords in the 1920s, some later entered the service of Manchukuo, either in the Russian detachments of the Japanese "mountain and forest police," created in 1935, or in the Asano Detachment (so named after its Japanese commander), a Russian unit of the Manchukuo army cloaked in secrecy and rumour, which was formed in 1938 and trained to infiltrate Soviet territory.[101] These forms of adaptation to the exigencies of Japanese rule would be classified as collaboration or treason by the Soviet Union and the Republic of China after 1945, with dire consequences for both Russians and Chinese who had worked with the Manchukuo administration.

In the winter of 1942, another writer for *National Geographic* reported that the Harbin Russians "scorned to adopt Chinese ways, or Japanese." The "largest white population under yellow rule," they were allegedly "too proud to work for yellow masters." The fear of losing racial prestige in Asia was clearly shared by the author, who had seen "smart White Russian girls" employed as waitresses in cars of the North Manchurian Railway (the former CER); he could have added that despite the racial pride he ascribed to them, they also worked as hostesses in Japanese bars.[102] Noticing Russians alongside the Chinese as "sleigh-taxi men," transporting passengers on the ice across the Sungari in vehicles that boasted Russian names, such as "Tamara" and "Bystryi" (Speedy), the same reporter included a group photograph of them. Russian memoirists of Harbin hardly wrote about Russian poverty, crime, or prostitution.[103] But they often described this exotic form of transport, famous for its amusing name in pidgin: *tolkai-tolkai*. In their recollections, the sleigh taxis were always driven by Chinese.

Beginning in 1943, all émigrés in Manchukuo were ordered to wear pins with their name and number. In response to protests against these "dog numbers," the Japanese had the badges for émigré Russians decorated with the colours of the tsarist flag (the bearer's number appeared on the reverse side). Soviet citizens had to wear Red Star pins.[104] A former professor at Harbin's Faculty of Law, Georgii K. Guins (1887–1971), who joined his sons in San Francisco in 1941, wrote in *The Russian Review* about the people he had known for twenty years. "The Russians in Manchukuo," he stated, "live in an environment of strange culture, strange customs and a strange, difficult language. All in all, their complete assimilation in Manchukuo would seem to be highly improbable." Located "at the very border of their native country but [knowing] that they cannot return there," they "feel their estrangement from the motherland as painfully as, perhaps, nowhere else in the world."

Nevertheless, "the final expulsion of the Russians from Manchuria would be a great injustice, and a loss for Russia." Guins concluded by recalling an opinion that "was met with enthusiasm" when it circulated in Harbin: the "best solution" would be if, "at some future time," Harbin was "proclaimed an international city."[105]

The Red Army in Harbin

When the Soviet army entered Manchuria in August 1945, the Communist poet Petr S. Komarov (1911–1949) accompanied it as a war correspondent. His cycle of poems, "A Manchurian Notebook," included in his collection *Under the Skies of Asia* (1947), helped earn him a posthumous Stalin Prize, Third Class.[106] Written in conformity with the assignment Komarov had received, these poems presented warfare in Manchuria just as the Soviet regime wished it to be interpreted.[107] The opening poem, "9 August 1945," resolutely positioned the current attack on Japan as retaliation for Japanese intervention in the Civil War in Siberia. This idea was restated in the following poems along with another historical throwback, as the poet described the Soviet Russian army returning to the battlefields of the Russo-Japanese War. The title of the poem, "Na sopkakh Man'chzhurii" (On Manchuria Hills), evoked a famous waltz from that time, and in the last lines of the closing poem, "3 September 1945," a Russian sailor was once again on watch in Port Arthur.

Everywhere the Soviet troops passed, the local inhabitants were grateful to them, so Komarov reported. The Russians had come as liberators restoring freedom and dignity to the Manchurians and their country, Manchuria (this recurrent idea of Komarov's was an echo of Manchukuo propaganda and would have surprised Chinese readers). As the intended Soviet readers of "Manchurian Notebook" turned the pages, they accompanied the poet from border villages and small towns to Ninguta and Mudanjiang, where Komarov heard Chinese children thank the Red Army soldiers with the pidgin "shango!" for treating them to a meal. Then the poet and reader reached Harbin, with a poem (the longest of the cycle) under that title.

Here, for the first time, they met Russians, who, however, were very strange. It was as if they lived in a different time from that of the author, the reader, and the Soviet soldiers. They wore old tsarist uniforms, "the relics of lost centuries." They rode in stagecoaches and rickshaws (the poet had failed to notice Harbin's automobiles and buses) and vegetated in decadent boredom. Yet even they could not help but be moved by the triumphant march of the glorious army of new Russia, their own flesh and blood, through the streets of their city now liberated from oppressive Japanese rule. The poet was excited too, confessing in another poem, "Evening on the Sungari," that he could not put out of mind "the girls singing the Russian 'Katyusha'" by the riverbank.

The second part of Komarov's "Harbin" poem was an almost accurate description. The majority of Harbin Russians were thrilled to see the victorious Soviet army. Ever since the German invasion of Russia in June 1941, most Russian émigrés worldwide had been prepared to set aside old scores by supporting the Soviet Union's defence of the motherland in a just war against the Nazis. In Harbin, some did more than cheer the parade of Soviet soldiers in front of St Nicholas Cathedral: in August 1945, while Soviet citizens were being swiftly arrested by the Japanese, some émigrés formed partisan units to fight Japan and assist the Soviet invasion; others, who had escaped execution for suspected treason by the Japanese, defected from the Russian detachments of the Japanese army. Still others formed self-defence units around rural Russian settlements in Manchuria, or using their familiarity with the city assisted Soviet intelligence in taking over Harbin. In such acts, patriotism combined with hope of erasing the record of past service in the White Army or the Manchukuo military. These expectations proved illusory. After Japan's capitulation on 14 August and the completion of the Soviet takeover of Manchuria by the end of the month, the émigré assistants of the Red Army in the Manchurian operation were mopped up and deported to Gulag camps.[108]

For a brief moment, Russians and Chinese in Harbin were united by a common interest as perhaps never before: while the former initially identified with "their own" army, most of the latter (with the exception of collaborators) were glad to see the defeat of Japan. Within a year, Harbin's 100,000 Japanese had been evacuated from the city, where by then they made up about one sixth of the population. No sooner had Japan's capitulation been announced than their property was looted by the city's Russians and Chinese.[109] Among the Japanese civilian settlers in Manchuria as a whole, there were numerous collective suicides by families who despaired of finding their way out of China; about 5,000 abandoned Japanese children became "war orphans."[110] More than 600,000 soldiers of the Kwantung Army became prisoners of war in camps in the Russian Far East, where they were put to hard labour.[111] Meanwhile, in August 1945, Chinese Communist units joined the Soviet forces in Manchuria in battles against the rapidly retreating Japanese. As the Chinese Communist Party fought to seize central power from the Nationalists, Manchuria became a periphery from which it could hope to advance toward decisive victory with Soviet support. Such support had to be clandestine, since on 14 August the Soviet Union had signed a friendship treaty with Nationalist China, promising that it would not interfere in Chinese politics. Nevertheless, that same month the Soviets allowed the Chinese Communist Party to establish its northeastern headquarters in Harbin.[112]

Among the ordinary Chinese population, joy upon seeing the end of Japanese occupation was soon mixed with fear of their Russian liberators. Although contact between Soviet soldiers and the local inhabitants was limited, reports of looting and rape spread across Manchuria. Such acts in China never came close to reaching the level of those associated with the victorious Soviet army in Germany. They did, however, repress the euphoria of liberation, reawakening old stigmas and rumours about the Russians.[113] For the Chinese, lasting political terror was to begin once the Chinese Communists replaced the Russians after less than a year, staging another liberation (*jiefang*) of their own as they took over Harbin in late April 1946.[114]

The Soviet period in Harbin proved most difficult for the local Russians – those who had not gone to Shanghai after 1932, but had lived through Manchukuo. Only the Soviet citizens among them found relative security in 1945, after long years of Japanese harassment. Indeed, in November, when the Soviet Union urged all Russians in Manchuria to apply for Soviet passports (a call extended to all Russians in China in January 1946), 31,730 applications were received by a committee established to consider them in Harbin. A total of 29,571 passports were issued, including 7,269 that were renewed.[115] The few young people who had studied Chinese found employment opportunities with the new authorities; after the Soviet departure, they would participate in the early reconstruction efforts under the People's Republic.[116] But whatever their legal status, Soviet or émigré, Harbin Russians were entirely at the mercy of the occupiers. They became targets for plunder and sexual assault by the representatives of Soviet power.[117]

The hunting down by Smersh, the Red Army counter-intelligence agency, of former White officers, actual and suspected collaborators with the Japanese, "class enemies," and all other persons who could be charged with anti-Soviet positions, ruined thousands of lives. The abbreviation Smersh stood for "Death to Spies," but people just said "Smert'" (Death) instead.[118] This ordeal would have made the advent of Chinese control of Manchuria in 1946 a true liberation for the survivors. Yet the complexity of the situation lay in the fact that the same people felt so strong a need to identify with their former country that they overcame their fears to approach the soldiers with questions about life in the new Russia. The Red Army soldiers were no less curious about the old Russia they found in Harbin, and some of them spent their free time in the CER library, or in the Orthodox churches. In one extraordinary case, a soldier took on himself to provide (from Japanese goods confiscated by the Soviets) for the ailing and destitute wife and sixteen-year-old son of a man whom Smersh had just arrested and deported to his death in the Soviet camps. Homesick and confused, because the encounter with Russian Harbin challenged the world view in which he had been brought up, all this soldier wanted was their hospitality, the woman's stories of "old Russia," and the chance to read the boy's uncensored history textbooks.[119] Many Russian girls in Harbin willingly took up love affairs with Soviet soldiers in the autumn and cold winter of 1945, and some gave birth to "trophy" children the following year. Even people who had been humiliated and assaulted applied for Soviet citizenship – whether they intended to repatriate or not, possession of these papers was now necessary for employment and survival.[120]

8

Kharbintsy and *Ha'erbin ren*

This book began with an encounter between sojourners. However, one of the two parties to that encounter in the newly founded city in Manchuria eventually left it, while the other stayed. It is now time to address the outcome and legacy of the contact between the Russian and Chinese societies in Harbin.

Kharbintsy

Most Russians coming to Manchuria before 1917 were imperialists by definition rather than by persuasion. The raison d'être of the Chinese Eastern Railway was economic. The idea of annexing Manchuria was never far from the minds of Russian statesmen in the capital and was periodically revived until the Revolution. But the sense of mission of Harbin's pioneers did not feed on dreams of conquest, nor was it markedly coloured by an imperialist ideology.[1] However determined they were to extend the Russian way of life into the new and unfamiliar country, mainly, the *man'chzhurtsy* ("Manchurians") were pursuing opportunities they felt life in Russia could not offer.[2] As assimilation into China was unthinkable, they maintained close links with the bordering Russian Far East while regarding Manchuria as merely a temporary abode. Early on, critical voices within Russian Harbin were warning compatriots that they needed to familiarize themselves with China; trade in Manchuria would only succeed, they argued, if Russians knew how the Chinese lived and what merchandise they required.[3] Nonetheless, a recurrent motif in writings by and about the first generation of Harbin's Russians is the word *polustanok*, literally a small railway station, but used metaphorically in the sense of a way station on life's journey. The mentality it denoted was passed on to children who, born in China, had been taught that they were growing up in a land they were fated to leave.

One Russian author, writing around 1912, found "no permanent population" in Harbin. "Who will call Harbin his motherland [*rodina*]? Who knows to whom this North Manchurian trading centre will belong in ten years' time?"[4] Two years earlier, the local journalist Nikolai P. Shteinfel'd had attempted to counter precisely such sentiments, both within Harbin and among outside observers of the Russian colony, when he wrote that the traders who settled in Harbin after the Russo-Japanese War no longer belonged to the earlier, rootless and profiteering kind, who had only wanted to make a quick profit and depart: rather, "they had set up their lives ... with the clear intention later to celebrate their twenty-fifth, as well as all successive anniversaries in Harbin or in other Russian towns of the railway zone, stipulating in their wills that their children should bury them in hospitable China, and carry on their fathers' work."[5]

The flood of newcomers to Harbin after the October Revolution turned it into a city of émigrés. The masses of refugees reminded Harbin's veteran settlers that they, too, no longer had a country. The Bolshevik government's decision to strip all Russians abroad of their citizenship confirmed this. Only proximity to the Russian border and Harbin's active role in the White Army's resistance kept alive the illusion of possible return, just as moving on to Shanghai or Tientsin symbolized a more irrevocable separation from Russia. The inner divisions within Harbin Russian society, which grew sharper during the 1920s, undermined the notion of a community. The term *man'chzhurtsy* was hardly used by that time. The only definition that united the Russians was *kharbintsy* (Harbinites). It was similar to the term Shanghailanders, used by the British and Americans in Shanghai, in that it excluded the Chinese (Shanghai's Chinese called themselves Shanghainese or *Szahaenin*, the Wu dialect pronunciation of *Shanghai ren*). The Mukden agreement on joint Soviet-Chinese management of the CER in 1924, under which émigrés lost their jobs on the railway, divided Harbin's Russians even further.

In 1928 a Soviet musician on a tour to the "emigrants' swamp" of Harbin saw a city "distinctly divided into four quarters, which had absolutely nothing in common": the Soviet-dominated Zhelsob, so named after the massive Railway Assembly building in Nangang; the bubbling commercial centre of town, Pristan'; the wholly Chinese Fujiadian; and the "White Russians' quarter," Modiagou (previously mentioned as an out-of-town settlement and the location of a racecourse, Majiagou was home to a large Russian population by the 1920s).[6] A former resident recalled no less than five distinct categories of Harbin Russians around this time: former subjects of tsarist Russia, settled in Harbin before the

Revolution; Soviet citizens delegated for work on the railway; veteran Harbinites and recent arrivals in the city, who had applied for Soviet citizenship to keep their jobs; members of the same group who had opted for Chinese citizenship; and stateless refugees. The "genuine" Soviets became known as *sovy* or *sovki* (literally, owls and dustpans, nicknames that were not limited to Harbin); the reluctant new Soviets as "radishes" (Red on the outside, White on the inside); the newly created Chinese subjects as *kity* (short for *kitaitsy*, "Chinese"); and the applicants for Soviet passports, who only got receipts (*kvitantsii*) in lieu of the passports until the time their requests were approved in Moscow, as *kvity*, short for *kvitpoddannye* ("receipt subjects") – a list that does not exhaust the sardonic depths of émigré black humour.[7]

Beyond the basic division between "us" (Europeans) and "them" (Asians), Harbin Russians did not necessarily consider themselves united by their roots in the former Russian empire. Despite some inevitable contacts, including intimate relationships between Soviets and émigrés, these groups were often ready to fight each other. Soviet youth joined so-called Otmol detachments (short for *Otriady molodezhi*), the nearest they could get to membership in the Komsomol, and fought with émigrés in Harbin's streets. The émigrés fought back by establishing a paramilitary "Musketeers' Union" in 1924 (this later became a monarchist party, which grew in strength in the 1930s). Assaults on Jews by Russian fascists after the establishment of Manchukuo led to the formation of Jewish self-defence squads.[8]

The fragmentation of Harbin Russian identity proceeded along with the loss of Russian privileges in Manchuria as administrative and judicial power passed over to the Chinese. Briefly in the mid-1920s, some members of the second generation of Harbin Russians, reconciled by that point to a long-term sojourn in China, were willing to accept the notion of professional assimilation (as distinct from cultural). Young people, mostly under twenty, enrolled in the two-year "Courses of the Chinese language, preparatory for service on the Chinese Eastern Railway," which the Society of Russian Orientalists began offering in April 1924. Demand for the courses in their first year of operation was twice as high as the number of students they could admit.[9] But the mere thought of having to master Chinese struck the mass of émigré youth, especially the recent refugees from Soviet Russia, as dauntingly unreal. This requirement radically limited the prospects for adapting to China at a time when young Russians were becoming part of their host societies in Europe and the United States. The Japanese occupation in 1932 demonstrated to Russians the uncertainty of their life in China; then the Soviet Union's sale of the CER to Japan in 1935 precipitated the first wave of return migration. Olga Bakich, the Harbin-born historian of the city, writes:

> China, a reluctant host country, had little effect on most Harbin Russians. A small number learned Chinese for professional reasons; some could communicate on everyday topics. But the majority knew next to nothing about Chinese history and culture. Intermarriages and friendships were rare. Most Russians, who generally had lived in Harbin for several decades or were even born there, maintained an entirely insular and Russian way of life. Though very few understood or loved China, their stepmother, many continued vainly loving and yearning for Mother Russia. As for China, the Russian presence was too small and too brief to bear any significant influence.[10]

This is true as generalizations go. Patriotism was taken for granted – as it still overwhelmingly is in contemporary Russia and China – and every person needed "a motherland." Some people could develop an emotional connection to more than one country, a disposition that made others suspicious of them, but attachment to none was inconceivable. These sentiments are distant from the guarded apprehension toward overarching political entities such as nations and states that is typical of attitudes in the liberal West today.[11] A certain sense of belonging to Manchuria (rather than to China) derived from the belief in Russia's modernizing contribution to the region through the railway and the founding of Harbin. In addition, colourful tales about Zheltuga, a gold mine in which Russian and Chinese gold miners worked alongside each other in the far north of Manchuria during the 1880s, circulated orally in Harbin until as late as the 1930s, offering an early example of peaceful cooperation between the nations. The story of Zheltuga was included in a textbook of Oriental Studies and taught at the Harbin Commercial School.[12] The annual ceremonies commemorating the defence of Harbin from the Boxers justified Russian presence in the city by giving it historical depth; they also united Russian residents by reminding them of the perils of life among the Chinese.

The professional and amateur archaeologists of the Society for the Study of the Manchurian Region, who organized expeditions to acquaint Harbinites with the unknown country that lay beyond the Russian city, identified some of the ruins they discovered there as abandoned Russian forts.[13] There was little general interest in the society's work and consequently in the efforts of its associates to date Russian settlement on the Chinese side of the Amur to as early as the seventeenth century. The common perception in Harbin was that the city had been an insignificant village prior to the Russian arrival and that it took the Russian-built railway to bring Chinese migrants to Harbin and the underpopulated parts of Manchuria. These opinions were not unfounded and indeed are being restated by local Chinese historians bent on celebrating Harbin as the conduit of modernity and progress to the northeast.[14] In their time, they flattered Russian self-esteem and buttressed assumptions about Russia's superiority in Asia.[15] A grade three Chinese-language textbook used in the Commercial School in or about 1912 reportedly contained these sentences: "Harbin is located in Jilin province. Before the construction of the railway this place was a large swamp."[16] A survey of Russian education along the CER line in 1922 opened with the image of the railway as a vehicle of Russian culture "in a completely barren and half-wild country" and never mentioned the presence of Chinese; it concluded by calling Harbin "a marvellous oasis" of Russianness after the Revolution.[17] In 1925, the director of the Polytechnic celebrated the railway's transformation of northern Manchuria (previously, "a wild and almost unpopulated country") in near identical terms, although, unlike the author of the earlier survey, he emphasized that the present "blossoming" of the region was the product of Russian-Chinese collaboration.[18]

In February 1929 the Chinese authorities closed down the Society for the Study of the Manchurian Region and took over its museum (renamed the Museum of Northern Manchuria, and later subordinated to a research institute in Changchun under Japanese rule, it is presently the Museum of Heilongjiang Province). Russian enthusiasts then created a Club of Natural Science and Geography, which lasted from 1929 until 1946 under the aegis of the Young Men's Christian Association in Harbin. In 1920 the YMCA opened the doors of its new three-storey building in Nangang; it housed sophisticated sports facilities and a large library. After 1925, Russian émigrés, alienated by the Sovietization of CER schools, preferred to send their children to the YMCA gymnasium. By the early 1930s the YMCA was offering education in Russian to pupils of all nations (including Chinese) from kindergarten to college level, with youth clubs and sections for chess and philately, among other things.[19] Between 1926 and 1933 it also hosted Russian Harbin's best-known poetry society, the "Churaevka." For émigrés, the YMCA's main attractions were the English classes it offered and its affiliation with the United States; the latter suggested that the YMCA was a potential bridge to America. The first *Annual of the Club of Natural Science and Geography of the YMCA* surveyed an impressive range of research on the geology, biology, zoology, geography, economy, anthropology, archaeology, and paleontology of northern Manchuria. It provided a list of scholars recently engaged in such work, including Russians and a number of visiting Europeans. On that list of thirty-nine, there were two women's names, two Chinese names, and one Japanese. It concluded, unusually, with a reference to Manchuria as "our country."[20]

Harbin's Club of Natural Science and Geography was shut down by the Soviets along with the YMCA. In March 1946 it was succeeded by a Society of Naturalists and Ethnographers, which made it known that reorganization had not affected its aims: "to unite persons working in Manchuria in the fields of the natural sciences, ethnography and other issues relating to the study of the local region." It had a membership of 141 (as of 1 July 1949), only one of whom was Chinese.[21]

The previous generation of sinologists had graduated from the Oriental Institute in Vladivostok and other institutions in Russia. But younger scholars had been initiated into research on China in Harbin. A number of them participated in the Society of Naturalists and Ethnographers – the last Russian organization in Harbin, disbanded by the Chinese Communist authorities in 1955. They included the aforementioned Professor of Chinese at Berkeley, Peter A. Boodberg; the Oriental librarian of Berlin University, Wolfgang Seuberlich (1906–1985); the son of a Transbaikal Cossack leader (a prime minister in the White government of *ataman* Semenov), who became a Soviet scholar of ancient nomadic peoples in China, Vsevolod S. Taskin (1917–1995); the Latvian sinologist and Japanologist Edgars Katajs (1923–2019);[22] the authority on Dunhuang manuscripts and the heritage of the Silk Road, Leonid I. Chuguevskii (1926–2000); the historian of late imperial China, later the main figure in Russian Harbin studies, Georgii V. Melikhov (1930–2019); and Svetlana Rimsky-Korsakoff (b. 1931; later known as Vieta Dyer), a grand-niece of the famous Russian composer, who, having graduated from Peking University, taught Chinese in the Department of Oriental Studies of Australian National University and published research on the Dungans, a Chinese Muslim minority in Kazakhstan and Kyrgyzstan.[23] Beyond academia, some Harbinites served as interpreters: Vladimir I. Storozhev (1907–1992) worked at the UN Secretariat in New York; likewise fluent in Chinese and Japanese, Georgii G. Permiakov (1917–2005) accompanied the deposed emperor Puyi during his postwar internment in the Russian Far East and at the international tribunal in Tokyo; Věra Sýkorová (b. 1931), the daughter of a Czech father and a Russian mother, was an interpreter from Chinese for the Czechoslovak government. The scholarly and mystical dimensions of the exploration of Manchuria became linked for ethnologist Vladimir S. Starikov (1919–1987), who, like the writer Kheidok, was inspired by meeting Nicholas Roerich as a youth in Harbin in 1934; he later taught at Peking University.[24]

Taskin, Permiakov, Katajs, Chuguevskii, Melikhov, and Starikov all repatriated to the Soviet Union, as did Ippolit Baranov, with whom some of them had studied. In Israel, the Vladivostok-born journalist Emmanuel Pratt (Pirutinskii, 1921–2015), who had lived in Harbin, Mukden, Tientsin, and Shanghai, compiled the only Chinese-Hebrew dictionary to date; and Harbin-educated sinologist Iurii K. Grause (1917–1999) produced Hebrew translations of Tang poetry, as well as the *Daodejing* (*The Book of Laozi*) and *The Book of Changes*.[25]

In the winter of 1933, the painter Antonin I. Sungurov (1894–1976), a Harbin resident from 1920 to 1934, exhibited more than one hundred paintings of Chinese people and cityscapes, including views of Fujiadian, Ashihe, and villages in Manchuria. He was described at the time as "painter-sinologist" (although he admitted to not knowing Chinese) and as "the first master of the brush in Harbin to turn his talent toward the systematic study of local Chinese life." Sungurov soon relocated to Tientsin and in 1940 repatriated to the Soviet Union.[26] When the painter Mikhail M. Lobanov (1891–about 1970) lived in Harbin, between 1931 and 1954, he also painted cityscapes, which included Chinese temples next to Russian churches. Then he immigrated again, this time to Brazil. As he prepared to settle in São Paulo, he displayed portraits of Chinese and Korean types and a painting titled "Sungari," which he considered his strongest work: it depicted *tolkai-tolkai* sleighs with their Chinese drivers on the frozen river.[27]

In March 1941, BREM organized a joint exhibition of Russian and Japanese painters at the Railway Assembly (Zhelsob). In December of that and the following year, the Club of Natural Science and Geography at the YMCA hosted exhibitions by Russian painters on the natural history and daily life of Manchuria.[28] Such exhibitions served the purposes of Manchukuo propaganda. Nonetheless, artists, whom no language barrier prevented from responding to the new landscape of China, and who after all were expected to paint what they saw around them, were freer than writers and poets of the demands of nostalgia for Russia. Some of them taught in Harbin, and although most of their students were Russian, they influenced a number of emerging Chinese watercolour painters.[29]

Russian musicians in Harbin were apparently uninterested in the kind of fusion between the Chinese and Western traditions that a nephew of General Khorvat's wife Camilla, the composer Aleksandr N. Cherepnin (Alexander Tcherepnin, 1899–1977), produced when teaching in Shanghai in the mid-1930s.[30] They did have Chinese students and through them made an impact on musical culture in Harbin, which has been the subject of a separate study.[31] Western music was also consumed popularly as a status symbol: in the later 1930s and '40s, Russians and other Westerners in Harbin were hired to play at the weddings and funerals of well-to-do Chinese.[32]

The outstanding poet of the Russian emigration, Valerii Pereleshin (1913–1992), learned Chinese as a law student in Harbin. After moving to Peking in 1939 and Shanghai in 1943, and resettling in Brazil in 1953, he published his Russian translations of the ancient Chinese classics, the *Daodejing* and the poem *Li Sao* ("Encountering Sorrow"), in the 1970s. China was a central theme in Pereleshin's own poetry. In being able to read Chinese, he was almost unique among fellow Russian writers, just as he stood out as being both an Orthodox monk (between 1938 and 1945) and a homosexual.[33] As only a few Chinese literary works were translated into Russian in China, and even then usually indirectly, via English or French, Pereleshin considered himself and was seen by many as "the first in translating from Chinese."[34] It also seems that he often felt like a discoverer of China.

Ha'erbin ren

Instances of cross-cultural engagement in the midst of general indifference or hostility existed on both sides. Harbin was far from the literary and publishing centres of Peking and Shanghai and thus was home to fewer Chinese intellectuals who were interested in modern ideas and foreign literature. Calls for Bolshevism in the city grew loud during the revolutionary reverberations of 1905 and again between 1917 and 1920, when Russian workers staged strikes, although the claims of PRC historians about Chinese participation in them are suspect as political propaganda.[35] The Russian Orthodox Church excluded those who were not Russian or Orthodox. By contrast, Russian literary culture, which flourished in the form of libraries, bookstores, literary circles, and many journals, cut across ethnic and political divisions within the Harbin Russian community. Being so prominent in Russian life, its pull was also felt by some Chinese: recall the two young men who had read a classical play in Russian before going to watch it performed in a Harbin theatre. There was a vogue for Russian literature in Republican-era China, and Shanghai journals were flooded with Russian fiction – usually retranslated via English or Japanese intermediary texts. Yet very few translations from Russian were made in Harbin.

One exception, an anthology of classical Russian verse published with a parallel Chinese text in 1933, was the work of an amateur translator who, though born in Liaoyang in the northeast, had studied law and Russian in Peking before getting a job in Harbin. In 1934, the same translator published Ivan Turgenev's famous novella *Asya* (1858).[36] A member of the following generation, Li Yanling was born in Bei'an in central Heilongjiang in 1940. He studied Russian with an émigré teacher from the age of twelve, graduated from Heilongjiang University in Harbin, and became a translator of Russian literature and professor of Russian at Qiqihar University. Because he wrote poetry in Russian, Li has been embraced in the Russian Far East: his first collection came out in Blagoveshchensk in 1994 under the title *I Love Russia*. A devoted collector of works by Russian émigré writers who lived in China, in 2002 he edited translations of these works into Chinese in five volumes. Now speaking for the émigrés, he titled a volume of their memoirs *China, I Love You*. Pursuing his chosen role as an agent of friendship and love between the two nations, Li has expressed such emotions in many interviews.[37]

The most durable legacy of the Russians was set in stone. These were the schools and institutes, churches, government buildings, and houses that for many years shaped Harbin's streets. Except for Orthodox churches, Russian architects in Harbin worked in the traditions of Art Nouveau, neoclassicism, and other European movements; the influence of Chinese aesthetics was limited to public parks and CER railway stations. Only moderately present in Harbin, Chinese architectural inspiration was more in evidence in early Russian construction in Dal'nii (Dalian).[38]

On the Chinese side, some efforts were made to redress the balance and make Harbin look "more Chinese." A Buddhist temple, the Jilesi, was constructed in 1924, and a Confucian shrine, the Wenmiao, was built in 1929. When funds for the Jilesi were being collected, Buddhist priests came knocking on Russian doors. Later, the lavish Confucius shrine necessitated outlays so high that pressure had to be applied on such unlikely disciples of the Sage as the owner of the Hotel Moderne, Iosif S. Kaspe (1878–1938), the international wheat and soybean magnate Semen Kh. Soskin (1881–?), and the timber merchant Władisław Kowalski (1871–1940).[39] The outrageously expensive Wenmiao (literally, Shrine of Culture) was a bid for legitimacy of a kind that had become fashionable among China's warlords.[40] The Jilesi (Temple of Ultimate Bliss) was strategically located to offset the damage that St Nicholas Cathedral had supposedly caused to Harbin's *feng shui*.

Perhaps more by coincidence than as a calculated affront, the Buddhist temple was situated close to the Orthodox New Cemetery.[41] As tourists rather than believers, some Harbin Russians visited these and other Chinese temples. One admiring visitor even thought she recognized the wooden figure of St Nicholas among the "Buddhas and Chinese religious objects" she saw in small shrines in the Harbin countryside.[42]

Harbin had begun to look more and more Chinese, yet the city administration continued to employ Russian architects for the construction of buildings and monuments in European style up to the early years of the PRC. Harbin's Russian past did not come under decisive attack until the Cultural Revolution. Its grandest representation, St Nicholas Cathedral, was razed, and few of the other city churches survived the Red Guards. Dwellings that had escaped the ideological campaigns of the 1960s and '70s deteriorated through years of neglect and seldom withstood the building boom, which began in the 1990s and has intensified ever since. A change in official attitudes came in the late 1990s, when some relics of Russian architecture were put under state protection. Now these Russian buildings, hotels, and private mansions (which in the PRC were diverted to administrative and Party purposes) are being exploited as tourist attractions – a source of local pride rather than a reminder of imperialist domination.

Between 1997 and 2006 the Cathedral of St Sophia was renovated, quickly to become Harbin's most recognizable visual symbol. No longer a house of worship, it functions as a museum and houses a permanent exhibition of photographs of old Harbin. New buildings erected in Harbin often copy "Western" style: columns, turrets, and cupolas proliferate, and there is even the occasional stucco cupid. In the early twentieth century, Chinese builders in the native quarter, Fujiadian, used cheaper materials and an adapted technique to imitate the European architecture of buildings they saw in Daoli.[43] But the formerly Russian buildings and mixed city had to become unquestionably Chinese, and indoctrinated hatred needed to subside, before the remnants of Russia in Harbin ceased to pose a threat to local Chinese identity. At that stage the fading traces of the city's past, now domesticated, became the object of nostalgia.

The growth of Chinese and international tourism in Harbin in the new climate of the 1990s was a major impetus behind the rediscovery of the Russian heritage. While a growing interest in exploring the Russian past seemed genuinely felt among people in Harbin, local history also became an industry, in which historians participated. Early photographs of Harbin streets, buildings, and churches, previously associated with émigré memorabilia, suddenly emerged from the albums of current Chinese residents, who contributed them for publication in a

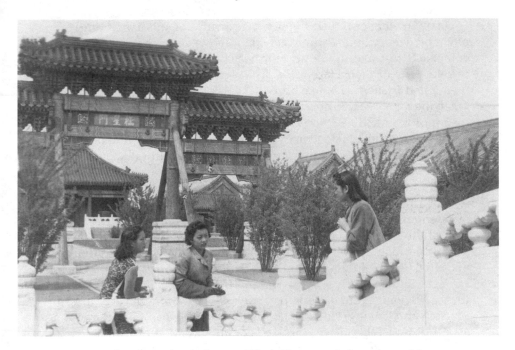

8.1. Jilesi (Temple of Ultimate Bliss). Photograph from the archive
of Vladimir Ablamskii, courtesy of the A.M. Sibiriakov Museum
of Irkutsk City History.

glossy album titled *Old Photos of Harbin*.[44] In one of the street photos,
an unidentified blonde woman is seen carrying her baby. She is in the
company of two other women, all unmistakably Russian. The editorial caption would have been hard to imagine when the Russian émigrés were still being condemned as intruders into China: "That child
in swaddling clothes is also a *Ha'erbin ren* [a Harbin person]."[45] The
images included in *Old Photos of Harbin* were exhibited in 2002 at the
Cathedral of St Sophia, where some were sold as postcards. In 2000,
the architect Hu Hong (b. 1951), whose mother was Russian, opened
a café on one of the streets adjacent to Zhongyang dajie. He called it
"Luxiya" (his old-style transcription of *Rossiia*, Russia) and filled it
to the brim with photographs of old Harbin, Russian antiques, and
paintings. A guest who sampled the Russian dishes and the Harbin
variations of Russian cuisine at Luxiya, still open today, would notice
an iconic photograph of the Harbin flood of 1932, and a private one
of a child in Harbin of the 1930s with the handwritten caption "Wo de
mama" ("My mum").[46]

On a smaller scale than the mass departure of Russians from Harbin, there were Chinese who, after spending years in the city, were also
compelled to leave it. Former northeasterners in Taiwan later wrote
recollections of their Harbin life. The writer Chen Jiying (1908–1997)
mentioned friends who, like himself, had to escape Harbin twice: first
when the Japanese army occupied the city, and again after the Communists took over.[47] Mixed Sino-Russian families fared the worst, and their
descendants who remained in China suffered harassment and discrimination, which became life-threatening during the Cultural Revolution.[48]

For decades, Chinese people who had left China were unable to
communicate with friends and relatives, and their fate became subject
to much the same speculations that Harbin Russians, in their places
of resettlement around the world, exchanged about former *kharbintsy*
behind the Iron Curtain. Associations of "Friends of the Harbin Polytechnic" sprang up among both Russian alumni in Sydney and California and Chinese alumni in Taipei, where their activities were sustained
by such figures as prime minister Sun Yunxuan and "Young Marshal"
Zhang Xueliang.[49] But these associations did not communicate: Russian
Kharbin and Chinese Ha'erbin cultivated separate pasts. An important
aspect of remembering the city, the commemoration of its dead, provides a compelling illustration of this mutual insularity.

Kharbin and *Ha'erbin*

Among Russian memoirists the idea is widespread that Harbin's Chinese authorities deliberately desecrated the graves of the Russians who
died and were buried there. The most often-mentioned grievance of
former Russian inhabitants of the city, next to the razing of St Nicholas Cathedral, is the creation of an amusement park on the site of the
New Cemetery, with some of the gravestones used to pave the path-
ways.[50] The Chinese counter that the émigrés are still being honoured
in Huangshan Cemetery, 20 kilometres outside Harbin, to which some
of the foreign graves were transferred when the New Cemetery in Nangang (commonly known as *lao maozi fen*, the Old Hairies' Cemetery)
was turned into a park. This took place as part of the Great Leap Forward in August 1958, and Chinese graves located next to the Buddhist
temple Jilesi were moved to Huangshan at the same time. Relatives of
the deceased were required to pay for the relocation within two to three
months. The result was the destruction of more than 20,000 graves of
émigrés, whose descendants lived abroad. Thanks to prompt action by
Jewish organizations, Jewish graves fared better than those of the Russian Orthodox and others in the transfer to Huangshan.[51]

The levelling of émigré graves was carried out with the approval of the Soviet Consulate, which insisted only on protecting the graves of Soviet soldiers.[52] When the Red Army swept through Manchuria in the summer of 1945, it demolished tsarist-era cemeteries as well as monuments to the Russo-Japanese War.[53] On what was then Cathedral Square (now Museum Square) in Nangang, directly opposite St Nicholas Cathedral, the Soviet authorities erected a monument to their dead by replacing a Manchukuo monument to "Fighters against the Comintern" (Russian émigré collaborators with Japan), which they had blown up. It still stands today, although the cathedral does not. The Russian inscription, dated 3 September 1945, proclaims "eternal glory to the heroes fallen in the battles for the freedom and independence of the Soviet Union." Just below this, the Chinese text says: "For the Soviet hero soldiers, fallen for the freedom and independence of China in the War of Liberation in the Northeast." The corresponding date, 3 September 1950, is written in Chinese characters rather than Arabic numerals; visitors able to read only one of the two languages would assume each inscription to be a literal translation of the other.

This monument was designed by the architect Mikhail A. Bakich (1909–2002), the son of the White general Andrei Bakich, whom the Reds executed at the end of the Civil War. He also created the landmark monument on the bank of the Sungari, "Victory over the Flood," commemorating the defence of Harbin from the floods of 1932 and 1957. Harbin's Chinese mayor at the time allowed the architect to include one Russian figure among the crowd of local Chinese citizens, who are shown protecting their city from the rising river: looking closely at the monument, the attentive tourist may notice it.[54] In 1959 (the year after the Bakich family left Harbin for Australia) a chapter on Harbin in a Soviet travelogue for young readers did not even mention that Russians had once lived in that Chinese city.[55] Soviet engineers arrived in Harbin in the 1950s to supervise the construction of industrial complexes.[56] Like Chinese Communist officials, they were under orders to avoid contact with the remaining "White Russians." It was the final bout of Russian involvement in Harbin: the Soviet experts were recalled from the People's Republic after Soviet-Chinese relations were severed in 1960.

Early in the Cultural Revolution, the Red Guards, who pulled down Harbin's Russian churches and ransacked the Jilesi temple the same day that they burned down St Nicholas Cathedral, also went to Huangshan cemetery. Traces of their visit can still be seen in the oval holes where images of the dead had once been fitted into the stone. Similarly, Red Guards smashed the faces of Buddha statues in China within the

Great Wall. The attack against the foreign dead was only one episode in a tragedy, the brunt of which was born by the living. Unlike the Russians, who regarded their last resting place in Harbin as eternal, many of the Chinese migrants, having buried family members in Manchuria, cherished hopes of carrying their remains back to their home villages.[57] The destruction of cemeteries that began during the Great Leap Forward thus constituted an even greater outrage to the Chinese population of Harbin than to the Russians, who had left China and often never learned that the peace of their deceased relatives had been disturbed. In 1963, breaking with ancient tradition, the Chinese government introduced compulsory cremation all over the country. In the Cultural Revolution more cemeteries and ancestral temples were razed, while the graves of Qing imperial officials became targets for sanctioned vandalism.[58] So the tomb of Song Xiaolian, who was buried in his native city of Jilin, was robbed, its stele used to support the wall of a livestock farm; Red Guards also ransacked the tomb of Ma Zhongjun, who had been buried in his Garden of Retreat.[59]

The shaping of a Harbin identity may be seen, at the risk of some simplification, through parallel images of rise and decline. Russian Harbin began as a colonial society, to become a centre of emigration after the Revolution and the Civil War. Chinese Harbin developed as the former Shandong migrants, their children and grandchildren, as well as new arrivals from the 1950s, put down firm roots in the city. Yet Kharbin did not just vanish, replaced by Ha'erbin. On the one hand, the identity lost as a result of the splintering and maltreatment of the Russian community between the 1920s and the 1950s (years that included the loss of legal rights and status, the Japanese occupation, the deportations to Soviet labour camps, and the final departure from Harbin) has been reconstructed in post-Soviet Russia by historians, memoirists, and tourists and pilgrims to Harbin. Through their efforts, Russian Harbin has been crystallized retrospectively in the image of the lifeboat that survived the shipwreck: a safe haven, where old Russia endured long after sinking at home. To be Chinese in Harbin today means, on the other hand, to be aware that the part played by Russians in the creation of the city makes it different from any other.

The local writer Ah Cheng has described the *Ha'erbin ren* as he sees them in a best-selling portrait of the city and its inhabitants, first published in 1995. The first five chapters of the book are dedicated to the "foreign flavour" (*yangqi*), which the author feels is inseparable from the Harbin identity.[60] He begins with the former Chinese Street, now Central Avenue, saying that Harbin residents proudly display it to every out-of-town visitor. Although Ah Cheng believes that most of the strollers on the old Chinese Street were foreigners, he comments that each of the nationalities represented in Harbin would have liked to lend their name to the most beautiful street in the city. Implicitly rejecting the official PRC view that for decades had equated Russian construction in Harbin with imperialist exploitation, Ah Cheng sees the people who built Central Avenue as ordinary Russians, who devoted their best efforts in an ultimately vain and tragic attempt to make the city their home.[61] Ah Cheng's investigation then leads him to the Russian beggars, who still played their musical instruments on the streets in the 1950s. He thinks that the special affinity of Harbin people for music is due to their influence.[62]

Ah Cheng appears to have no doubt that both the past and the present of his city belong to him and his compatriots. Kharbin and Ha'erbin are the essential building blocks of this city, neither of them complete without the other. The destruction of old Harbin, be it in the name of nationalist causes or of commercial interests, accordingly becomes an act of violence, not against the memory of foreigners, but against him, the *Ha'erbin ren*, who still remembers St Nicholas Cathedral:

In my childhood, our family was very poor. I often went out to the street pulling a small cart, to earn a bit of money. My route often passed there, and I frequently could see neatly dressed priests, clergymen and old ladies filing in and out. To me, a poor child doing a coolie's work, it exuded a true sense of mystery and the pleasure of beauty. Moreover, its very existence stimulated my power of imagination and my interest in architecture. This makes me wonder whether my father's becoming a master builder may have had to do with his roaming in that part of town in his early days as a young intellectual. That Cathedral, which everybody in Harbin used to call "the Nangang lama tower," no longer exists. It has "passed away." During the "CultRev," it was demolished by the Red Guards. On the day when the Cathedral was pulled down, I too went there. Frankly speaking, I had an ineffable feeling toward it, as did many middle-aged and old people in Harbin.

On that day the city was shrouded in misty rain. Looking from beyond the Cathedral's iron railing, I saw the Red Guards carrying out books, which appeared to be Bibles, piling them on the flowerbed in the courtyard and then setting them on fire. With a coarse rope, a group of Red Guards pulled the cross on the Cathedral's onion dome until it came tumbling down with a thud. Observing all this next to me was an emigrant, aged probably above fifty, wearing a faded Zhongshan suit and a red medallion on his chest. His hands were agitatedly clenching the iron railing, his mouth mumbling something, his eyes brimming with tears. He must have been a devout believer. This sight made me very sad at heart, and as long as I live I shall not be able to forget it.[63]

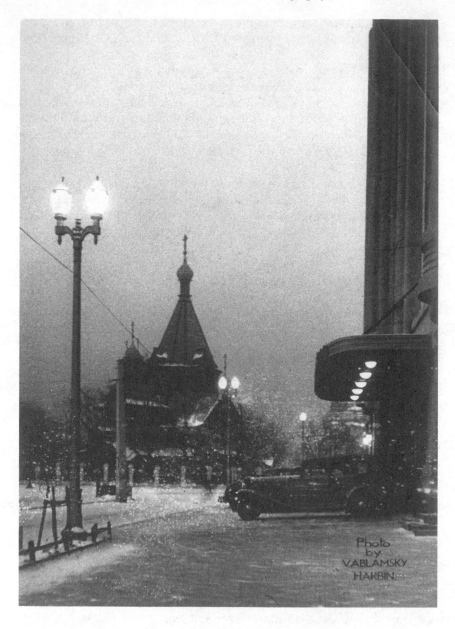

8.2. An evening view of St Nicholas Cathedral. Photograph from the archive
of Vladimir Ablamskii, courtesy of the A.M. Sibiriakov Museum
of Irkutsk City History.

Contemporary Russian and Chinese writers about Harbin agree on the need to preserve the cultural heritage the two countries share in that city. The existence of a confident Chinese Harbin makes it difficult for Russians to overlook the fact that the relic of tsarist Russia was after all located in China; ignoring the Chinese side of the Harbin experience, as was done by memoirists describing "an essentially Russian city," will no longer do. China must be fitted into the narrative of Russian Harbin, and Russia into that of Chinese Harbin. However, beyond the much-rehearsed politically motivated claims regarding Russia's role in Harbin's modernization, the history of the mixed city is now too often garbed in nebulous references to a mutually enriching mingling of cultures, or friendship between nations, that supposedly developed there. This book has argued that the encounter in Harbin resulted in only limited and reluctant contact between the populations on both sides. Yet from its foundation in 1898 to the end of the 1950s, Harbin was not solely "Russian," or solely "Chinese": it was both – which a minority among its Russians, Chinese, and other residents actually took as an advantage rather than a regrettable and transitory reality.

Epilogue: The General and the Particular

The Logic of Blood and Birth

The period during which we have observed the Russian colonizers and émigrés in Harbin and examined their relations with their host environment, the first half of the twentieth century, was a time of voluntary migration and forced expulsion on an enormous scale. It was marked by the loss of roots, the collapse of hierarchies, and mass extermination culminating with the Holocaust. The nineteenth century, which had seen the rise of nationalism, was still the age of empires, within which multiple identities were possible, even natural. Thus, the Habsburg Empire, "that many-nationed crucible," left behind "a profound feeling of not belonging to any precise world, but also the conviction that that elusive identity – composed of mixtures, suppressions and elisions – was ... a general historical condition, the being of each and every individual."[1] However, such convictions rapidly lost out to the belief that a single identity, derived from belonging to a nation and an ethnic group, was the norm, to which all other forms of self-identification constituted an exception. The First World War was followed by the destruction and displacement of minority communities by the states that had previously hosted them.[2] People came under unprecedented pressure to understand themselves and others in terms of race, and racial categories were invoked to determine their present or prospective allegiance to the nation.

Though their status deteriorated, Russians in China did not face expulsion in the 1920s or '30s, because they lived at the margins of a weak state. However, in the peace settlements of 1945, as in those of 1918, countries again cleansed their border areas and forcibly exchanged populations as a means to ensure loyalty through ethnic homogeneity. The Chinese Communist regime, continuing the policy initiated by

Manchukuo, treated the Russians collectively as a national group rather than as individuals, who might disagree about where they belonged. When deciding whether to repatriate during the 1950s, most Russians thought in the same terms and relied on the same logic – living outside the nation of one's birth and ethnicity was unnatural.

Here is what happened to one extended family, which entered the twentieth century as part of a privileged estate within a small minority in the Russian empire and was persecuted relentlessly after the October Revolution because of its ethnic and class background and its presumed or actual political positions. Of the seven children of Annette Budberg, the young beauty who married Roger Budberg's great-uncle, all four sons perished between 1917 and 1921. Nicolaus, Anatol, and Andreas (since the family was Russian Orthodox, they were better known as Nikolai, Anatolii, and Andrei) had served with the Dragoon Guards Regiment in Saint Petersburg; Alexander, too, had been a career officer.[3] In February 1945, Soviet soldiers shot and killed Count Alexander Keyserlingk, seventy-five years old, together with his second son, also named Alexander, on their estate, Condehnen in East Prussia, which, after the expulsion of the Germans, soon became the Soviet Kaliningrad *oblast*.[4] These were the husband and son of Roger Budberg's maternal cousin Margarethe (1876–1941). Also in 1945, another seventy-five-year-old, the widow of Roger's cousin Heinrich Keyserlingk, Johanna, "went missing," *vermisst* being the legal formulation for persons whose bodies were never recovered. So did another Heinrich Keyserlingk, an eighteen-year-old grandson of Alexander and Margarethe.[5] Many more of Roger Budberg's relatives met a violent and unnatural death.

During the Civil War in Siberia, Joseph, the brother who was closest to Roger, was shot on the street; and brother Gotthard died soon after being arrested . At the same time, Luis Bubnik, a refugee from Ufa, told Roger Budberg in Harbin that Wilhelm, his long-lost youngest brother, had died in that city ten years earlier and that he, Bubnik, and his wife had done all they could to help him in his last days. Yet in 1930, Wilhelm Budberg attempted to come back from the dead.

Wilhelm's military career ended before it had even begun. Because of poor performance, the Nicholas Cadet Corps (Nikolaevskii kadetskii korpus) in Saint Petersburg expelled him, assigning him to serve as a non-commissioned officer in the Dragoons.[6] Like his brother Gotthard, he seems to have acquired no profession and fell into poverty. Not having Joseph to take him under his wing and probably receiving no support from his father's cousins, the Dragoon Guards officers in the capital, Wilhelm ended up as badly as Gotthard, or worse. Aged twenty-five, he became a permanent resident in Uspenskoe, then a village of about 230 people on the river Kerzhenets in the Governorate of Kostroma. The Kerzhenets, a tributary of the Volga, had been known as a refuge of Old Believers, who had come to its banks in the late tsarist era to escape state control.

This information emerges from an archival file of a police investigation in the winter of 1896, which resulted in Wilhelm Budberg being sentenced to a month in prison for insulting the tsar during an altercation with the village blacksmith. This was already his third trial: he had previously been charged with poaching and disorderly conduct. The prosecutor described the baron as having no fixed occupation, noting that "during his stay in the village Budberg never read books, but, socializing only with peasants, has been spending his time in idleness, hunting and hard drinking."[7] Remarkably, thirty-four years later, when Wilhelm Budberg provided his address in documents he submitted in the Soviet Union, he indicated two villages in the same area. He could hardly have spent the entire period between 1896 and 1930 in the countryside by Kerzhenets River, but he did return there. In January 1930, he wrote to the Minister of Foreign Affairs of Latvia from Bogoiavlenie village, only 30 kilometres south of Uspenskoe in Semenovskii district of Nizhny Novgorod *oblast*. In August, he gave his address as Klyshino, a village neighbouring Uspenskoe, which had been his home in the 1890s.

He wrote by hand, in halting Russian, saying that in the past fifteen years he had tried in vain to return to Latvia and referring to that country as his motherland (*rodina*). Though not daring to use his title, which the Bolsheviks had abolished, he did claim to be the heir to the two family estates, Magnushof near Riga in the Governorate of Livland and Gemauert Poniemon in the Governorate of Courland, and he wished to travel to Latvia so as "not to lose the property of [his] late father."[8] He also addressed the police department of Bauska, asking who was presently the manager of Poniemon and whether his brother Joseph still lived there.[9] By April, an entry visa valid for 120 days awaited him at the Latvian Consulate in Moscow. He did not collect it, however, and in August applied for another visa, which was again approved in December. This was the last communication from him that survives in the Latvian archives. So far as can be known, he never went back to Latvia. Had he returned to his old home, he would have learned that the Budberg estates had been expropriated long ago, that none of his surviving siblings lived in the country, and that the Republic of Latvia was far from willing to serve as a motherland for the Baltic barons.

Shortly before his attempted "return to the motherland," Wilhelm Budberg managed to contact his sister Antoinette Raczynski.[10] When she received the first letter from the region of Nizhny Novgorod,

Antoinette could not believe that her brother was alive after all. She consulted her sisters Marie in Italy and Cecile in Germany, and together they wrote back to the purported Wilhelm in Soviet Russia, challenging him to prove his identity by answering questions on details of their common childhood. Once he had passed this test convincingly and had sent the sisters his photograph, Antoinette wired him travel money through the British embassy in Moscow (it is unclear from the family version of this story whether they wanted Wilhelm to join Antoinette in Poland). He got the money, but a few weeks later wrote from Moscow that, on arriving there to obtain the permit to travel abroad, he had had his papers confiscated and was turned away. In late 1929, in response to the rural collectivization campaign, many ethnic Germans, most of whom were Mennonites (a religious Protestant community, whose roughly 120,000 members in Russia at the time lived in hundreds of German-speaking villages across the country), came to Moscow to apply for exit visas from the Soviet Union. After the first group of under 6,000 was allowed out, finding temporary refuge in Germany, the Soviet government changed its position. The remaining applicants were either returned to their places of residence, where they had been branded as kulaks, or exiled to labour camps.[11] Wilhelm was never heard from again. Since his name is not on the available incomplete lists of victims of political repression, perhaps he did find his way back to his village. By then, even the Kerzhenets River was not a safe retreat for someone of his background, but he may have died there before the worst purges of class enemies, other counter-revolutionary elements, and "foreign agents" unfolded nationwide in 1937.

Luis Bubnik was an impostor and grifter with a complex past. In 1902, he was on record as a "German subject" employed as the forester by a cast iron factory in Verkhneural'sk County, southeast of Ufa (today's Beloretskii district in the Republic of Bashkortostan). His name appears on police records as being involved in an incident: to force Bashkir villagers to surrender hay they had mowed on factory land, he had shot at them. The Bashkirs gave Bubnik a sound beating, and for this were arrested for attempted "revolt."[12] Bubnik later managed a similar factory for a French company on the Inzer River in the same region.[13] His claim to have nursed Wilhelm Budberg was a lie, but as lies sometimes do, it had a grain of truth. A Baron Sergei Pavlovich Budberg, no relative of Roger Budberg's, had been an assistant forester in Ufa when he died there, aged only twenty-four, in 1899.[14] If Bubnik was already in Ufa then, this would have been the Baron Budberg whose death he witnessed. Through Sergei, he would have learned about the Budberg family; he might even have come across Joseph, who was a judge in Ufa

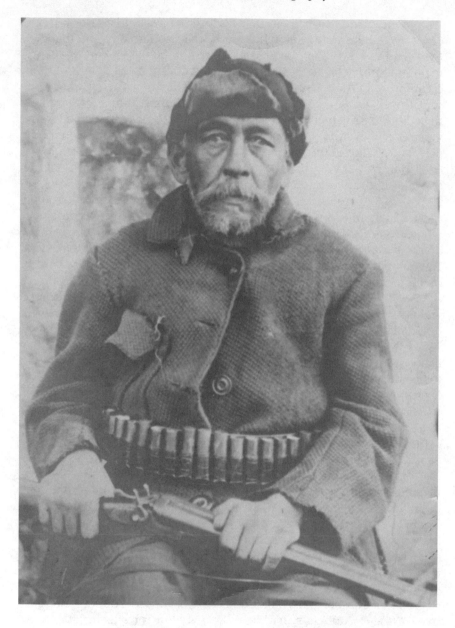

E.1. Wilhelm Budberg. Photograph in Köhler family album.

in 1898 and 1899. More than twenty years later, in Harbin, Bubnik was probably able to make the story he spun about burying Wilhelm in Ufa "around 1911" sound more plausible by including some details about the Budbergs that he remembered.

In 1923 a Russian commercial partnership in Harbin warned the public through the local press that it no longer recognized Luis Bubnik as its trustee.[15] In 1926, shortly after Roger Budberg's death, Bubnik married a recently widowed Russian, the affluent owner of a large flour business and a horse-breeding farm: the same Aleksandra Zamesova who along with Bubnik had placed a mourning notice about Baron Budberg in *Russkoe slovo*. Bubnik was described in that newspaper as "treasurer of the Horse-owners' Committee" when he died in Harbin in May 1932.[16]

For several generations, members of the Raczynski family could not and did not have to decide whether they were German or Polish.[17] After September 1939, Obrzycko by Poznań, where the Raczynski castle was situated, again became Augustusburg by Posen, as it had been until the end of the First World War. Under the Nazi occupation in the newly created Warthegau, the Poles were expelled, while *Volksdeutsche*, ethnic Germans brought from other parts of Europe, including 51,000 Baltic Germans, were resettled in the region to replace them and the local Jews, who were exterminated. In January 1945, however, the German army evacuated Posen, and the widowed Antoinette Raczynski left Augustusburg. In February, her son Andreas Raczynski (alternatively, Andrzej Raczyński, b. 1910) went missing in the war.[18] By May, Poland was forcibly evicting all non-Polish populations from its eastern border area while the Soviet army advanced. Around this time, a relative from the Polish branch, Count Edward Bernard Raczyński (1891–1993), represented the Polish government-in-exile in London. As the war neared its end, more than 12 million ethnic Germans ("up to a tenth of whom did not even speak German") were expelled from central and southern Europe for resettlement in Germany.[19] The decision that the Raczynskis who had identified with Germany no longer belonged in their native places in Poland had been made for them.

Antoinette Raczynski's two daughters were married to German aristocrats, one of whom was a senior Nazi officer. She first went to Germany, but in 1950 she joined her son Sigismund (1901–1980) and his family to live at "the end of the world," the *finis terrae* of Chile. That country, where the youngest of the Raczynski siblings, Joseph Alexander, was the first to settle in 1948, became a refuge for them and a home for their next generation. Roger Budberg's faithful correspondent died in Santiago, aged eighty-two, in 1952. More than thirty years later,

Joseph Alexander transcribed Uncle Roger's letters, which had unexpectedly come into his possession. In 1984, he had travelled to Poland with his family and contacted an aged former employee of their castle. That man handed him a folder he had found in 1945 in the park near the house, where Antoinette stayed before her departure. The folder contained Budberg's letters from Harbin.[20]

Latin America was also the last destination of many Harbinites. The poet Marianna Kolosova (1901–1964), for example, whom the Japanese had expelled from Manchukuo, lived in Shanghai until being evacuated along with the last 6,000 "White Russians" on the eve of the Communist takeover in 1949. The only country that agreed to accept these refugees temporarily was the Philippines. The UN Relief Organization transported them to Tubabao Island. After two years in a tent camp, Kolosova and her husband moved to Brazil and then on to Chile; she died in Santiago.[21]

The longest-lived of the eight Budberg siblings proved to be the eldest sister, Marie. Having gone to Italy to study painting, she remained in Rome until her death, aged eighty-eight, in 1953. The first of her three sons, Giulio Andrea Belloni (1902–1957), became Secretary of the Italian Republican Party in the 1940s and was later a member of the Chamber of Deputies. He was exceptionally devoted to his mother, writing her letters from the fascist prison in 1932, extracts of which were published after his death.[22] Perhaps because descent from the Baltic German nobility was inappropriate for a leftist public figure, or just difficult to explain, Belloni's supporters remembered him as "Roman to the core (but the son of a Russian mother)."[23]

Between October and December 1939, around 65,000 Baltic Germans sailed from Tallinn and Riga in about one hundred ships in response to the recall of ethnic Germans to the Reich, the "Umsiedlung" (resettlement) announced by Adolf Hitler in October.[24] Although some had already left Estonia and Latvia when the standing of Germans there deteriorated in the 1920s, most were only persuaded to depart from the region by alarmist Nazi propaganda, threats to be forever severed from the German nation if they refused to be resettled, promises of a dignified new life among their own people if they mobilized to do their part for the Fatherland by cultivating the newly "recovered" territories in Poland, and, if that was not enough, rumours that the Bolsheviks were coming. Indeed, they were coming, since the Baltic states had been declared a part of the Soviet sphere of interest in the secret protocol of the Molotov-Rippentrop Pact, signed in Moscow in August.

Like the Russians in Harbin and the region they called "Manchuria," the Baltic Germans had attempted for as long as possible to preserve their "Baltikum" in the form familiar to them, calling cities and streets by their German rather than Latvian or Estonian names.[25] After losing their privileged status by the early 1920s, both Baltic Germans and Russians in Manchuria became threatened minorities (indeed, both appealed for protection to the League of Nations). Expelled by the rise of Latvian, Estonian, and Chinese nationalism, and driven by their perceptions of national identity, most of them then "repatriated" collectively to an ancestral land, which national ideology and political propaganda celebrated as *Vaterland*, or "motherland" (*rodina*). Both groups joined the population transfers that marked the first half of the twentieth century and that forced individuals to reinvent their homes in new places.

The Manchus, too, experienced a dramatic transformation from rulers to beleaguered underdogs, although few of them left China. After the revolution of 1911 they were massacred in garrisons around the country (although not in Peking or Manchuria). The Republic of China nationalized Manchu land. Some Manchus, who had lived within the Great Wall for generations, began thinking of Manchuria as their homeland, and some "repatriated" there, either after the fall of the Qing or once a "Manchurian state" was proclaimed in 1932.[26] There were, of course, great differences in the circumstances and time spans: seven centuries had passed since the first Germans settled in the Baltic; the Manchus had spent two centuries and a half in Peking, and the Russians only a few decades in Harbin. Yet Baron Nikolai Budberg, for one, erased the centuries as if they were a mere parenthesis.

No direct relation, he had begun writing to Roger Budberg in Harbin as a needy student in Tartu in 1922.[27] Before enrolling for medical and then zoological studies at the university, neither of which he finished, Nikolai Budberg fought against the Bolsheviks with the Baltic forces of Colonel Prince Anatol Lieven (1872–1937), which drove the Reds from Latvia in 1919. He then participated alongside the Estonian military in a failed attack on Petrograd by the White Northwestern Army, leaving memoirs about these campaigns in Russian.[28] About twenty years later, he was transplanted with other *Volksdeutsche* to occupied northern Poland, which had become Reichsgau Danzig – West Prussia. He was soon mobilized and fought as a German officer in the Second World War from 1941 to 1945. By 1949, a retired educational councillor at a *Gymnasium* in Detmold, he had cast himself as the genealogist of the Budberg family. Living in North Rhine-Westphalia within 200 kilometres of the ancestral Budberg village, in a leap of faith unhindered by his Russian Orthodox birth, he had fully embraced the narrative of return to Germanic roots.[29]

History is what happens to people, individuals with names and biographies. And it is through people that everything connects. Eight kilometres to the north of Roger Budberg's birthplace, Gemauert Poniemon, was another manor belonging to the extended Budberg family: Brunowischek, now Brunava parish.[30] When the Soviet state annexed Latvia in August 1940, it launched the deportation of more than 15,000 people, mostly ethnic Latvians, but also people of other nationalities. Families were broken up: the men were sent to the Gulag, rarely to return, while women and children were resettled in inhospitable parts of Siberia and the Russian Far North. Laima Āriņš (1919–1985) was taken from Brunava with the last deportees on 16 June 1941, only a week before the Soviet army retreated from Latvia in the face of the Nazi invasion. In 2011 her daughter Nadezhda, born in Igarka above the Arctic Circle, travelled to see the ravines in Kirov Region where her maternal grandfather, an agronomist from Brunava, was probably buried in a mass grave. Speaking better Russian than Latvian, she repatriated to Latvia after 1991; by then, her mother had died in her place of banishment after a lifetime of deprivation.[31]

These snippets of life stories offer the possibility of thinking through the dilemmas of identity in the twentieth century against the increasingly brutal intervention of the state by following the threads emerging from a single biography, the life of Roger Budberg. Their other common theme is the Second World War as the watershed beyond which nothing could continue as before.[32] Not only were millions of lives lost in that war, but so many ways of life, which had survived cataclysms earlier in the twentieth century, were dealt an irreparable blow – either by the war itself or by its aftermath. In Harbin on 17 November 1925, Budberg signed a copy of his new book, the *Memoirs* in Russian, with this inscription in German: "To Mr Senator John Kalatz, the righteous judge, who lives on (with such sympathy) in the author's memory, in recollection of the times of tsarist jurisdiction in Manchuria, presented by the author in deep honour and gratitude."[33] The receiver was Jānis Kalacs (1868–1947): born to a family of farmers in Trikāta parish in northern Latvia, he was educated at Saint Petersburg University and served as a judge in western Siberia and Sakhalin between 1897 and 1905, then in the Border Circuit Court in Harbin from 1906 to 1918. He returned to Latvia in 1920 and two years later was elected to the Latvian Senate (the High Court of Justice).[34] Like Budberg, Kalacs had attended the Governorate Gymnasium in Riga; as chance would have it, he was one of the judges before whom Budberg appeared in August 1916.[35] Having spent his life among three cultures, Latvian, Russian, and German, in 1944 Kalacs joined the 200,000 refugees who left Latvia for Germany and Sweden before the return of the Soviets. He died in a camp for displaced persons in Detmold, one of the locations where the Baltic German "repatriates" of 1939 were surprised to encounter their former Latvian neighbours.[36]

Another connection of Budberg's from his time in Tartu was the ophthalmologist Friedrich Akel (b. 1871). As young medics, Budberg and Akel inspected an Estonian kindergarten together.[37] Later both physicians left Tartu at the same time for the Russo-Japanese War in Manchuria.[38] A diplomat and political figure, Akel served three terms as Estonia's foreign minister and was briefly head of state in 1924. In October 1940, during the Soviet prewar invasion of the Baltic, the NKVD arrested Akel in Tallinn, where by then he had resumed work as an eye doctor. He was shot in July 1941, and his family members were deported to the Kirov region.[39]

In Harbin in 1945, as the Soviet military went on a rampage of terror amid the helpless "Whites," former tsarist positions of power and prestige similarly became death sentences, which few were lucky enough to avoid. Among those who did, some chose to continue their lives in emigration in any other part of the world that would accept them rather than "repatriate" to a menacing Russia, which had driven them from their homeland after 1917, exterminated the railway employees who had been compelled to return from Manchuria in 1935, and persecuted them even on Chinese soil ten years later. Yet in the imagination of those who had been born in China but were still considered "émigrés," Russia was a myth that had been inculcated since childhood.[40] It was they who most wanted to "return" to the idealized home of their parents, which they had never seen for themselves. Between 1945 and 1954, they had gotten to know the Soviets in Harbin and had eagerly watched Soviet films and read Soviet journals. Merging the dreams of the emigration with the message of Soviet propaganda, they had learned to identify their lost motherland with the powerful state that had defeated Germany and Japan.[41]

Often, the older generation was prepared to forgive and forget why they had left Russia, or to act as if they forgave and forgot, so as to bestow a "motherland" on the young. Pavel Severnyi, the popular writer on exotic China, who had enlisted in the White Army after his parents and two sisters were executed by the Bolsheviks, and who concealed his previous identity as Baron Olbrich, took Soviet citizenship and in 1954 repatriated from Shanghai with his wife and son to be settled in Chkalov (now Orenburg) in the southern Urals. He was allowed to keep his pen name and to continue writing, and he went on to publish more than thirty books, mostly for young readers, including a short novel about Lenin and another, set in the Manchurian taiga, in which Chinese ginseng gatherers and tiger trappers resisted Japanese imperialists.[42]

Some of the returnees internalized the Soviet discourse – or played their part by mouthing it – according to which they had betrayed the motherland by living abroad, especially during the ultimate trial of the world war, and now they had to spend years apologizing and proving themselves worthy of readmission. One such was the singer and composer Alexander Vertinsky (1889–1957), the most famous performing artist of the Russian emigration, who repatriated as early as 1943. After a career in Europe and the United States, he spent a short time in Harbin and about six years in Shanghai. Until his death he publicly wore the persona of a repentant sinner.[43] There is every indication that Vertinsky had wanted to return to Russia, as did other Russians from China in the 1950s. But many "repatriated" by yielding to the combined persuasion of the Soviet consular officials and the Chinese Communist administration and because they had no other choice, as leaving China for any destination other than the Soviet Union involved a far more complicated, prolonged, and costly procedure with an unpredictable outcome.[44]

After a declaration on repatriation was made by the Soviet Consulate in Harbin on 26 April 1954, almost 9,000 Soviet citizens left the city on trains for the Soviet Union between late May and August. Then the process was suspended without prior notice; and in September, when Nikita Khrushchev himself passed through Harbin en route to a state visit in Beijing, some impatient local Russians questioned him in Churin's department store on when repatriation would restart. When it did, in April 1955, another 8,100 people joined the exodus. In January 1958, the Soviet Consul in Harbin reported that "the Chinese friends" were pressuring him to remove all the Soviet citizens remaining in Heilongjiang province. He recommended that the Chinese "buy up the Russian houses, as they had done in 1954 and 1955." In 1960, the next Soviet consul reported "that the Chinese had discontinued the life-long pensions promised to former CER employees, even though the Japanese had paid them regularly until 1945." By October that year, Harbin had only 2,764 Russians, many of whom were elderly or married to Chinese citizens.[45]

Individual attitudes were mixed: in Harbin in the 1950s, Russians heard from Chinese friends that they were sorry to see them go, or that they envied the opportunity foreigners had of leaving the country. But Russians also encountered the rise of chauvinism on the streets and in Chinese institutions.[46] The "repatriation" of all foreigners from China amounted to a Maoist policy of ethnic cleansing by deportation.

Population transfers in Europe in the 1940s ran into difficulties when it came to untangling the ancestry of an individual: to establish, for example, whether a person was really a Pole (and so should naturally live in Poland), or a Lithuanian (and should therefore remain in Soviet Lithuania).[47] No such ambiguity existed with regard to Russians and other Westerners in China, who were visibly set apart from the Chinese and earmarked for relocation to "their own country." Those who had become Chinese citizens were treated no differently from the mass of foreign citizens and émigrés, and in any case, by the 1950s, most of the Chinese identity papers given to Westerners from the 1920s had either been revoked by the Chinese authorities or surrendered by the people concerned. Chinese living among whites in the United States, Canada, or Australia were just as visible, of course, as whites in China, but despite racial discrimination and exclusionary policies against Chinese immigrants, no Western country deported them on an ethnic basis under the pretext of repatriation. The rare exceptions were the violent evictions of Chinese from the Russian Far East: in 1900, and again when the Soviet borderlands were cleansed of "suspect nationalities" between 1937 and 1939.

Having treated Russians abroad as traitors from the early 1920s, after the Second World War the Soviet state wished to bring them back into the bosom of the socialist motherland much as Nazi Germany had collected "the splinters of the German nationality" in 1939.[48] Similarly, the Soviet Union settled its repatriates from China in colonized territories, although in less agreeable conditions than Baltic Germans enjoyed when resettled on Polish lands in the Reich. The postwar repatriation drive was far more successful with the Russians in China than anywhere else. In 1945 and 1946 the Soviet Union was able to forcibly repatriate more than 4 million of its POWs and displaced persons from Europe under the terms of the Yalta Conference. But once the Allies stopped cooperating, the persistent efforts and large resources invested by the Soviet Union from 1947 to 1952 to convince people with Soviet passports to repatriate from DP camps achieved that purpose with only about 2 per cent. All the others used every possible excuse, including the falsification of identity papers, to remain in Western Europe or move to the United States. Nor did the announcement, made in 1946 to the post-revolutionary ("first-wave") émigrés in France, that the Soviet Union had now restored their citizenship, which it had cancelled in 1922, trigger an exodus from Paris.[49]

The situation for Russians in China in 1954 was very different, however. Although no physical violence was used to compel them to leave, moral and economic coercion to repatriate was actively applied toward them by both the Soviet and the Chinese authorities.[50] And the pressing need to leave China was plain to all: as ethnic Poles left for Poland, and

Russian Tatars departed for Turkey, "foreign" Harbin quickly shrank.[51] Harbin's Russians had cultivated nostalgia for Russia over decades and were largely alienated from China. After a xenophobic regime came to power in their "reluctant host country," they saw no future for themselves there.[52]

Cosmopolitan Cities in the Age of Nations

Roger Budberg admired the racial and religious tolerance he believed he had found in China. In an age of stringent identification by criteria of race and nation, he stood out in wanting to learn from China and adopt Chinese ways, yet he was also fully a European of his time in the racial and hierarchical patterns of his thought (and almost a caricature of a Baltic baron in his resentment of Russians). This was the salient contradiction about him. He cannot be evaluated by liberal standards that were alien to all the societies in which he moved; it would be wrong to enlist him as a present-day believer in multiculturalism. Profoundly conservative in his respect for the rigid principles of the society of his birth, he also was strikingly modern in the choice he made to become somebody else: to live as both Baron Budberg and Bu daifu.

Far from advocating cosmopolitanism, Budberg made the characters of nations a defining factor in the way he ordered and understood the world. Not many people in Harbin would have disagreed with him on this principle (although few shared his conclusions). Nevertheless, and even if its inhabitants did not use the word, Harbin was a cosmopolitan city. It was the often reluctant meeting place of ethnicities, minorities, and individuals, who were more than only "Russians," or "Chinese."[53] At the time, those who defined identities and allegiances primarily in ethnic and national terms, believing that these essentialist denominations made coherent groups, might describe others as "sinicized" Manchus and Mongols; "Manchufied" and "Mongolized" Chinese;[54] "Russianized" Ukrainians, Cossacks, Jews, Poles, Georgians, and Germans; "Germanized" Estonians and Latvians. These terms were seldom used in self-definition, so Budberg's calling himself a sinicized German was an act of defiance against Russians, who meant to deride him by that label.

Budberg's friend, Luis (Alois) Bubnik, was referred to as a German in Russian Bashkiria in the 1900s; Budberg called him a Bavarian. Of Bavarian descent, he was born in 1871 in southern Bohemia, which was part of the Habsburg Empire until the end of the First World War and thereafter a part of Czechoslovakia; later it became known as part of the Sudetenland.[55] Before the turn of the century, he immigrated to

Russia. When he left Ufa around 1920, he brought with him to Harbin two Russia-born children, who after about a decade in China repatriated to Czechoslovakia.[56] The tsarist-period Russian settler in Manchuria, Aleksandra Zamesova, received Czechoslovak citizenship through her marriage to Bubnik, which she traded for a German one after her late husband's home region was incorporated into the Protectorate of Bohemia and Moravia in 1939.[57] Such composite identities were not only a matter of personal or collective choice, or of being born into an environment where, contrary to the logic of nationalism, more than one sense of identity existed, but also the outcome of political events and government policies.

In the Baltic and elsewhere in the Russian empire, "Russification" in the second half of the nineteenth century aimed at replacing ethnic and confessional loyalties with identification with Russia and Orthodoxy. With the possible exception of Ukrainians, it generally failed to impact cultural orientation inasmuch as assimilation went both ways. At its western borders, the empire's officials combated the "Polonization" of Lithuanians and Belarusians.[58] In the Russian Far East and the frontier regions of China, groups have been described as Russianized Buryats, but also as Buryatized Tungus and Cossacks, and Mongolized Russians. All of these appear in an excellent recent study of Baron Roman Ungern-Sternberg, which opens by introducing him as "a Russianized Baltic German" and closes by proposing that he be considered not quite "German, Russian, European, Asian [or] Eurasian"; rather, "say that he belonged to the tsarist empire and leave it at that."[59] Indeed, the trouble with such ethnic definitions is that analytically they lead into the nationalist fallacy, according to which a person's first and natural identity is determined from birth by membership in a nation. Leaving the group one is presumed to belong to, be it by adopting another language, by marrying a member of another ethnicity, or through emigration, is criticized as denationalization and miscegenation. Although a Western historian may feel uneasy about these assumptions, they are still widely accepted in Russia and China. During the first half of the twentieth century, race and nation were meaningful for everyone, including people who transgressed their "original" identities. On the basis of the same categories, states began to pursue the "geopolitical logic [of] trying to make territory and identity coincide" by violent measures.[60] The Soviet Union and Nazi Germany implemented such geopolitical concerns through population transfers, which they justified by the needs of state security in the one case and by a racial theory in the other.

Sinicization (*Hanhua*) of the Manchus and other ethnicities in China under the civilizing leadership of the Han was already a tenet of

Chinese state ideology in the Republican period. It was pursued in the PRC along with promotion of the ideal of "the Chinese nation" (*Zhonghua*). Manchus were classified as an ethnic minority, *Manzu*, in 1952; the descendants of Han Chinese members of the banners were allowed to claim this status, but fearing repression in the Mao era, most former banner people of either ethnicity registered as Han.[61] Roger Budberg's wife was considered Manchu by some, although he described her as Chinese. Her dressing as a Manchu could hold a clue to her "true" identity, or it could offer an illustration of Manchu influence over the Han in Manchuria. We shall never find out how she thought of herself, but it is safe to assume that this would have been very unlike any official definitions of "ethnic consciousness." In any case, as time went by, Li alias Baroness Budberg preferred to wear Western dresses, which her husband unsurprisingly did not approve of, arguing that they did not fit her (and were sometimes "immodest"); he attributed her change of taste in clothes to pernicious Russian influence and never photographed her in such attire.[62]

Under Manchukuo rule, ethnic and racial classifications proved flexible to the point of absurdity as the Chinese, who made up the absolute majority of the population in Manchuria, were counted as "Manchurians," or as "Manchus" (depending on the translation of *Manzhou ren*) to support the fiction of a state ruled by the last scion of the Qing dynasty.[63] The Chinese had learned that Russians were divided into Red and White but understood little else about the divisions and loyalties of their neighbours. The Russians regarded the Chinese as an indistinguishable mass. They usually saw the Cossacks as part of the Russian community but kept them at arm's length in other situations. In different senses, this was also the case for Russian religious dissenters and for Jews. These minority groups within the Russian-speaking society in Harbin and Manchuria collectively, and their members as individuals, went through their own phases of wishing to be accepted as equals and of emphasizing their separate identity.

In Harbin, even people whose ethnic, national, and religious backgrounds were unambiguously clear – whose names had one stable version rather than two or three, with variations depending on cultural context – had important affinities to places they had come from before reaching that city: places in Shandong, or perhaps in Ukraine. Their ties to Harbin developed slowly and were often severed by departure from it, be they émigrés from Russia who moved on to Shanghai or Tientsin, repatriated to the Soviet Union, or left China for another country, or Chinese migrants, who returned for good to their home villages after a period in Manchuria. An observation made about another place, Hong Kong, is valid for Harbin as well: "both the British and the Chinese ...

were equally migrants. Yet the principle of cultural separation seemed to deny that shared migrant role."[64] Beyond China and the obvious comparison with Shanghai, beyond the treaty ports and Chinese-Western relations, Harbin may be compared with such cosmopolitan cities as Alexandria, Thessaloniki, Beirut, Baku, and the places mentioned here as part of the biography of Roger Budberg – Riga and Tartu.[65]

Yet during the time of actual cohabitation in the city, "cosmopolitanism" was ridden with tensions and limited by insularity. In that sense, Russian life in Harbin was typical of the lot of foreigners in China. A historian of the diaspora communities in Shanghai notes that the Jews "lived in a kind of bubble, with little regular contact with the other foreign communities in the city"; Russians and Chinese "shared the same physical spaces," but "lived very much apart."[66] As one urban historian points out, "a central question concerning cities as promoters of cultural exchange is whether within individual cities cultures were transferred, exchanged, intermixed, absorbed or simply juxtaposed." He suggests that "cultural transfer is often, perhaps even usually, both partial and selective and, far from being straightforwardly imitative, can involve the reinterpretation of borrowed traits in ways that their original practitioners may not recognise. Such processes are familiar to those who observe the relationship between 'history' and 'myth.'"[67] It is the myth not the reality of the cosmopolitan past that becomes enshrined in nostalgic memory.

The Networks of Nostalgia

Russian graduates of the Harbin Polytechnic in Australia were resolved to remember their time in China and their alma mater. They published their reminiscences in a journal named *Polytechnic*, sixteen issues of which came out between 1969 and 2004. In 1985, a Sydney-based union of former students of the YMCA schools in Harbin also launched a journal in Russian, *Druz'iam ot druzei iz dalekoi Avstralii* (To Friends from Friends, Out of Distant Australia). As the title implied, the alumni had in mind reconnecting with the cross-national diaspora of former Harbin residents, which, after *perestroika*, could include those living in Russia. After being silenced or vilified throughout the Soviet period, the émigrés and their history became all the rage in Russia in the 1990s. In Moscow in 1988, a Harbin Association was established, and branches soon opened in other cities. In 1993, the Harbinites in Novosibirsk began publishing a newspaper titled *Na sopkakh Man'chzhurii* (On Manchuria Hills), which by February 2018 had reached its two hundredth issue. In 1995, Ekaterinburg followed with *Russkie v Kitae* (Russians in China), and in 1998 *Russkaia Atlantida* (Russian Atlantis) was started nearby in Chelyabinsk. These print platforms reanimated the aging community of Russians from China. With the advent of the internet, portals have emerged in which it has become possible for descendants and amateur historians to discuss Russian life in China and to post photographs and queries on family history.[68]

Harbinites still share their memories, respond to one another's publications, celebrate Russian and Chinese festivals, and meet for reunions. Along with the Russian *zemliak*, for "compatriot," they might call each other *losian*, after the Chinese term *laoxiang*.[69] Using selected Chinese words, eating Chinese dishes on special occasions, and playing mahjong are all signs of belonging to this community.[70] The first books on Harbin to be published in Russia in the 1990s, by Harbinites Elena Taskina (1927–2020) and Georgii Melikhov, were written primarily for this audience and helped foster pride in the Harbinite identity. In 1998, conferences on the centenary of Harbin were hosted in Moscow and Khabarovsk, although a conference planned in Harbin itself was vetoed by Beijing, which did not want to acknowledge that the city had been founded by Russians.

The Association of Former Residents of China in Israel, established in 1951, has published ever since a quarterly *Bulletin* in three languages, Russian, English, and Hebrew, which is received by subscribers in Israel and around the world. In 2007, the association's charismatic chairman Teddy Kaufman (1924–2012) challenged his readers to answer a remarkably detailed quiz of thirty questions under the title, "Do You Remember and Know the Past of Harbin?"[71] Naturally, *Bulletin* readers still refer to the Russian rather than the Chinese street names of the city they left. Besides helping elderly *kharbintsy* and a smaller contingent of *shankhaitsy* (the Russian equivalent of Shanghailanders) remember their Harbin and Shanghai, and influencing the ways in which they remember them, the association supports people in material need and distributes university scholarships to members' descendants. As it takes one of its missions to be promoting friendship between Israel and the PRC, it frequently hosts Chinese delegations.

Over the past twenty years, the association's delegates and many of its members have travelled to Harbin, either individually or to take part in large reunions, which the Chinese side has hosted. Jewish "repatriation" to Israel has been part of the process by which homelands in the twentieth century have been invented by acts of faith and ideology and the need for an imagined community. Some of those who repatriated to Israel from China later moved again, but most of them accepted the Zionist ideal of Israel as the motherland that Jews had regained after

2,000 years of exile. Thus they were reluctant to revisit the places they were born, or where they passed significant parts of their lives, until the moral grip of this conception had weakened.[72] At about the same time, travelling to China or to Eastern Europe became possible politically and financially.

Nostalgia among the former residents of the mixed Baltic cities brings them and their descendants back to the now thoroughly changed Riga or Tallinn much as it attracts Harbinites to the new Harbin. In the capital of Heilongjiang province, as a historian has said of Alexandria, "the cosmopolitan cityscape remains, inhabited by a largely homogeneous 'native' population."[73] Books about formerly cosmopolitan cities that lost a part of their residents to exile, expulsion, or extermination, or a combination of all three, often end with cemeteries and the ghosts of the forgotten and disrespected dead. These places are presented as repositories of authenticity, symbols of the city as it once was and as it should have stayed.[74] A historian of Tartu (former Dorpat and Iur'ev) makes a stronger case by concluding that despite the ravages of the twentieth century, today's Tartu belongs to its new residents "who are no strangers to this city and its past."[75]

The graves of Baron Budberg and his wife Li in Harbin are long gone, and so are their cemeteries, foreign and Chinese respectively. No original buildings survive on Harbin's former Kavkazskaia Street (now Xi sandao jie), where the Budberg house once stood. Similarly, no traces remain of the section of Turu Street (Marktstrasse, or Rynochnaia ulitsa), where Roger and Joseph Budberg lived in Tartu: it was destroyed by bombing in the Second World War. During the last phase of warfare in the Baltic, the battles between the Soviet and German armies in the so-called Courland Pocket, the Budberg manor Gemauert Poniemon suffered the same fate. It is exceptional that the father of the Budberg siblings, who remained on his estate at the twilight of empire, still has an inscribed gravestone in Budberga village – and that even the resting place of the Moor, whose life of fantastic travels and role changes seemingly had so little to do with his own choosing, is still known, although only in memory.

Some former residents of Harbin have refused to recognize the modern Chinese city, limiting their nostalgic feelings to the Harbin of their past.[76] Yet having lost or driven out its "foreign" population, Harbin lives on as a sprawling metropolis with many other concerns besides its international heritage, and even today it extends some limited space to Russians. The members of the Russian emigration remaining in Harbin had dwindled to less than a dozen by the 1990s. Together with the descendants of mixed families, they congregated around the last functioning Russian church, where services were given by a Chinese priest, Father Grigorii (Zhu Shipu, 1925–2000), a convert to Russian Orthodoxy in Peking, who had barely survived the Cultural Revolution in Harbin.[77] Before the last Russian Harbinite died in the city aged ninety-six in 2006, she had become the object of intense curiosity as a relic of a bygone era: interviews with her by Russian and Chinese visitors had appeared in Russia as well as in Harbin. However, among those most nostalgic about "old Harbin" at present are newcomers to the city: Russian citizens, who settled there as ex-pats beginning in the 1990s and in 2005 founded the "Russian Club in Harbin."

Club members meet for social activities, often tied to preserving the Russian language and culture among their children. On Victory Day (9 May), they make a pilgrimage to the graves of Red Army soldiers, who, in the narrative they espouse, liberated Manchuria in 1945. They are closely engaged in commemorating Harbin's Russian past and cultivate connections with Harbinites abroad and their descendants. In 2015, the head of the club's historical section published *Beloved Harbin*, sketches on "the most Russian of all Chinese cities."[78] In June 2018, with the permission of Harbin's municipal authorities, the club hosted a Russian-language conference under the title "Beloved Harbin: The City of Russia's and China's Friendship." The event was officially tied to the 120th "anniversary of Russian history in Harbin" – a diplomatic formulation meant to avoid controversy on whether a "Chinese history" had predated the Russian.

While some of these expressions of Russian nostalgia for Harbin clash with the approved Chinese version of how the city came to be, among educated Chinese residents there is wide interest in Harbin's history that is often just as nostalgic. Non-academic enthusiasts of local history are rarely able to read documents in Russian. Instead, many find their connection to "old Harbin" through artefacts, especially photographs and other relics that can still be found in private possession and that come up for sale in flea markets.[79] The journalist Zeng Yizhi (1954–2017), who came to Harbin as a child, sought out and interviewed the last Russian Harbinites beginning in the 1990s, and campaigned fearlessly for the preservation of the city's architectural heritage. This campaigning earned her harassment from local administrators and the real-estate developers, whose joint interest was to have old buildings demolished and who usually prevailed in the end. Like Ah Cheng, having witnessed the pulling down of St Nicholas Cathedral, Zeng Yizhi "could never forget" that day, 23 August 1966.[80] By now there are few buildings to be saved: from the perspective of the twenty-first century, the city of a mere hundred years ago seems irretrievably lost.[81]

However, between 2015 and 2017, a decade after completing the restoration of St Sophia Cathedral, the Harbin municipality demolished the city's main railway station, which had replaced the old tsarist station in 1959. Now arrivals to Harbin by rail are greeted by a modernized replica of the original railway station, which Russian architects had constructed in Art Nouveau style between 1899 and the Russo-Japanese War. Beyond the museified façades of select buildings in the Harbin city centre, which too are exploited by the tourist industry, the notion of "Russian Harbin" has been transferred to Sun Island, on the north bank of the Songhua River. There, in the so-called Russian Village and Russian Golden Theatre, staffed by migrant workers from the Russian Far East, Russianness is consumed as fake Orthodox churches and *izbas* (rural log cabins), oil paintings of Russian motifs, vodka, and sexual titillation. On the banks of Ashihe River, in 2006, a Chinese businessman launched another theme park and hotel complex, the Volga Manor. Next to copies of tsarist castles, marble sculptures, cafés called "Misha" and "Masha," the Russian village "Alenka," and a fake Protestant church for fashionable wedding ceremonies, there is a life-size copy of St Nicholas Cathedral, designed by the historian of architecture from Khabarovsk, Nikolai P. Kradin.

Pictures of Harbin city streets from foundation to 1932 – often enhanced by adding colour to black-and-white photographs – are used abundantly in marketing and entertainment. They sustain local nostalgia for what is perceived as the benign age before the Japanese occupation, a time when erstwhile imperialists turned into refugees and became the objects of Chinese charity. Nostalgia for "old Harbin" echoes that for "old Shanghai," a source of influence for the northeast. But the recovery of any reliable information about that past for Harbin residents today is fraught with difficulty. The language gap obstructs access to "foreign" Harbin by largely monolingual Chinese-speakers. Even more decisively, the Chinese Communist discourse and world view shape the ways the past may be conceptualized and spoken about. The concerns of the present, determined by the changing priorities of the Party and the market, take precedence over truthful reporting, while low standards of history writing make filling in the blanks by uninformed guesswork a usual practice.

These problems are reflected in the complete disappearance of Roger Budberg from historical memory in Harbin and in the form of some recent efforts to rediscover his life and writings. A copy of *Bilder aus der Zeit der Lungenpest-Epidemien in der Mandschurei 1910/11 und 1921* was donated to the Memorial Hall of Dr Wu Liande (Lien-teh) when it opened in the former building of the North Manchuria Plague

Prevention Service in Harbin's Daowai quarter in autumn 2008. Wu had ascended to the status of an officially sanctioned hero in Harbin; all credit for plague prevention in Manchuria is ascribed to him as the Chinese physician who fought against the deadly epidemics of 1910 and 1920 and who safeguarded China's national interest. The encomiums for Wu fail to mention that, upon arriving in Harbin in 1910, he worked closely with the Russian medical administration instead of resisting it. Moreover, labelling him as a Chinese patriot ignores his dual allegiance. Wu kept his British nationality; after leaving Manchuria for Peking and Shanghai in 1931, he moved to Hong Kong during the Sino-Japanese War and returned to his native Penang in 1946.[82] At the permanent exhibition on Wu Liande in Harbin, Budberg's book on the plague has attracted visitors' interest because of the dramatic visual images it contains. In April 2018, the daughter of the person who donated the book to the Memorial Hall told the story behind it in an article posted on the internet.[83]

In the 1920s, the grandfather of the online author was already proficient in Japanese, English, and Russian when he decided to learn German, too. His language teacher then brought him the Budberg book as a gift from a home visit to Germany. Settling in Harbin in 1929, the grandfather, a physician from Shenyang, was soon appointed director of the Harbin Municipal Hospital and later filled other top positions in the Harbin medical establishment. He was so fascinated by the German book on plague in Manchuria that he kept it until the end of his life and in 1975 passed it on to his son, with the hope that it might be translated. Accordingly, in the 1980s, Harbin paediatrician Jia Shuhua (b. 1922) began translating the book into Chinese together with a colleague, who knew German. Yet as the author of the article in 2018 put it, "for reasons that everybody understands," their translation remained unpublished.

As she does reproduce the intended preface of the manuscript, it emerges that the translators considered "Baron" to have been the book author's surname. They regarded him as a German, who entered CER service and "in 1910" married "Li Shuzhen" (the Chinese characters, which the translators chose, amount to a reverse translation from the German transcription), supposedly an actress of Peking opera (a guess based on the photographs). Baron called his daughter "The Flower of Germany and China" (a telling reversal of the order of nations in Zhong-De-Hua's name), and he eventually repatriated to Germany (as assumed from the author's ethnicity, or the book's place of publication). Moreover, the translators claimed that Li died of the plague at Dr Wu's hospital (she died of relapsing fever, at home), and they made up and "quoted" praise allegedly found in the book for Wu's "deep knowledge and spirit of national patriotism." In the actual work, Budberg saw Wu as one of the abhorred reformers of traditional China and denigrated him as a servile follower of the West and a stranger to the country of his ancestors (he also had harsh criticism for Wu's hospital).[84] He certainly never called him, in the recognizable style of PRC propaganda, "a good son of the Chinese nation, who with the highest professional dedication, at the risk of life and limb, busily worked day and night to rescue the dying and support the wounded at the front line of the epidemic of pneumonic plague."[85]

Harbin as it was in the first half of the twentieth century is still being reimagined, idealized, and dreamed about by former inhabitants of that city, spread over many countries. As mentioned in the last chapter, some Harbin Chinese evacuated with the Nationalist Party to Taiwan in 1949 (a Russian family who also went to Taiwan were the Chistiakovs: the senior CER official, initiated into the Rosicrucian Order in Baron Budberg's cellar, moved there with his wife and daughter in 1956).[86] Nostalgia for the northeast has persisted on the island, uniting ethnic Manchus and Han Chinese.[87] Feelings for Harbin become especially complex in Japan by being mixed with guilt about the army's conduct in the war; Japanese returns to "Manchuria" are therefore partly attempts at redemption.[88] One unusually independent person, however, the poet Kumiko Muraoka, who was raised in Harbin and transported to Japan with her family at the age of ten in August 1946, resisted so-called repatriation to the country of her parents as a terrible "misunderstanding" and a "deportation." She used the first opportunity to re-emigrate to France in 1966 and there, too, never stopped considering Harbin her true and perfect home. She missed everything: the views, the streets, the mix of languages, the food (both Russian and Chinese), and a Chinese domestic named Vassili.[89]

A Home in China

In his last known letter to his sister, Roger Budberg wrote that his home in Harbin had been built on sand. He did not mean this metaphorically: the house on Kavkazskaia Street had been constructed without foundations, of half-brick laid on plain wooden boards. By autumn 1925, as his life neared its end, his house, too, was collapsing.[90] Budberg's story is exceptional, in that he made China his permanent home and a second homeland. China became central to his sense of self soon after his arrival there and remained so to the very end. Although profoundly attached to his aristocratic German origins, he illustrated the argument that "to acquire a new identity does not mean betraying the first one, but

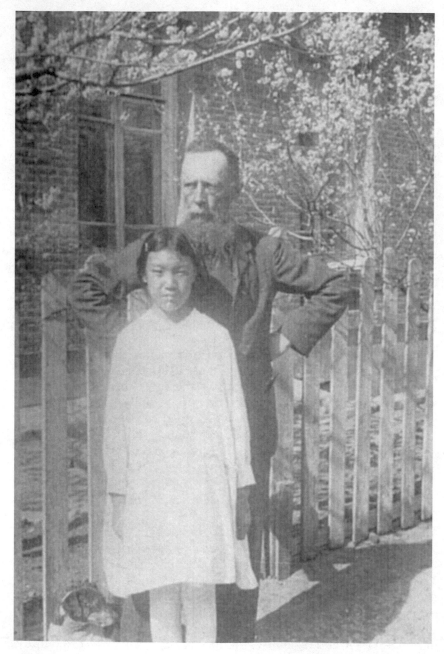

E.2. Roger Budberg and his daughter Zhong-De-Hua in front of their house on Kavkazskaia Street. Photograph in Popoff family album.

enriching one's own self with a new soul."[91] The glimpses that his biography provides into the lives of individuals like Johan W.N. Munthe, and even August Stöffler, show that, although untypical, he was not a lone case. Beyond the Budberg story, we have seen how China became important to the peripatetic thinker Vsevolod Ivanov, and to a small group of young intellectuals in Russian Harbin.

The Russians in Harbin did not develop a "hyphenated identity" while living there. But they did begin viewing themselves, and begin to be viewed by others, as a special group defined by their past life in China, once they repatriated to Soviet Russia or re-emigrated from China to other destinations. In the Soviet Union, to be a "Harbinite" was to be a "traitor" during the purges of the 1930s and was still a background many preferred not to divulge to strangers, until, suddenly in the late 1980s, it became a badge of honour. Among Harbinites, a collective sense of belonging had been fashioned by this secrecy as well as by the strangeness of their Chinese experience when seen in retrospect from the Soviet Union, which made them feel apart from ordinary Soviet citizens.[92] Some of the Harbinites had absorbed elements of China, to varying degrees, depending on the vagaries of their biographies. Often people didn't realize in what ways living in China had influenced them. The same may be said about Russian influence on the Chinese who remained in Harbin after their Russian neighbours had departed.

Hardly any of the former subjects of the Russian empire in the Chinese emigration dared to accept China as both their present and future. Most would never admit that thought, believing that they would inevitably go to Russia or move elsewhere. The temptation at last to acquire a home for good – which the Chinese called *luodi shenggen*, "fall to the ground and put down roots" – does appear in lyric poetry. In "The Refugee," the homeless poet Leonid Eshchin, a converted Jew, who had crossed the borders between Harbin and Fujiadian, begged the Russian Orthodox icon of the Mother of God for "fanza, kurma and chifan" (home, clothes, and food) "in that land, guarded by dragons." She understood his pidgin and granted him his wish, insofar as he died and was buried in the land about which he wrote.[93] Valerii Pereleshin imagined being born as the son of a scholarly Chinese clan, "in Baoshan or Chengdu," to grow up "in the intricate web/of Chinese characters and poems," only to conclude that he was "to the bone marrow a Russian/ lost Argonaut."[94]

Although not a border city in the conventional geographical sense, Harbin nonetheless lay between Russia and China. Committing oneself to life in China after the protective shell of "Russian Harbin" no longer existed would have taken unusual courage and the effort of mastering a difficult language along with the rules of Chinese society. And of course, it would have required the readiness of the Chinese state and society to accept foreigners. Even the few persons who made that choice were to discover by the 1950s that their homes in China had been "built on sand." One of them, Pereleshin (ethnically Polish and Belarusian), said in a poem written in Brazil under the title "Three Motherlands" that he had been "expelled from China/Like from Russia – forever."[95] Still, together with the Russia of his birth and Brazil, which had accepted him, China remained "a motherland" and the place where, in another poem, he saw his soul returning in the end.[96] Another Russian poet (of Georgian and Polish extraction), who, like Pereleshin, was raised in Harbin and who later lived in Dairen, Tientsin, and Shanghai, Lydia Khaindrova (1910–1986), wrote in the Soviet Union about having "three Fatherlands," counting China along with Russia and Georgia.[97] Unlike Pereleshin, she had not learned Chinese, and in her old age she regretted (as did some other Harbinites) having missed an opportunity to get to know and even "love Manchuria and China."[98] It was an opportunity, perhaps a chance forgone, but by no means a duty. No moral judgment has been implied in this book about people who preferred to identify with a single country and culture – to live among their own and not to admit others.

It is a paradox that history is explained collectively but that historical explanations may only be partly and inadequately applied to individual cases. Few people (and fewer ordinary people) commit their thoughts and memories to paper or leave caches of letters that may be read many decades later. The ideas and feelings we find expressed in writing (and documents, published and archival, remain our main sources) were originally bound to a specific occasion and intended audience; their meaning did not remain constant even for their authors, but rather swayed with time and under the influence of changes in political and personal circumstances. Switching from the general to the specific, one discovers that the threads cannot be fully tied and the questions neatly answered, since every person's life is a riddle, first to him- or herself and all the more so for us, looking through a glass darkly, from the great distances of time and space. The historian's task is to allow you, the reader, to come closer to the people of the past and to understand the circumstances and constraints of their lives. Unlike historical novelists, historians do not pretend either to solve the riddles of their subjects or to bring them back to life by writing about them. What we can do for the few we select is to save them from generalization by respecting their uniqueness.

Notes

Introduction

1 The earliest version may have been *Man'zhuriia*, still used in Russian texts of the 1860s and 1870s. *Mandzhuriia* and *Manchzhuriia* were employed interchangeably in the 1890s.

2 "Man'chzhuriia," in *Entsiklopedicheskii slovar' Brokgauz i Efron*, vol. 18a (1896), 574–81. The entry was divided between the two leading Russian specialists on the region, Aleksei O. Ivanovskii (1863–1903) and Dmitrii M. Pozdneev (1865–1937). In the following year, Pozdneev published his pioneering monograph, *Opisanie Man'chzhurii*.

3 Andrei Belyi, *Peterburg* (Moscow: Respublika, 1994), esp. 271, 381. The hats also refer ironically to the Russian boast about the ease with which they would defeat the Japanese enemy: *shapkami zakidaem* ("we'll only need to throw [our] hats at them!"). The red flags, associated with the hat wearers in the novel, harked back to China's Boxers as much as to the first Russian Revolution. Compare the use of *Mandzhuriia* by Ivan Bunin (1870–1953), in his stories "Derevnia" (The Village, 1909–10) and "Sootechestvennik" (The Compatriot, 1916). In 1914, the inspector of schools Pavel E. Sokolovskii (1860–1934) reported in his *Russkaia shkola v Vostochnoi Sibiri i Priamurskom Krae* from a region he spelled as *Manzhuriia* on one occasion, *Mandzhuriia* on another, and *Manchzhuriia* on a third (2, 110–11, 278).

4 For Russian-Chinese diplomatic relations in the Far East, from the Treaty of Aigun to the Russo-Japanese War, see Paine, *Imperial Rivals*, pts 1 and 3.

5 Quested, *"Matey" Imperialists?*, 100.

6 Xue Lianju, *Ha'erbin renkou bianqian*, 52–4.

7 Christie, *Thirty Years in Moukden*, ch. 20, "Suffering of the Innocent."

8 Salogub, "Stanovlenie smeshannykh sudov."

9 Bakich, "Russian Émigrés in Harbin's Multinational Past," 86–8.

10 See, on these events, Quested, *"Matey" Imperialists?*, ch. 16; and Belov, "Bor'ba za KVZhD v kontse 1917–nachale 1918 g."

11 Figures for May 1922: Melikhov, *Rossiiskaia emigratsiia v Kitae*, 58.
12 Figures rounded from Bakich, *Harbin Russian Imprints*, 2. The official figure for the total population of Harbin in 1929 is given here as 160,670.
13 Ablova, *KVZhD i rossiiskaia emigratsiia v Kitae*, 158–60; Melikhov, *Belyi Kharbin*, 390–405.
14 Nazemtseva, "Peredacha KVZhD v sobstvennost' SSSR."
15 Only three seats on the council were kept by Russians, with another seven being given to representatives of foreign business firms. Smirnov, *Rossiiskie emigranty v Severnoi Man'chzhurii*, 38.
16 Oblastnik, "Trekhrechenskaia golgofa"; Sibiriakov, "Konets zabaikal'skogo kazach'ego voiska," 216–19.
17 See Krotova, *SSSR i rossiiskaia emigratsiia v Man'chzhurii*, 194–220.
18 These acts are described at length in Vespa, *Secret Agent of Japan*. See also Gamsa, "The Many Faces of Hotel Moderne in Harbin."
19 According to archival data collected by the late historian Bruce Adams and published in Wolff, "Returning from Harbin," 97, the repatriation of 1935 included 21,343 persons (making up 7,400 families), who departed from Harbin in eighty-four trains.
20 This is the main theme of Moustafine, *Secrets and Spies*. See also Merritt, "Matushka Rossiia, primi svoikh detei!"
21 Kuznetsov, "'Arestu podlezhat vse,'" 142.
22 Meyer, "Garden of Grand Vision," 331, citing data from *Outline of the Manchukuo Empire, 1939*. Cf. Xue Lianju, *Ha'erbin renkou bianqian*, ch. 4, on the period between 1932 and 1948.
23 Ablazhei, "Russkie emigranty iz Kitaia," 24–5.
24 Manchester, "Repatriation to a Totalitarian Homeland," 354.
25 The Harbin Jewish community reached about 12,000 in the early 1920s; it then declined when Jews left Japanese-occupied Harbin for Shanghai and other Chinese cities. It diminished further after the sale of the CER to Japan in 1935. About 2,000 Jews still lived in Harbin in June 1949; by April 1962, only 48 remained. Altman, "Controlling the Jews, Manchukuo Style," 315; Agranovskii, "Evreiskaia obshchina Kharbina 1948–1962," no. 381, 54.
26 Khisamutdinov, *Rossiiskaia emigratsiia v Kitae*, 104–5.
27 For a review of later research on Harbin, in Russian and Chinese, see Gamsa, "The Historiography of Harbin."
28 Quested, *"Matey" Imperialists?*, 156. Cf. ibid., 3–4; ch. 7, "A Foetal Yellow Russia?"; and 277–84.
29 Alan Bullock, *Hitler and Stalin: Parallel Lives*, 2nd rev. ed. (London: Fontana, 1993).
30 Wu Hung, *Remaking Beijing: Tiananmen Square and the Creation of a Political Space* (London: Reaktion Books, 2005), 13. His book is constructed as two parallel narratives, one historical and the other autobiographical.

31 Quoted in James D. Houston, "Where Does History Live?," *Rethinking History* 11, no. 1 (March 2007), 51–60 at 59. The California writer James D. Houston (1933–2009) used the "double-track narrative" himself in *Snow Mountain Passage* (San Diego: Harcourt, 2002), a novel of the Donner Party.

32 In advance of the book's publication, preliminary versions of excerpts from chapters 1 and 3 appeared in *Ab Imperio* 3 (2019).

33 Readers interested in these thoughts may want to consult Mark Gamsa, "Challenges to Generalization in Historical Writing," *Storia della Storiografia* 63 (January 2013), 51–68; and idem, "Biography and (Global) Microhistory," *New Global Studies* 11, no. 3 (December 2017), 231–41.

1 Of Ethnicity and Identity

1 Crossley, *The Manchus*, 103, 122–5. For an introduction to the region, see Gamsa, *Manchuria: A Concise History*.

2 The ecological dimensions of Qing border policy are highlighted in Schlesinger, *A World Trimmed with Fur*.

3 Young, "Chinese Immigration and Colonization in Manchuria," 335.

4 Zhao Zhongfu, "The Role of the Government in Inter-regional Migration," 220–1, therefore calls the official ban on Han settlement in Manchuria "a myth."

5 Morrison, "Russian Settler Colonialism," 316–17.

6 Waley-Cohen, *Exile in Mid-Qing China*, 56–60; cf. Lee, *The Manchurian Frontier*, 79–87.

7 Thus Lobza, "V Mandzhurii," 282, observed that in Ninguta not a single Han Chinese could be found even in the lowest echelons of the local administration.

8 "Man'chzhuriia," in *Entsiklopedicheskii slovar' Brokgauz i Efron*, vol. 18a, 576.

9 Cf. Lee, *The Manchurian Frontier*, 113–15.

10 Shan, *Taming China's Wilderness*, 80–7.

11 Lee, *The Manchurian Frontier*, 42–9.

12 For much more information on all the ethnic groups mentioned in these paragraphs, see Janhunen, *Manchuria: An Ethnic History*, 50–1.

13 Lee, *The Manchurian Frontier*, 15–16, 34, 51.

14 According to Kachanovskii, "Kak zaselialsia Dal'nii Vostok," 11,700 indigenous people passed under Russian rule with the cession of land; their numbers reached 17,900 by 1897 but declined in later years due to recurring epidemics, of which smallpox claimed the heaviest toll.

15 Kim, "Saints for Shamans?," 192–3.

16 Vasily V. Ushanoff (1904–1989), "Recollections of Life in the Russian Community in Manchuria and in Emigration," 2, 5–6.

17 Sablin, *Governing Post-Imperial Siberia and Mongolia*, 33, 80.

18 The main study is now Park, *Sovereignty Experiments*.

19 Zhao Zhongfu, "The Role of the Government in Inter-regional Migration," 219, 227.

20 Idem, "Qingdai dongsansheng beibu de kaifa yu Hanhua," 2–4.

21 Gottschang, "Economic Change, Disasters, and Migration," 480, 484. For the larger context, see Li, *Fighting Famine in North China*, which cites the same data on page 301.

22 Zhao Zhongfu, "Qingdai dongsansheng," 11–12.

23 Gottschang, "Economic Change, Disasters, and Migration," 487n6.

24 Shan, *Taming China's Wilderness*, 17, 44.

25 Kachanovskii, "Kak zaselialsia Dal'nii Vostok," 187.

26 Aleksandrov, "Argun' i priargun'e," 286.

27 Ibid., 282–4. Cf. 296, 301 on Cossack cruelty toward Mongols in the area; quotation on page 302. On a Cossack ataman near Sretensk who ordered subordinates to shoot at a group of Chinese workers to test a gun, see A.A. Kaufman, *Po novym mestam*, 6. Karpov, "Sbornik slov," 16, confirms the use of *tvar'* by Cossacks as "the derisive nickname of all Manchus and Chinese."

28 Lindgren, "An Example of Culture Contact Without Conflict," based on fieldwork between 1929 and 1932.

29 See Remnev and Suvorova, " 'Russkoe delo' na aziatskikh okrainakh," 174–7; and Remnev, "Russians as Colonists at the Empire's Asian Borders," 134–5, 140.

30 On the Ems Edict and the earlier circular by Minister of the Interior Petr A. Valuev, which banned the publication of books in Ukrainian in 1863, see Alexei Miller, *The Ukrainian Question: The Russian Empire and Nationalism in the Nineteenth Century* (Budapest: CEU Press, 2003).

31 Hosking, *Russia: People and Empire*, 26–7.

32 Cipko, "Ukrainians in Manchuria," 156.

33 Chernolutskaia, "Ukrainskaia natsional'naia koloniia v Kharbine," 95–7. Another contribution by the same author, in *Rossiiane v Aziatsko-Tikhookeanskom Regione*, ed. Chernolutskaia et al., 30, estimates there were about 22,000 Ukrainians in the whole of Manchuria by 1917, when they would have made up about 10 per cent of the total Russian population. According to data collected by Ukrainian associations, more than 15,000 lived in Harbin from the 1920s to the 1930s. See Chernomaz, "Obshchestvenno-politicheskaia deiatel'nost'," 34.

34 Chernolutskaia, "Religious Communities in Harbin," 94.

35 Mao Hong, "Ha'erbin Zhong-E renmin shenghuo zhuangkuang," 116–17.

36 Hosking, *Russia*, 237–9.

37 Kaufman, *Po novym mestam*, 57, called them "the best pioneers of the Siberian and the Amur taiga" (cf. 153). Another example of such praise is Blagoveshchenskii, "Zapiski o Sibiri," 300–25.

38 Report by Sergei M. Dukhovskoi (1838–1901), quoted in D.E. Buianov, "Dukhovnye khristiane v Sibiri i na Dal'nem Vostoke," 66.

39 Quested, "A Fresh Look at the Sino-Russian Conflict," 489–92. Cf. Lensen, *The Russo-Chinese War*, 68–125, for an early study. T.N. Sorokina, "'The Blagoveshchensk Panic,'" 111, proposes the lowest estimate – 2,000 dead. See also Datsyshen, *Voina v Priamur'e*; and Petrov, *Istoriia kitaitsev v Rossii 1856–1917 gody*, 328–38. Zatsepine, "The Blagoveshchensk Massacre of 1900," is a one-sided interpretation, restated in idem, *Beyond the Amur*, 120–4.

40 Sun Rongtu, ed., *Aihui xianzhi, juan* 8, s. 6, 321–3, "Gengzi nian E-nan" (The Russian calamity of 1900.)

41 Testimonies about the killings of Chinese and Manchu farmers by Russians and the looting of their property are in Kaufman, *Po novym mestam*, 68–72, 83–4.

42 Guzei, *'Zheltaia opasnost','* 65–80, 104–26. The ubiquitous panic and wild rumours in Blagoveshchensk in summer 1900 were a prominent motif in the promptly issued chronicle of the siege by the local newspaper editor, Kirkhner, *Osada Blagoveshchenska i vziatie Aiguna*.

43 *Kharbinskii vestnik*, 1903, no. 17, quoted in Ermachenko, "'V Kharbine vse spokoino,'" 87.

44 Grauze, *Kitaiskie fragmenty*, 78–83.

45 V., "Blagoveshchenskaia 'utopiia.'" The article's author was Nikolai P. Vishniakov (1871–1937), at that time a colonel in the Military Judicial Administration, later a tsarist major-general and military judge.

46 On the use of the Blagoveshchensk massacre during the anti-Soviet campaign of 1975, see Cohen, *History in Three Keys*, 277–80; on the subsequent period, see Fromm, "Invoking the Ghosts of Blagoveshchensk." On memory in Russia, see Dyatlov, "The Blagoveshchensk Drowning," originally published in Russian in 2002. See also idem, "'The Blagoveshchensk Utopia,'" which compares reactions to his above article in Russia to the larger debate initiated in Poland by the publication of Jan T. Gross, *Neighbors: The Destruction of the Jewish Community in Jedwabne, Poland* (Princeton: Princeton University Press, 2001).

47 Sokolova, "Vospominaniia o pogrome v Manchzhurii," 826.

48 Stephan, *The Russian Far East*, 67–8; E.V. Buianov, *Dukhovnye khristiane molokane v Amurskoi oblasti*, 57–8.

49 Sokolova, "Vospominaniia," 828.

50 This is quoted approvingly in Dubinina, *Priamurskii general-gubernator N.I. Grodekov*, 237. Kirkhner, *Osada Blagoveshchenska*, 19–20, 37, asserted that the Chinese in town, as well as the Manchus of the "64 villages," had foreknowledge of the Qing attack against Russia. Several apologetic Russian accounts claimed, like Pozdneev, that fire was opened on the Chinese in the river from the Qing bank of the Amur. Anon., "Khronika

vnutrennei zhizni," 219, cites a letter about this from Blagoveshchensk
by a woman who added that she had saved her family cook, "a Chinese
from Chefoo," by having him christened on the day of the round-up. If
indeed the desperate swimmers could have been mistaken for an invading
Russian force, visibility across the river would not have allowed a glimpse
of Cossack "knives and axes," as depicted in the Aigun gazetteer.

51 See Sonin, "Bombardirovka Blagoveshchenska kitaitsami"; Deich, *16 let
v Sibiri*, 284–88 (the English version of these memoirs is in Leo Deutsch,
Sixteen Years in Siberia [London: J. Murray, 1903]); idem, *Krovavye dni*.
Having carried out political propaganda among Molokans in Ukraine
in the 1870s, Deich would have been attentive to their doings in
Blagoveshchensk, yet he never connected them to the massacre.

52 See the reports of the Blagoveshchensk Chief of Police dated 29 July and
7 September 1900, translated in Sorokina, " 'The Blagoveshchensk Panic,' "
105–8.

53 Meakin, *A Ribbon of Iron*, 6–7. On Meakin's impressions of the handsome
and urbane general, 240.

54 Kaufman, *Po novym mestam*, 22, 50–1. See entries on the novel *Amurskie
volki* and its main author, Aleksandr I. Matiushenskii (1862–1931), who
spent his last years in Harbin, in *Entsiklopediia literaturnoi zhizni Priamur'ia
XIX–XXI vekov*, ed. Urmanov, 28–30, 254–9. Cf. Buianov, *Dukhovnye
khristiane molokane*, 217, 315–18.

55 On the razed village, see Kirkhner, *Osada Blagoveshchenska*, 101–2; like
Nikitina's memoir cited below, Kirkhner's account ended with the sight of
Sakhalian in flames as it was observed from Blagoveshchensk.

56 Nikitina, "Osada Blagoveschenska kitaitsami v 1900 godu," 221.

57 Kirkhner, *Osada Blagoveshchenska*, 29, acknowledged that some Russians
plundered the corpses in the river. Weulersse, "Au Petchili et sur les
frontières de Mandchourie," 121–32, is an extensive description of razed
villages and floating corpses by a pro-Russian traveller bound from
Khabarovsk to Blagoveshchensk. A Belgian reporter and a Russian
officer saw the same sights while sailing in the opposite direction:
Tytgat, *Un reportage en Chine*, ch. 5, "Les massacres de Blagovetschensk";
Vereshchagin, *Po Manchzhurii 1900–1901 gg.*, pt i, 116–18. Cf. Galambos,
"The Blagoveshchensk Massacre of July 1900."

58 Aigun had been founded by the Ming on the left bank of the Amur and was
built anew on the right bank by the Qing in 1684. Summaries of its history
are in Kirkhner, *Osada Blagoveshchenska*, 99–101; and Qi Xuejun, "Aihui de
bianqian." Heihe was known unofficially as Sakhalian until the 1950s.

59 The text is quoted from the Blagoveshchensk press in Anon., "Khronika
vnutrennei zhizni," 224–5.

60 Shirokogoroff, *Social Organization the Manchus*, 3–4.

61 A rich literature exists on Yuan Chonghuan (1584–1630), whose ancestral home was in Dongguan, Guangdong; in English, see Becker, *The City of Heavenly Tranquillity*, ch. 18; and Swope, *The Military Collapse of China's Ming Dynasty*, ch. 3. According to Zhang Jiangcai, *Dongguan Yuan dushi houyi kao*, 234–5, the general's son Yuan Wenbi joined the White Banner stationed in Ninguta, Jilin province; the Yuan family moved to Heilongjiang once Yuan Wenbi's son, Yuan Erhan, was appointed to the Aigun garrison in 1684.

62 Crossley, *The Manchus*, 80.

63 Shao, *Remote Homeland, Recovered Borderland*, 32.

64 This was a break with the traditional practice that prevented officials from serving in their home province. Shou Shan was appointed on the express request of his predecessor, having distinguished himself on the battlefield. See the biographical entry on Shou Shan in *Qingshi liezhuan*, vol. 61, 4824–7.

65 A.I., "Poslednie dni v Man'chzhurii," 147, describes "general Sheu" as "a young, energetic man, a good military commander, who had often been to Blagoveshchensk and was far from a sympathiser of the Russians." This article of 1900, by the wife of the Russian commander at Fularji station near Qiqihar, portrays Shou Shan as the villain in the story. By contrast, Datsyshen, "Shou Shan,'" 153–4, stresses Shou's knowledge of Russian and friendly relations with Governor Gribskii.

66 Liu Shude, "Wo suo zhidao de Shou Shan jiangjun zhi si." The story of the golden tablet is also in Vereshchagin, *Po Manchzhurii*, pt ii, 595. Bannermen killed their families and themselves after defeats in the Opium War and the Taiping Rebellion. Crossley, *Orphan Warriors*, 110–13, 131–3.

67 *Qingshi liezhuan*, vol. 61, 4827. Analysing this text, Li Xiangchen, "Shou Shan de kenhuang shibian sixiang," argues that Shou was ready to go further than any of his predecessors in confronting the court's deep resistance to permitting Han Chinese competition in the territory, which had long been a Manchu reserve.

68 See Crossley, *A Translucent Mirror*, esp. 45–50. Descendants of Shou Shan in the twentieth century would have been counted as Manchu (Manzu) by the modern Chinese state. Elliott, "Ethnicity in the Qing Eight Banners," 50–1.

69 The suicides in August 1900 of the Manchu governor of Zhili province and the former Han governor of Shandong are mentioned in Esherick, *The Origins of the Boxer Uprising*, 310.

70 Quested, "A Fresh Look," 494. On Jin Chang, see Ross, *The Boxers in Manchuria*.

71 Lee, *The Manchurian Frontier*, 140–1.

72 Quested, "A Fresh Look," 496–7, praises this as a feat of pragmatism. In the *Qingshi* (History of the Qing, published on Taiwan in 1961), too, Chang is lauded for having spared his province the retributions the enemy forces exacted in Heilongjiang.

73 Ermachenko, "'V Kharbine vse spokoino,'" 91.
74 Harbin's Molokans also published their own journal, *Vestnik dukhovnykh khristian* (The Herald of Spiritual Christians, 1934–40).
75 See, for example, the beginning of Sokolova's "Vospominaniia," a part of her memoirs that should be dated to 1899 (81–2); see also Kaufman, *Po novym mestam*, 113.
76 Note the title of the main study in English, Gottschang and Lary, *Swallows and Settlers: The Great Migration from North China to Manchuria.*
77 Bix, "Japanese Imperialism and the Manchurian Economy, 1900–31," 426, 431. On the *wopeng*, cf. Zhao Zhongfu, "Qingdai dongsansheng," 55–6. These aspects of the Chinese migration are emphasized in Reardon-Anderson, *Reluctant Pioneers.*
78 Figures from Wolff, *To the Harbin Station*, 31–3, 43. The mechanics in coolie recruitment in Chefoo are described in T.N. Sorokina, "Kitaiskaia immigratsiia na Dal'nii Vostok Rossii."
79 "A significant and curious fact is that, despite the recent massacres not only in Manchuria but to a smaller degree in the neighbourhood of Vladivostock, Chinese coolies are proceeding in large numbers to Southern Manchuria and to Port Arthur, where, by working under the Muscovites, they are actually assisting the Russification of their own country." Colquhoun, "Manchuria in Transformation," 60. The explorer Paul Labbé, on a visit to Dal'nii, was similarly puzzled; see his *Les Russes en Extrême-Orient*, 160. Weulersse, "Au Petchili," 99, 102, 104, wondered what a Chinese service crew was doing aboard a German ship preparing to join the Allied forces against the Boxers, and why the Chinese in Chefoo supplied coal to the enemy fleet (105).
80 See, for example, Lobza, "V Mandzhurii," 276–7; see also the concluding paragraph of Runich, "V Man'chzhurii," 270–1.
81 See Young, "Chinese Immigration and Colonization in Manchuria," 349–52. "Each home in the pioneer community includes the *lares* and *penates* of the former abode ... And over every community hovers the memory of the ancestral village" (352).
82 Cf. Bayly, *The Birth of the Modern World, 1780–1914*, ch. 6, "Nation, Empire, and Ethnicity, c. 1860–1900". See also the introduction in Naimark, *Fires of Hatred*, on the links between ethnic cleansing and modern conceptions of nation and race.
83 All quotations are from Sokolova, "Vospominaniia," 93.
84 Ibid., 88.
85 Ibid., 101. It was Mme Roganova who had thrown "beads, sweets and nuts" at the raging natives in Lahasusu; "the little horned god" was in the end awarded to her for these efforts. Ross, *The Boxers in Manchuria*, 13, noted that "Manchurian dust saturates the air in dry and windy weather."

86 Vereshchagin, *Po Manchzhurii*, pt i, 136; and Heretz, *Russia on the Eve of Modernity*, 150.

87 Among the shallow Russian stereotypes of the Chinese, one early settler disparagingly listed "eating garlic and millet [*chumiza*]." Semigorov, "Ocherki Girinskoi provintsii," 393. A physician at the Russian embassy in Peking, who thought that the Chinese "stood immeasurably higher than the civilized Western nations" in many aspects of daily life, explained the medical uses of garlic and other pungent herbs in the Chinese tradition. Korsakov, "Verovaniia i sueveriia u kitaitsev," 656, 658–60. A strongly pro-Chinese diary kept by a military physician during the Russo-Japanese War, first published in 2016, described Chinese peasants (and their villages) as cleaner than their Russian counterparts but their body odour as unbearable. Kravkov, *Voina v Man'chzhurii*, 49. See also Mo Yan, *The Garlic Ballads*, trans. Howard Goldblatt (1988; New York: Viking, 1995). A comparative angle on the odour of garlic, as a marker of national and social distinction, is offered in Mark S.R. Jenner, "Civilization and Deodorization? Smell in Early Modern English Culture," in Peter Burke, Brian Harrison, and Paul Slack, eds., *Civil Histories: Essays Presented to Sir Keith Thomas* (Oxford: Oxford University Press, 2004), 138–43.

88 "The funeral rites are… the binding force that holds together the family and the clan as a religious corporation throughout the generations." Thompson, *Chinese Religion*, 51.

89 During the Russo-Japanese War, the physician of the French embassy in Peking and scholar of China, Jean-Jacques Matignon (1866–1928), reported on dogs fighting over bodies pulled out of coffins that had been left to lie on the open ground near Mukden. Matignon, "Moukden, capitale de la Mandchourie," 241–2. Similar scenes were recorded by Kravkov, *Voina v Man'chzhurii*, 28–30, 38, 141. Another sympathetic observer of Chinese customs in Manchuria described public executions and the discarded bodies being consumed by dogs and pigs. Rotshtein, "Manchzhurskie ocherki," pt ii, 496–9, 503–5.

90 Khvostov, "Russkii Kitai," pt i, 662–3, 675. The article's optimistic title failed to predict, in 1902, the consequent loss of southern Manchuria to the Japanese.

91 Grulev, "Iz poezdki v Man'chzhuriiu," 946–8.

92 Lattimore heard from the Hezhe that their burial customs were like those of the Manchus, but his Chinese informant was uncertain whether "a temporary shelter for a coffin awaiting burial" that they saw was Gold or Chinese. Lattimore, "The Gold Tribe," 6, 7, 51. A garrison post was established in Sanxing in 1714. From 1732 to the mid-nineteenth century, the town was the principal site of tribal and Manchu commercial exchange, regulated by the Qing tribute system in Jilin (in Heilongjiang, the same function was fulfilled by Qiqihar). Lee, *The Manchurian Frontier*, 15, 34, 45–8.

93 Sokolova's "Prince Kh-ov" is Stepan N. Khilkov (1866–1916); see Melikhov, *Man'chzhuriia dalekaia i blizkaia*, 64–5. On his instructions, in 1898, the future factory manager Roganov explored the environs for clay deposits. See Sokolova, "Vospominaniia," 100, on the "removal" of the Chinese village with compensation paid and the immediate launch of brick production by hired Chinese workers.

94 See more in Xiao Hong, *The Field of Life and Death*, esp. 55–60.

95 Coltman, *The Chinese, Their Present and Future*, 77. Cf. Wolf, "Gods, Ghosts, and Ancestors," 147–8. There is brief mention of the same practice in Manchuria in the memoirs of other physicians; see Botkin, "Svet i teni russko-iaponskoi voiny 1904–5 gg.," 70; Christie, *Thirty Years in Moukden*, 37; Kravkov, *Voina v Man'chzhurii*, 311; and Böttcher, *Die Kolonne Ihrer Majestät*, 127–8.

96 Lobza, "Kitaiskie sektanty," 16–17; for the same discoveries in Harbin of the late 1930s or early 1940s, see Nikolaeva, *Iapontsy*, 65.

97 Lobza, "V Mandzhurii," 278–9.

98 The American missionary Justus Doolittle, in his *Social Life of the Chinese*, vol. 2, 369, offered this reason as well as the extinction of the families who would normally have tended to relatives' remains to explain a similar phenomenon, which he observed in mid-nineteenth-century Fuzhou, the port capital of Fujian province in southern China. Temporary burial sites were also described on the basis of Fujian material by De Groot in *The Religious System of China*, vol. 1, 129–32. De Groot wrote that "sending the dead to their ancestral home, there to be buried, is indeed very common with the well-to-do," but that on his walks in the Fujian countryside he often saw the earth "studded with corpses awaiting interment," the coffins either lying in the fields or piled up in small huts – probably of the type that Lobza described as "burial vaults." An early travel account by James, *The Long White Mountain*, 140–1, 305, made note of coffins being shipped home, and of neglected coffins left to rot on the ground, in different locations in Manchuria.

99 Contrary to the practices of temporary burial, the importance that Chinese migrants attached to transporting their dead home impressed Russian observers: see R.F., "Vospominaniia iz zhizni na Amure," 357–8; Baranov, "Po kitaiskim khramam Ashikhe," 199.

100 Becker, *The City of Heavenly Tranquillity*, 26–7; and, for childhood impressions of a Chinese cemetery, my interview in Ogre, Latvia, on 22 September 2018, with Natalia Nikolaeva (Laletina), born in Harbin in 1931.

2 Beginnings

1 The shared grandmother of Roger Budberg's parents Alexander and Alexandrine was Anna Magdalene, née Baranoff (1777–1845), mother

of Andreas Budberg by her first marriage and of Cecile Elmpt by her
second. Genealogical and biographical data are drawn from many
sources, the most important of which (not separately cited below) have
been the family genealogy by Roger's father, Alexander Baron von
Budberg-Gemauert-Poniemon, *Beiträge zu einer Geschichte des Geschlechtes
der Freiherrn v. Bönninghausen genannt Budberg*; the self-published
pamphlets by Nikolai Baron von Budberg, *Budbergiana. Beiträge zur
Familiengeschichte*; and the genealogy of Barons von Bönninghausen gen.
Budberg, the extinct line Gemauert-Poniemon, by Klas Lackschewitz
(ms received from the author and gratefully acknowledged). I gained
unique insights into the family lore, surroundings, and atmosphere of
the Budberg household from the memoirs of Roger's sister Antoinette,
written between 1945 and 1948 with commentary by her son, the art
historian Joseph A. Raczynski, *'Lebenserinnerung' meiner Mutter. Notizen
zur Geschichte der Familie Budberg* (unpublished typescript, Munich, 1980–1,
hereafter cited as *Lebenserinnerung*). I would have been severely impaired
in my interpretation of Roger Budberg without the privilege of accessing
his private letters from Harbin, which miraculously survived war and
emigration: *Roger Budberg: Briefe an seine Schwester Antoinette 1903–1925*,
with commentary by Joseph A. Raczynski (unpublished typescript,
Munich, 1986; hereafter cited as *Briefe*, followed by letter date, with
commentaries indicated by page number). For German Baltic biography,
the first port of call is Feest, ed., *Baltisches Biographisches Lexikon digital*, the
online entries in which are hereafter indicated by the abbreviation BBL;
for information on place names, Feldmann and von zur Mühlen, eds.,
Baltisches historisches Ortslexikon.

2 Amalie's grandmother, Countess Eleonore Caroline zu Leiningen (1771–
1832), was one of the four children born to Duke Carl Theodor of Bavaria
(1724–1799) and his mistress, the actress Maria Josepha Seyffert, later
Countess von Heydeck (1748–1771). *Lebenserinnerung*, app. 2, 18–28;
cf. Otto Freiherrn Stockhorner von Starein, *Die Stockhorner von Starein*.

3 Following standard practice, the German term Livland is used here for
the tsarist period. The name Livonia, which is more natural in English, is
associated with an earlier polity (Old Livonia, 1207–1561).

4 Entry on Andrei Ia. Budberg in Shilov, *Gosudarstvennye deiateli Rossiiskoi
imperii*, 95–6; and more in Grigorash, "Budberg Andrei Iakovlevich."

5 Quested, "Further Light on the Expansion of Russia in East Asia," 341–2;
Oxana Zemtsova, *Russification and Educational Policies in the Middle Volga
Region (1860–1914)*, PhD diss., European University Institute, Florence,
2014, 45.

6 Shilov and Kuz'min, *Chleny Gosudarstvennogo soveta Rossiiskoi imperii*, 90–1.

7 The Russian strategy led to the dispatch of a naval expedition under
Admiral Putiatin and the signing of the Treaty of Shimoda in 1855, a year

after the treaty negotiated for the United States by Commodore Perry. On the role of ambassador Budberg in the scheme, see Edgar Franz, *Philipp Franz von Siebold and Russian Policy and Action on Opening Japan to the West in the Middle of the Nineteenth Century* (Munich: Iudicium Verlag, 2005), 94–105.

8 Mednikov, "Rossiiskii posol v neitral'noi Ispanii."

9 Shilov and Kuz'min, *Chleny Gosudarstvennogo soveta Rossiiskoi imperii*, 88–90; on the chancellery, and Alexander Budberg as its head, see Alpern Engel, "In the Name of the Tsar."

10 *Lebenserinnerung*, 1–2 (which wrongly refers to "Alexander I"), 47; and, on Alexander Theodor Budberg, entry in BBL. Anna (Annette) Fuhrmann was born in 1837 according to the above memoir, or in 1832 according to standard genealogies, which do not mention the putative royal connection. She died in 1907.

11 Karl Vasil'evich, by his German name Carl Ludwig von Budberg. See BBL. Along with the entire gallery of more than three hundred portraits of Russian generals, Budberg's portrait was made by the English painter George Dawe (1781–1829); a German artist portrayed Tsar Alexander.

12 See Domnin, ed., *Voennyi al'bom generala A.P. Budberga*.

13 On Peter A. Boodberg, see esp. ch. 11 in Honey, *Incense at the Altar*.

14 The poem begins with the words: "I don't remember when Budberg died." Its protagonists are three foreign academics at Berkeley: Peter Boodberg, the Chinese literary scholar and poet Chen Shih-Hsiang (Peking, 1912–Berkeley, 1972), and Miłosz himself: "What a procession! *Quelles délices!* / What caps and hooded gowns! / Most respected Professor Budberg, / Most distinguished Professor Chen, / Wrong Honorable Professor Miłosz / Who wrote poems in some unheard-of tongue. / Who will count them anyway." See "A Magic Mountain," trans. by the author and Lillian Vallee, in Czesław Miłosz, *The Collected Poems: 1931–1987* (New York: The Ecco Press, 1988), 317–18. Miłosz was awarded the Nobel Prize in Literature in 1980.

15 On Moura Budberg (née Mariia I. Zakrevskaia, 1892–1974), see Deborah McDonald and Jeremy Dronfield, *A Very Dangerous Woman: The Lives, Loves, and Lies of Russia's Most Seductive Spy* (London: Oneworld, 2015).

16 See entry in BBL. Roger Budberg supplied materials for an article on his great-grandfather, published in Riga in 1904. See Stackelberg, "Heinrich Reinhold von Anrep," 23n1.

17 Krebs, *Niederau-Krauthausen und die Herrschaft Burgau*, 128.

18 *Briefe*, 9 June 1922 and 13 June 1922.

19 Lamping and Lamping, "Die Australienreisen von Reinhold Graf Anrep-Elmpt," 188–9, 197–8.

20 Obst, "Reinhold Graf Anrep-Elmpts letzte Reise."

21 *Lebenserinnerung*, 7, and commentary by Joseph A. Raczynski. The date and place indicated in secondary sources (which do not give the cause of death) are 26 August 1888 in Main-Ling-Gyll (Siam). I am grateful to Professor Dhiravat na Pombejra for deciphering the latter for me as a corrupt transcription for "Maing-lon-gyi" in Burmese, or "Moeng Loen Long" / "Muang Loen Luang" in Siamese. It is the present-day town of Mae Sariang, Mae Hongson province, in the far north of Thailand along the Myanmar border.

22 Anrep-Elmpt, *Reise um die Welt*, vol. 1, 247–8, 262–3, 268–71, 274, 279. Anrep-Elmpt became best-known for his travels in Hawai'i and Australia: see entry in Howgego, *Encyclopedia of Exploration*, vol. 3: *1850 to 1940: The Oceans, Islands, and Polar Regions*, 35.

23 Photographs of the tomb, made in 1937, are in the Raczynski family album.

24 Stockhorner von Starein, *Die Stockhorner von Starein*, 94.

25 The birthplaces of Joseph and Cecile, not indicated in other sources, are given as Gemauert Poniemon in *Lebenserinnerung*, 4 (commentary).

26 *Lebenserinnerung*, app. 2, 2. Grigorash, "Budberg Andrei Iakovlevich," 49, discusses Magnushof as the birthplace of foreign minister Andreas Eberhard Budberg in 1750. His mother was granted perpetual lease of this manor a year after the death of her husband, Andreas's father, the Russian colonel Jacob Wilhelm Budberg, in the Battle of Kunersdorf against Prussia in August 1759, a pivotal event in the Seven Years' War (1756–63).

27 Russian State Historical Archive (hereafter RGIA), f. 1344, op. 19, d. 1547.

28 Telephone interview with Mrs Velta Belmane, Riga, 27 July 2004.

29 Interviews in Budberga village, 21 October 2008.

30 Ancelāne, ed., *Latviešu tautas teikas*, 384; cf. 405–6. Velta Belmane and informants in Budberga village in 2008 told me similar stories, which also featured the cruel baroness. The local landlord in the early nineteenth century appears to have been Baron Diedrich Otto Karl von Grotthuss (1789–1839), marshal of the nobility in the Courland governorate between 1828 and 1836. See Erik-Amburger-Datenbank, "Ausländern im vorrevolutionären Russland."

31 *Lebenserinnerung*, 18, and photographs in the Raczynski family album (nos. 72–98).

32 This and the following paragraphs draw on *Lebenserinnerung* (here 11–12). Aunt Lonny was Helen Anrep-Elmpt (née Baroness Stackelberg, 1845–1931).

33 *Album Curonorum* (1903 edition), ed. Räder and Bettac, 203, lists Alexander Budberg's travels after graduating from university between 1859 and 1861.

34 See the entry on "professional education" in *Entsiklopedicheskii slovar' Brokgauz i Efron*, vol. 50 [25a], 563–74 at 573; and the chapter on Ponevezh County in Shul'man, *Goroda i liudi evreiskoi diaspory*, 20.

35 Interview with Kārlis Āzis in Budberga, 21 October 2008. Antoinette Raczynski also recalled her mother's reckless spending habits, in *Lebenserinnerung*, 62.

36 *Lebenserinnerung*, 18 (commentary).

37 Death announcement in *Rigasche Zeitung*, no. 232 (1876), copy among the Budberg family files in the Latvian State Historical Archives (hereafter LVVA), 4011/1/676/37.

38 Haltzel, "The Russification of the Baltic Germans."

39 *Lebenserinnerung*, 16. Information on his primary education in the Bergmann-Schultze school, Doblen, comes from Roger Budberg's papers at the Estonian Historical Archives (hereafter EHA), 402/2/3277.

40 The building, dating to the 1780s, until recently housed the Museum of Literature and Music.

41 *Lebenserinnerung*, 3, 5–6. Executions were carried out on the Town Hall Square (Latvian: Rātslaukums).

42 A school certificate survives as well, although the Gymnasium initially registered him, by the first of his four given names, as Andreas Budberg. LVVA 244/1/426, 427. I am most grateful to my research assistant Georgijs Dunajevs for locating this archival source and many others.

43 Only in his memoirs, published in Harbin in 1925, did he recall his expulsion from school in Riga, explaining it by his "striving for personal freedom": *Memuary Doktora-Meditsiny R.A. Barona Beningsgauzen-Budberg* (hereafter Budberg, *Memuary*), pt ii, 21.

44 On his studies at the school of Baroness Léocardie Freytag von Loringhoven (1842–1912) in Adiamünde (misprinted as "Freitag-Loringhofen" and "Abbiamünde"): *Lebenserinnerung*, 16–17. Cf. Goertz, "Beiträge zur Geschichte der baltischen Internate," 209–10.

45 His graduation was reported in the local press, filed under news from Goldingen: "Inland," *Libausche Zeitung*, no. 297 (21 December 1887), 2.

46 Entries on Alexander, Joseph, and Roger Budberg in the biographical dictionary of Dorpat University graduates, *Album Curonorum 1808–1932*, 91, 168–9, 187–8. For Roger's graduation diplomas from the Gymnasium zu Goldingen, in both Russian and German versions, see EHA, 402/2/3276. The restored two-storey building of his school, constructed in the 1840s in the red brick masonry of the German Romanesque revival, is now Kuldiga's pedagogical seminary.

47 *Personal der Kaiserlichen Universität zu Dorpat*, 14. After the Russification of the university, these registers of faculty, staff, and students were published in Russian, as *Lichnyi sostav imperatorskogo Iur'evskogo universiteta*. I am indebted to Dr Toomas Hiio of the Estonian Institute for Historical Memory, University of Tartu, for his kind help with these and related sources.

48 Joseph Budberg was originally sentenced to two years' imprisonment for his first duel and another year for his second. The trial verdicts and petitions to the tsar are collected in RGIA, f. 1405, op. 92, d. 5812.
49 Roger Budberg's grades in the Law Faculty are in EHA, 402/2/2343.
50 *Briefe*, 24 April 1924.
51 *Lebenserinnerung*, 10.
52 *Sitzungsberichte Naturforscher-Gesellschaft bei der Universität Dorpat* 10, no. 1 (1892), 2. His brother Gotthard participated in a similar society in Riga: see *Korrespondenzblatt des Naturforscher-Vereins zu Riga* 38 (1895), 13; 40 (1898), 67.
53 CV (probably dating to 1902) in EHA, 402/2/3277 (Russian and German versions). An attestation by the Faculty Dean (issued 14 February 1894) confirms that Roger Budberg had lost half a year of study due to work in cholera-infected localities. Cf. *Album Curonorum 1808–1932*, 187; Budberg, *Memuary*, pt ii, 5.
54 CV by Budberg in EHA, 402/2/3277; CV by Koch, with Budberg's name included on the list of the doctorates he supervised, in G.V. Levitskii, ed., *Biograficheskii slovar'professorov i prepodavatelei*, vol. 2, 290–4.
55 *Lebenserinnerung*, 17.
56 This clinic of Tartu University continued to function in the same location until as late as 2008. Salupere, *Tysiacheletnii Tartu*, 87.
57 Roger Freiherrn v. Budberg, "Zur Behandlung des Nabelschnurrestes," *Zentralblatt für Gynäkologie* (Leipzig) 22, no. 47 (26 November 1898), 1288–9. A Russian version, "K voprosu ob ukhode za pupkom posle pererezki pupoviny," appeared in the midwives' journal *Akusherka* (Odessa) 9, nos. 23–4 (1898), 378–9; the article was summarized in *Gazette hebdomadaire de médecine et de chirurgie*, 3rd series, 4, no. 1 (1 January 1899), 9–10; and in *La Presse médicale* 3 (11 January 1899), 19.
58 *Postimees* 254 (13 November 1898).
59 See Mertelsmann, "Tartu–Dorpat–Jur'ev," 212, on this pidgin.
60 Dr. med. gynäkol. R. parun Budberg, *Nõuuandmised noortele naestele ja emadele* (Advice for Young Ladies and Mothers) (Iur'ev: K. Mattiesen, 1902), copy in Estonian Literary Museum, Tartu.
61 EHA, 402/2/193.
62 This note reviews Budberg's scholarly output during his years in Dorpat and its international dissemination. His doctoral dissertation was printed there in 1901 as Roger Frh. von Boeninghausen-Budberg, *Über den Dickdarm erwachsener Menschen und einiger Mammalien, welcher dem Dickdarm des dritten menschlichen Entwicklungsmonates ähnlich ist.* Earlier articles were published jointly with his supervisor: R. Budberg-Boeninghausen and Wilh. Koch, "Darmchirurgie bei ungewöhnlichen Lagen und Gestaltungen des Darmes," *Deutsche Zeitschrift für Chirurgie* 42 (1896), 329–423; and by the same authors, in the same journal, "Grössere

Darmresectionen wegen eingeklemmter Hernie, Dünndarmvolvulus
und Invagination," 43 (1896), 118–27. Budberg's inaugural lecture was
published as "Sposob vyzhimaniia posleda: vstupitel'naia lektsiia,"
Zhurnal akusherstva i zhenskikh boleznei 17, no. 3 (March 1903), 283–9; it was
summarized as "A New Method of Expressing the Placenta" in *Progressive
Medicine* 6, no. 3 (September 1904), 240; and in *Zentralblatt für Gynäkologie*
29, no. 7 (18 February 1905), 212–13. Budberg first presented his method,
while still an assistant in the women's clinic in Dorpat, in "Methode
der Placentaexpression," *Deutsche medizinische Wochenschrift* 24, no. 43
(27 October 1898), 683–4, with a Russian version, "Sposob vyzhimaniia
posleda," in *Vrach* 19, no. 44 (31 October 1898), 1278–9. On the use of green
soap, see "Upotreblenie zelenogo myla dlia dezinfektsii ruk," *Akusherka* 10,
nos. 9–10 (1899), 129–32; German version, "Grüne Seife für Desinfektion
der Hände," *Allgemeine Deutsche Hebammen-Zeitung* 15 (1900), 60–1.
Budberg's articles in *Zentralblatt für Gynäkologie*, the main journal in his
field, include "Zur Alkoholbehandlung des Nabelschnurrestes," 25, no. 39
(28 September 1901), 1080–1; "Über einige wesentliche Grundsätze bei
Dammschutz und Expression," 27, no. 24 (13 June 1903), 721–9; and "Ist
das Ödem der Vulva während der Geburt ein natürliches Schutzmittel für
den Damm oder steigert es gar die Gefahr des Zerreißens?," 28, no. 8
(27 February 1904), 245–9.

63 *Postimees* 107 (17 May 1903). For his address at 12 Grosser Markt:
    Nordlivländischer Kalender 1901 (Jurjew/Dorpat: H. Laakmann, 1901),
    90; and *Schnakenburg's Kalender für das Jahr 1905* (Jurjew/Dorpat:
    Schnakenburg's, 1904), 116, 136 (with the precision: "temporarily in
    Manchuria").

64 *Briefe*, 22 June 1903.

65 He recalled his art collection many years later: *Briefe*, 9 June 1924.

66 Russian State Archive of Military History (hereafter RGVIA), f. 12651,
    d. 1392, l. 94. Budberg's application was turned down. On travelling to
    Germany in 1893, see Budberg, *Memuary*, pt i, 21.

67 Letter of the Russian Red Cross to Rector of Iur'ev (Dorpat) University,
    21 February 1904, EHA, 402/2/192. The press agencies reported from Saint
    Petersburg that "Baron Budberg is starting for the far east to organize a
    flotilla of ten hospital barges on the Amur river." *Boston Globe*, 25 February
    1904. On Budberg's appointment, see also *Revel'skie izvestiia* (Tallinn) 241
    (25 February 1904).

68 RGVIA, f. 12651, op. 12, d. 128, ll. 9, 164, 166. On the workings of such
    aristocratic networks, illustrated by a Russian family in Riga whom
    Alexandrine Budberg would have known, see Winning, "The Empire as
    Family Affair." The professor of medicine was the father of Boris Anrep
    (1883–1969), who became a famous British artist, and of Gleb Anrep

(1891–1955), a prominent physiologist, who spent most of his career in Egypt.

69 Budberg, *Memuary*, i. Cf. *Lebenserinnerung*, 10. An essay from Manchuria published in *Düna Zeitung* (Riga) 297 (30 December 1904) attested that Budberg assisted the column in Harbin; a member of the flying column also mentioned Budberg among other Baltic physicians present in Manchuria during the war. See Hohlbeck, "Professor Zoege und die Fliegende Kolonne," 133; on Werner Zoege von Manteuffel (1857–1926), see entry in BBL.

70 Instruction letter to Baron Budberg, dated 22 February 1904. RGVIA f. 12651, op. 12, d. 128, ll. 7–8. Cf. "Inland," *Düna Zeitung* 46 (26 February 1904).

71 Telegram from nurse Else Riemer, dated 18 March 1904; reply from the Red Cross on 19 March. RGVIA f. 12651, op. 12, d. 128, II. 51–2.

72 Telegram by Prince Vasil'chikov in Harbin to the Red Cross in Saint Petersburg, dated 16 March 1904. RGVIA f. 12651, op. 12, d. 128, I. 43. On him, see entry in Shilov, *Gosudarstvennye deiateli Rossiiskoi imperii*.

73 "Neueste Nachrichten," *Düna Zeitung* 126 (7 June 1904); and another report from Blagoveshchensk, *Düna Zeitung* 133 (15 June 1904).

74 The false report first appeared in *Rizhskie vedomosti* (Riga Records) and was picked up by the Latvian paper *Baltijas Vēstnesis* (Baltic Herald; Riga) 153 (9 July 1904).

75 On Budberg's supposed death in Manchuria and superlative praise for his medical work in Tartu, see *Postimees* 151 (10 July 1904) and 153 (13 July 1904); for his own "greetings from the battlefield," 174 (7 August 1904). On the disproved rumour and the success of Budberg's floating hospitals, see *Ristirahwa Pühhapäewaleht* (Christian Sunday Mail; Tallinn) 37 (12 September 1904).

76 Havard and Hoff, *Reports of Military Observers*, 66. Ibid., 100, describes the same "flotilla" as having consisted of "17 two-decked barges and 7 tugs, with total capacity of 2,000 beds."

77 Report on the floating hospitals of the Russian Red Cross on the Sungari and the Amur, by [Sergei P.] Shlikevich; dated by context. RGVIA f. 12651, op. 12, d. 117. More descriptions of the medical barges, with photographs of them, are in Kuznetsov, *'Gol'd' ukhodit v Kharbin*, 48–55.

78 It remains unclear how this complaint was submitted and handled or what exact charges Budberg made. *Lebenserinnerung*, 10–11, cannot be trusted on this point, for Antoinette lionizes her brother. Intriguingly, she implies that as a physician in Dorpat, Roger had saved the life of Prince Vasil'chikov's wife. In memoirs written during the emigration and first published in 2003, Vasil'chikov dismissed the allegations of corruption, which, he said, the press spread about all Red Cross officials; see *Vospominaniia*, 158–60. The suspicions of false bookkeeping against Sergei A. Aleksandrovskii

(1863–1907), Chief Plenipotentiary of the Russian Red Cross with the army in Manchuria between March 1904 and January 1905, are echoed in Kravkov, *Voina v Man'chzhurii*, 131, 188, 212 (cf. 26n1).

79 The following relies on letters by Alexander Budberg to his wife and daughters from November 1905 to February 1906, as reproduced in *Lebenserinnerung*, esp. 83, 87, 94–9.

80 *Lebenserinnerung*, 22–5, with photograph of Abdallah (no. 103) in the Raczynski family album. Engaged as chief housekeeper on the Poniemon estate, Abdallah was later downgraded to servant and jester and eventually to garden worker on account of his heavy drinking. In 2012, the granddaughter of a governess at Poniemon remembered hearing that Abdallah used to offer her grandmother roses from the garden in exchange for vodka (Anna Sudmalnece, in conversation in Budberga village on 23 May 2012). The Budbergs were not the first aristocrats in the region to take a black servant: the princely Radziwiłł family brought twelve African slaves to Riga via London in 1752. Adam Teller, *Money, Power, and Influence in Eighteenth-Century Lithuania: The Jews on the Radziwiłł Estates* (Stanford: Stanford University Press, 2016), 163. The Duchy of Courland possessed a colony in Gambia between 1651 and 1661, and imported slaves from it.

81 Konstantin von Kochendörffer (1875–1941) was an architect and civil engineer; see B.M. Kirikov, ed., *Arkhitektory-stroiteli Sankt-Peterburga serediny XIX–nachala XX veka* (Architects-Constructors of Saint Petersburg, Mid-Nineteenth to Early Twentieth Century) (Saint Petersburg: Piligrim, 1996), 174–5. He left Russia for Finland in 1920 after fighting in the White Army, then immigrated to Canada with his family in 1930. "Czarist Officer Dies in Montreal," *The Gazette* (Montreal) 305 (22 December 1941).

82 Lieven, "… I teni tekh, kogo uzh net," pt i, 166, described Budberg in these late recollections of the 1950s as "having deep respect for the teaching of Confucius and all things Chinese, and speaking their language." The memoirist's sister Maria Lieven (1877–1907) was also in Manchuria with the Livland lazaretto, one of the many aristocratic Russian and Baltic German women who had volunteered as nurses during the Russo-Japanese War.

83 *Lebenserinnerung*, 11; cf. "Vmesto vstupleniia. Ot izdatelia" (In Lieu of an Introduction: From the Publisher), in Budberg, *Memuary*, i, iii.

84 Misspelled as Shai-sha-kai in the publisher's introduction in Budberg, *Memuary*, iii, the only source of information on this period. See the mention of "Maimakai" in Kravkov, *Voina v Man'chzhurii*, 287, which includes an excellent commentary on Chinese place names during the Russo-Japanese War; and Bo Yang, "Lishu diming tanyuan."

85 Budberg, "Vom Seelenleben der Chinesen," 62.

86 Ostrovskii and Safonov, "15–17 oktiabria 1905 g."

87 Baron Otto Bernhard Budberg (1850–1907), justice of the peace and
    marshal of the nobility. See BBL; on his death two years later, see "Russian
    Noble Murdered," *New York Times*, 3 March 1907; also *The Times*, 4 March
    1907, under "Murders and Robberies"; and *The North China Herald*,
    8 March 1907, under "Russia: The Crusade of Terrorism." In 1921, Moura
    Budberg obtained her surname, her Estonian passport, and her title of
    baroness through a marriage of convenience to his son Nicolai.
88 Gotthard Budberg leased the Magnushof estate from his father after 1889.
    Richter's Baltische Verkehrs- u. Adreßbücher, vol. 1, *Livland* (Riga: Adolf
    Richter, 1900), pt iii, "Güter und Pastorate Livlands," 9.
89 See ch. 8, "The Russo-Japanese War and the 1905 Revolution in
    Manchuria," in Quested, *"Matey" Imperialists?*; and Grüner, "The Russian
    Revolution of 1905 at the Periphery."
90 RGVIA f. 12651, op. 2, d. 94.
91 Budberg never mentioned the unsuccessful application. See more on this
    in Gamsa, "China as Seen and Imagined by Roger Baron Budberg," 12–13.
92 *Briefe*, 23 and 25 July 1906.

3 Intermediaries and Channels of Communication

1 Quested, *"Matey" Imperialists?*, 146; also Katajs, *Zem desmit valstu karogiem*, 8.
2 Quested, *"Matey" Imperialists?*, 31, 135–7.
3 Recouly, "En Mandchourie."
4 Quested, *"Matey" Imperialists?*, 132. Ross, in *The Boxers in Manchuria*,
   which emphasized the evil doings of the Zaili sect, noted that former
   participants in the uprising became "interpreters and policemen in Russian
   employment" (17). On the Zaili, cf. Lobza, "Kitaiskie sektanty"; Drake,
   "Religion in a Manchurian City," 15.
5 A critic of the Russian involvement in Manchuria, Golovachev, in *Rossiia
   nu Dal'nem Vostoke*, 134, argued ironically that "concern for the edification
   of the natives" as of 1904 was limited to "two bad Russian-Chinese schools
   in Piziwo and Jinzhou," both founded to train interpreters. See Khvostov,
   "Russkii Kitai," pt i, 673, on the school in Piziwo (now Pikou, in Pulandian
   District of Dalian City), which opened in 1898.
6 Quested, *"Matey" Imperialists?*, 118. Cf. the 1908 court case of an interpreter
   of mixed Chinese and Russian descent, in Nesterova, "Kitaitsy na
   rossiiskom Dal'nem Vostoke," 11–13.
7 See Karttunen, *Between Worlds*.
8 Luke S.K. Kwong, "The T'i-Yung Dichotomy," 264–7.
9 See Sokolova, "Vospominaniia," 445, 814, on the execution of interpreters
   by the Boxers. A.I., "Poslednie dni v Man'chzhurii," 151, 161, mentions by
   name an interpreter in Fularji who fled with the Russians to Khabarovsk

in the summer of 1900 and returned with them to serve in the Harbin administration after the uprising had been crushed a few months later. Another interpreter warned the author's husband that the Qiqihar governor general (i.e., Shou Shan, discussed in ch. 1) had ordered his arrest.

10 On Japanese executions of Chinese interpreters previously employed by the Russians, see Recouly, "En Mandchourie," 211. Cf. Quested, *"Matey" Imperialists?*, 182–4, on the Chinese measures.

11 From a report by Liuba, cited with no indication of a year in Datsyshen, "Inkou," 81.

12 See entry on Liuba in M.Iu. Sorokina, *Rossiiskoe nauchnoe zarubezh'e*, 122.

13 Wrangel, "Manchzhurskie pis'ma," 380–1.

14 See Marks, *Road to Power*, ch. 9.

15 Quoted in Brower, "Islam and Ethnicity," 132.

16 Quested, *"Matey" Imperialists?*, 91–2. For more on the *khunkhuzy* in reality and imagination, see Gamsa, "How a Republic of Chinese Red Beards Was Invented in Paris."

17 Colley, "Going Native, Telling Tales," 186.

18 Cf. Recouly, "En Mandchourie," 210, on the hostile native reaction to interpreters' appearance.

19 Ch'en, *China and the West*, 224.

20 Quested, "An Introduction to the Enigmatic Career of Chou Mien."

21 Petrov, *Istoriia kitaitsev v Rossii*, 127, 130 (I have added the census data for 1897).

22 Ibid., 142.

23 Ji would have owed his Russian name and patronymic to a Russian godfather. For previous research in English, cf. Quested, *"Matey" Imperialists?*, 134–5; Wolff, *To the Harbin Station*, 14–16; Zatsepine, *Beyond the Amur*, 93–5.

24 On the possible year of his birth, and his rise in the 1870s, see Nesterova, "Kitaitsy na rossiiskom Dal'nem Vostoke," 16–17. The above version of his arrival in Russia is from Su Su, *Liuguang suiying* (Flittering Lights and Fragmented Shadows) (Dalian: Dalian chubanshe, 2008), 191–5.

25 R.F., "Vospominaniia iz zhizni na Amure," 360.

26 Grulev, "Iz poezdki v Man'chzhuriiu," 947.

27 Jordan, "Notes on a Journey from Vladivostock to Irkutsk," 326. On interpreters becoming contractors, and on some being christened and cutting off their queue, see Matveev, "Kitaitsy na Kariiskikh promyslakh," 32–3.

28 Nesterova, "Kitaitsy na rossiiskom Dal'nem Vostoke," 7–8.

29 Ibid.; cf. Petrov, *Istoriia kitaitsev v Rossii*, 400–1.

30 Koz'min, *Dal'nii Vostok*, 66–8. In 1910 the writer Vasilii Nemirovich-Danchenko (1844–1936; brother of the famous theatre director Vladimir), who had met Tifontai as a military reporter during the Russo-Japanese

War, wrote about him in a similar vein under the title "Russkii kitaez" (A Russian Chink); see excerpts in Petrov, *Istoriia kitaitsev v Rossii*, 398–404.

31 Letter by Tifontai (containing the reference to "500 mounted *khunkhuzy*"), signed in Kuanchengzi on 16 May 1905, to Major-General Vladimir A. Oranovskii; and report of 1 September 1905, "Tainaia razvedka cherez kitaiskikh agentov" (Secret Intelligence through Chinese Agents), by Junior Captain Blonskii, both in Derevianko, ed., *'Belye piatna' Russko-iaponskoi voiny*, respectively 328–30, 306–12.

32 See Quested, *"Matey" Imperialists?*, 135, and Nesterova, "Kitaitsy na rossiiskom Dal'nem Vostoke," 23, on the Japanese death sentence. Tifontai is described betraying Russia to the Japanese in Stepanov, *Port-Artur*, 216–20.

33 I thank Qu Changliang of Dalian University of Foreign Languages for information on Ji Fengtai's former properties. An architect's sketch of the residence in Port Arthur decorated a wall in the modest Moscow apartment of journalist Natal'ia Tifontai, a great-granddaughter, whom I interviewed in October 2007.

34 On the theatre in Dal'nii, see Labbé, *Les Russes en Extrême-Orient*, 208. Built in 1902, it was turned into a public hall by the Japanese in 1908, but was revived as a theatre in the PRC until demolition in the 1990s. Yu Zhiyuan and Dong Zhizheng, eds., *Jianming Dalian cidian* (Concise Dictionary of Dalian) (Dalian: Dalian chubanshe, 1995), 741, 872; Ji Ruguang, *Jiyi: Dalian laojie* (Memories: Old Streets in Dalian) (Dalian: Dalian chubanshe, 2012), 266–7.

35 Chinese plays performed in "Tifontai's Chinese Theatre" in Harbin, in 1906, are listed in Diao Shaohua, *Literatura russkogo zarubezh'ia v Kitae*, 179. See Botkin, "Svet i teni russko-iaponskoi voiny," 58–60, on a performance arranged by the wife of General Khorvat, and a reception at the theatre held by Mr and Mrs Zhou Mian.

36 Nesterova, "Kitaitsy na rossiiskom Dal'nem Vostoke," 24–6.

37 A London resident when naturalized in 1938, she died there, aged seventy-eight, in 1968. National Archives of the United Kingdom, Kew, HO 334/150/12443 on her naturalization; *England and Wales Civil Registration Indexes* (General Register Office), on her death in Hounslow, London.

38 The following information on Zhang Tingge is drawn from a biographical sketch by Jin Zonglin, translated in Clausen and Thøgersen, *The Making of a Chinese City*, 69–74; Ji Fenghui, *Ha'erbin xungen*, 229–30; and Nesterova, "Kitaiskii torgovyi dom 'Shuankheshen.'"

39 Ivan S. Stepanov, "Pervaia russkaia shkola v Man'chzhurii" (The First Russian School in Manchuria), in *Nachal'noe obrazovanie na Kitaiskoi Vostochnoi zheleznoi doroge*, 131. Cf. Vasilenko, "Shkol'noe obrazovanie v polose otchuzhdeniia KVZhD," 94.

40 Kosinova, "Organizatorskaia i pedagogicheskaia deiatel'nost'," 61–2.
41 Gintse, *Russkaia sem'ia doma i v Man'chzhurii*, 50–2, 56–60.
42 Bakich, "Russian Education in Harbin," 273.
43 "Etong ru Woguo xuexiao" (Russian Children Enter Chinese School),
   Yuandong bao, 18 September 1919. Here and below, my references to
   Yuandong bao are based on the selection published as twelve inner-
   circulation (*neibu*) supplements to *Ha'erbin shizhi congkan*, from no. 4 (1983)
   to no. 8 (1984).
44 Ermachenko, "'V Kharbine vse spokoino,'" 83, 90.
45 The fundraising was announced and promoted by articles in the CER
   newspaper *Yuandong bao*; for example, "Hua-E gu'eryuan zhi mujuan"
   (Chinese-Russian Orphanage Collects Donations), 8 September 1918. See
   also Gintse, *Russkaia sem'ia doma i v Man'chzhurii*, 83–4; *Polytechnic*, jubilee
   issue, 206.
46 By then, the Soviet administration of the railway was presenting
   the expansion of CER schools for Chinese employees as proof of its
   progressive policies while denigrating the tsarist regime for ignoring the
   Chinese population. Filippovich, "Sovetskie i kitaiskie shkoly na KVZhD,"
   32–3, 36, 38.
47 One example is the Soviet-leaning "Mixed Russian-Chinese Realgymnasium
   of G.A. Las," which advertised in the Harbin press in 1924; see
   Ekonomicheskii vestnik Man'chzhurii 35 (31 August 1924), 16. The "mixed"
   in its name indicated that it was co-educational, but it is doubtful whether
   Chinese were included; the school had closed by the following year.
   See Peremilovskii, "Russkaia shkola v Man'chzhurii." An orphanage
   and school for Russian boys, founded as the Russian Home in 1920 and
   modelled on tsarist navy schools, with the children wearing sailors'
   uniforms, was later renamed the Russian-Chinese Asylum for political
   reasons. It became the Alexander Nevsky Lyceum in 1945. See Bakich,
   Harbin Russian Imprints, no. 4121; *Polytechnic*, jubilee issue, 122–3; and
   Smirnov, *Rossiiskie emigranty v Severnoi Man'chzhurii*, 150, 154–5.
48 Cf. Hsu, "Railroad Technocracy."
49 [Shchelkov], *Kratkii ocherk vozniknoveniia i deiatel'nosti*, 2–3; idem, "Russko-
   Kitaiskii Politekhnicheskii Institut."
50 N.P. Kalugin, "Iubileinaia data kharbinskogo Politekhnicheskogo
   instituta" (The Anniversary Date of the Harbin Polytechnic Institute, 1972),
   in Taskina, *Russkii Kharbin*, 57–60.
51 *Istoricheskii obzor i sovremennoe polozhenie podgotovitel'nykh kursov
   Kharbinskogo Politekhnicheskogo Instituta*, 3–7.
52 Ibid., 90; A.N. Kniazev, "Vyderzhki iz dnevnika Politekhnika" (Excerpts
   from the Polytechnic's Diary), in *Polytechnic*, jubilee issue, 50–4 at 51;
   Fialkovskii, "V ego stenakh my vse byli molody."

53 Cf. Eropkina, "Russkie i kitaiskie shkoly na KVZhD."
54 See Bakich, "Russian Education in Harbin," 280; and a historical sketch of the Faculty of Law by the Harbin educator Nikolai P. Avtonomov (1885–1976), collected in Taskina, *Russkii Kharbin*, 50–7.
55 Ratmanov, *Vklad rossiiskikh vrachei v meditsinu Kitaia*, 144–50.
56 Even a historian as appreciative of the Russian heritage in Harbin as Ji Fenghui offered this explanation in his *Ha'erbin xungen*. The term *Zhongxue* was coined in the late Qing to signify Chinese education, as opposed to Western-introduced methods.
57 Deng Jiemin and his school come under close scrutiny in Carter, *Creating a Chinese Harbin*, 31–65. On the choice of English as the school language, cf. Shi Fang and Gao Ling, *Chuantong yu biange*, 335–6.
58 That was the educational background of most of the Chinese students whom Mordechai Olmert (see below) met at the Harbin Polytechnic in the late 1920s.
59 Abe, "The Movement to Restore Educational Prerogatives," 20–1. In response to the Japanese refusal to comply with its demands, the Chinese Educational Association in Mukden turned to the schools' Chinese teachers and the pupils' parents: the former were urged to resign and the latter to withdraw their children under threat of severe sanctions; ibid., 23, 25.
60 Lee, "The Foreign Ministry's Cultural Agenda for China," 294, 296. Wang Fengrui, *Wang Fengrui xiansheng fangwen jilu*, 15–18, 26.
61 See Chen, *State-Sponsored Inequality*. The Harbin sinologist, Georgii G. Avenarius (1876–1948), described this area as a rare success of the Qing policy of resettling Peking Manchus in Manchuria, commenting that "the national composition of Shuangcheng County presents a high degree of interest for the ethnologist, the student of daily life and the linguist alike." Avenarius, "Shuanchenpu i Shuanchensian'," 115.
62 Olmert, *Darki bederekh harabim*, 33–45. Olmert was the founder of the settlement Amikam, established in 1950 by a nucleus of twenty-eight families, most of them from Harbin, and a member of the Israeli Parliament. His son Ehud became mayor of Jerusalem and later Prime Minister of Israel.
63 Yang Aili, *Sun Yunxuan zhuan*, 16–17. When he was still a student of the Polytechnic, Sun participated in protests against the Soviet Union during the Sino-Russian conflict in 1929. Most of his Chinese fellow students chose to stay in Harbin and enter the CER service after their graduation; Sun declared he did not want to remain under the Japanese occupation. Ibid., 21–2.
64 Shi Fang, Gao Ling, and Liu Shuang, *Ha'erbin Eqiao shi*, 510, list the names of the students and of their hosts, on the basis of *Yuandong bao* of 17 September 1911. On their arrival in Harbin, see also "Eren huanying

Fengpai nannü xuesheng" (Russians Welcome Male and Female Students Sent by Fengtian), *Yuandong bao*, 31 August 1911.

65 For elaboration on this case and on other intermediaries in Harbin, see Gamsa, "Cross-cultural Contact in Manchuria."

66 Li Sui'an, *Ma Zhongjun ji Ha'erbin Dunyuan*, esp. ch. 3.

67 Ben Chi, "Guanyu Songbin yinshe."

68 See Xin Peilin, "Ma Zhongjun xiansheng shilüe," 9–13, on life in the garden and in the castle; on the garden, cf. the recollections of Ma's son Ma Weiquan, "Yi Dunyuan (dai xu)," in Li Sui'an, *Ma Zhongjun ji Ha'erbin Dunyuan*. Li Shuxiao et al., *Ha'erbin jiuying: Old Photos of Harbin*, 52, has a photograph of the castle, since 1956 a fortified hotel for visiting Party leaders and foreign statesmen.

69 Li Sui'an, *Ma Zhongjun ji Ha'erbin Dunyuan*, 20–3. The mission to Alekseev was a more ambiguous matter than Ma cared to remember: see Quested, *"Matey" Imperialists?* 54–5.

70 Quested, *"Matey" Imperialists?* 246. Cf. Chen Yuan, *Wolfgang Seuberlich (1906–1985)*, 41–2. Mikhail Hintze knew the Ma family well through his father, the senior CER official; see ch. 49 of Gintse, *Russkaia sem'ia doma i v Man'chzhurii*.

71 "Tielu renyuan xuexi Eyu" (Railway Personnel Learns Russian), *Yuandong bao*, 22 May 1920; "Tielu fushe Eyu jiangxisuo" (The Railway Creates a Russian Language Institute), *Yuandong bao*, 27 June 1920.

72 Chiasson, *Administering the Colonizer*, ch. 4.

73 *Xunyue dongsheng tielu jilüe* (Brief Record of an Inspection Tour of the Chinese Eastern Railway), in *Song Xiaolian ji*, 117.

74 For example, Wang Peiyue, "Kuayue liang ge lishi shiqi de Heilongjiangsheng xingzheng zhangguan"; Lü Huifen, "Weihu zhuquan cuntu bizheng de Song Xiaolian."

75 *Yuandong bao*, 10 and 13 August 1920.

76 Qu Qiubai, *Exiang jicheng*, 265–7.

77 See Carter, *Creating a Chinese Harbin*, 145–7; Li Shuxiao, "Ha'erbin jieming xiao kao."

78 N.I. Abrosimov, "Izuchenie kitaiskogo iazyka i KVZhD," 7.

79 Pavlovskaia, "Vostokovedenie v Institute Oriental'nykh i Kommercheskikh Nauk v Kharbine"; eadem, "Vostokovedenie na Iuridicheskom Fakul'tete Kharbina." See also Koretskii, "Epopeia russkogo emigranta," 127–33, 137–8, on the Faculty of Law and on Usov's teaching; and advertisements in the Harbin Russian press.

80 Galia Katz, "Kharbin," 35–6; M. Sorokina, "Moi KhPI"; and the memoir of Edgars Katajs, a teacher at North Manchuria University: *Zem desmit valstu karogiem*, here 153–7, 160–2.

81 Wolff, *To the Harbin Station*, uses the *vostokovedy* and their societies and publications in Manchuria to support his main thesis that Harbin was a haven of liberalism and inter-racial tolerance. Russian Orientalists in Manchuria are also addressed in Kovalevskii, *Zarubezhnaia Rossiia*, 88–98; Taskina, "Sinologi i kraevedy Kharbina"; and numerous publications by Khisamutdinov, such as his *Kak russkie izuchali Kitai*.

82 By 1911 the society had members in Hankou, Qiqihar, and Peking as well as in Seoul, Tokyo, and the Russian Far East. Branches were also established in Saint Petersburg and Vladivostok. See Khisamutdinov, "Obshchestvo russkikh orientalistov v Kharbine," 104–5; Kanevskaia and Pavlovskaia, "Deiatel'nost' vypusknikov," 74.

83 See Wolff, *To the Harbin Station*, 156–7; and entries in Baskhanov, *Russkie voennye vostokovedy do 1917 goda*.

84 Among a total of 252 articles in *Vestnik Azii*, the division was as follows: 119 on China, 33 on the Russian Far East, 30 on Japan, and 28 on Manchuria. Kanevskaia and Pavlovskaia, "Deiatel'nost' vypusknikov," 76.

85 A. Baranov, "Zadachi sektsii etnografii," 14; idem, "Doklad Predsedatelia Istoriko-Etnograficheskoi sektsii O.I.M.K.," 7, 8. The full list of members was published in no. 2 of the *Izvestiia*, 39–42.

86 Jones, *Harbin as a Russo-Chinese City*, 87. Some of the monograph publications of Harbin sinologists did reach Chinese readers through translations undertaken in the 1930s; but the systematic translation of archaeological articles had to await the 1990s, when they began to appear in the Harbin journal *Beifang wenwu* (Northern Antiquities).

87 Ng, "The *Yuandongbao*," 115–16.

88 See Gamsa, "Cross-cultural Contact in Manchuria," for a brief discussion.

89 The 1926 edition is in the British Library. The modern edition, Ivanov, *My na Zapade i na Vostoke*, bears an expanded title. This author should not be confused with the Soviet writer Vsevolod V. Ivanov (1895–1963), who also wrote on the Far East.

90 See Glebov, *From Empire to Eurasia*.

91 The Russian typescript of the essay by P.N. Savitskii, "Geograficheskie i geopoliticheskie osnovy evraziistva" (The Geographical and Geopolitical Foundations of Eurasianism) is collected in Ponomareva, ed., *Evraziia*, 110–18 at 110, 113.

92 See the exchange between Ivanov and Vasilii P. Nikitin (1885–1960), excerpted in ibid., 77–80. Cf. Gamsa, "Asiatics and Chinamen."

93 Ivanov, *Bezhenskaia poema*, 5–6, 35–40, 85. The printed "Dedication" of the work was signed in Mukden on 5 December 1922.

94 The quoted editorial is Ivanov, "Ot redaktsii." All five issues of *Vestnik Kitaia* are available in the National Library of Israel. On Ivanov and his

journal, see ch. 5, "Tientsin," in Yakobson (née Elena A. Zhemchuzhnaia, 1913–2002), *Crossing Borders*. Yakobson knew Ivanov well and was a contributor to *Vestnik Kitaia*.

95 Ivanov, "Logika Evropy i Kitaia." The Li Bai poem is analysed in Ivanov, "Poeziia i ieroglif Kitaia."

96 Part One of *Dar messii* (Messiah's Gift, 1912) by Nikolai F. Oliger (1882–1919), subtitled "Kitaiskaia povest'" (a Chinese novel), was serialized in *Vestnik Kitaia*, no. 5.

97 Cf. Kobzev and Serbinenko, "Iz naslediia russkogo filosofa Vl. Solov'eva."

98 Setnitskii, "Russkie mysliteli o Kitae." This includes Fedorov's essay "Chemu nauchaet drevneishii khristianskii pamiatnik v Kitae" (What the Most Ancient Christian Monument in China Can Teach Us), first published in a Moscow journal in 1901. The mission of resurrecting the Russian ancestors in China is also espoused in Ivanov, *Bezhenskaia poema*, 43. On Setnitskii at the head of a circle of Fedorov disciples in Harbin between 1925 and 1935, see Hagemeister, "Neue Materialien zur Wirkungsgeschichte N. F. Fedorovs."

99 Makarov, "Russkii filosof Nikolai Setnitskii," 137, 139, 149.

100 The first part of Setnitskii's principal philosophical work *O konechnom ideale* (On the Final Ideal, 1932) is collected in Gorskii and Setnitskii, *Sochineniia*.

101 Serebrennikov, *Ocherk ekonomicheskoi geografii Kitaia*, Introduction.

102 Wrangel, "Manchzhurskie pis'ma," 384.

103 Stern, "Russische Pidgins," 2. Runich, "V Man'chzhurii," 622–4, comments on a pidgin conversation between a Russian batman and a Chinese hawker, writing that the former "mangled his language in a way that our common folk almost invariably does when speaking to foreigners." Silin, *Kiakhta v XVIII veke*, 115, acknowledged that the Russian merchants in Kiakhta never addressed their Chinese counterparts in correct Russian.

104 Stern, *Saitensprünge*, 57, 68 (Stern's autobiography appeared in Chinese translation in 2003). For similar reasons, Wolfgang Seuberlich, born in Berlin and brought to Riga in 1910, acquired Russian, Chinese, and Japanese when he lived in Harbin between 1914 and his repatriation to Germany in 1937. Chen Yuan, ed., *Wolfgang Seuberlich*.

105 Cf. Anderson, *Imagined Communities*, 148n12: "The logic here is: 1. I will be dead before I have penetrated them. 2. My power is such that they have had to learn my language. 3. But this means that my privacy has been penetrated. Terming them 'gooks' is small revenge."

106 Tellingly, Botkin, "Svet i teni russko-iaponskoi voiny," 62, thought the word Chinese. Quested, *"Matey" Imperialists?*, 137, notes that the friendly colouring of *khodia* was not lost on the Chinese, who in appropriate

circumstances gave it back to the Russians. However, Russians would have felt more comfortable with the ingratiating *kapitan* (ibid.). Cf. Vereshchagin, *Po Manchzhurii*, pt ii, 611; Veresaev, *Zapiski vracha*, 358 (a Chinese person using *khodia* to address a Russian), 431, 444.

107 General Aleksei Budberg's diary entry of 17 June 1918, in his *Dnevnik 1917–1919*, 236. Another diarist made a nearly identical observation in 1924; see entry of 24 July in Lyandres and Wulff, eds., *A Chronicle of the Civil War in Siberia and Exile in China*, vol. 2, 219.

108 Mao Hong, "Ha'erbin Zhong-E renmin shenghuo zhuangkuang," 119.

109 I. Abrosimov, *Pod chuzhim nebom*, 34, mentions other nicknames for the Chinese: *fazan* (literally: pheasant), *kitaeza* (which comes close to the English "Chink"), and *khodun* (a derogative form of *khodia*).

110 The connection of *manza* to "Manchu" is made erroneously in Stephan, *The Russian Far East*, 73. The Russian word for China, "Kitai," did evolve from an ethnonym: the Qidan (also: Khitan) people, founders of the Liao state (916–1125), which ruled over a vast territory that included Manchuria.

111 James, *The Long White Mountain*, 123; on the use of *qiren*, cf. Rhoads, *Manchus and Han*, 18. As James and others indicate, *manzi* was used as a curse for the Chinese by Manchu armies during the conquest of China.

112 The eminent Russian missionary sinologist in Peking, Archimandrite Palladii (1817–1878), argued in his "O Man'tszakh i koreitsakh" and "Usuriiskie Man'tszy" (369), that Chinese settlers in the Ussuri district received the name *man'tszy* from Manchurian natives, who thought of them as "southerners." They did not mind being called that, although they preferred to call themselves *paotuizi* or *paotuir de*, that is, walkers, runaways, or vagrants. In the 1930s, Lattimore, *Manchuria*, 66, glossed *paotuir de* as "distinctly a pejorative term"; he also wrote that *manzi* was "still used in Manchuria for non-Manchurian Chinese" (62n2). Zhao Zhongfu, *Qingji Zhong-E dongsansheng jiewu jiaoshe*, 147, transcribed *manza* as a Russian word, offering no etymology for it.

113 For example, *waiguo gui* was applied to the Russians in a popular song, which, according to Xia Chongwei, "Aihui xuehuo," no. 6, 75, was sung in the Aigun area after the conflict of 1900.

114 On "big" and "small" noses, see, for example, Wang Fengrui, *Fangwen jilu*, 6. Stern, *Saitensprünge*, 60, specified that since Russians were known as *lao maozi*, the nickname "big noses" was reserved for other foreigners in Harbin, such as himself. On "stink noses," as a Chinese nickname for the Mongols, cf. Lindt, *Im Sattel durch Mandschukuo*, 231.

115 Lattimore, *Manchuria*, 175. A former German official in Qingdao, the ethnologist Ernst Grosse, wrote that "the Chinese could not bear our smell." See his *Ostasiatische Erinnerungen*, 38.

116　Curiously, some Harbin memoirs interpret *lamoza* as "old hat": see, for example, Taskina and Sel'kina, *Kharbin*, 209; Stern, *Saitensprünge*, 60; cf. Nikolaeva, *Iapontsy*, 313–14. This was probably how the Chinese preferred to explain *lao maozi* when asked about its meaning. Li Rong, *Ha'erbin fangyan cidian*, shows that *maozi* of "hat" had no such associations and that "hairy ones" was indeed used for Russians (it continues to be so used in internet forums today).

117　Liaozuo sanren (Liu Jingyan), *Binjiang chenxiao lu*, 134, cites many examples. These terms, which are now obsolete, were used in Soviet Russia until the switch to the metric system in 1927. On the use of Russian and pidgin terms by the Chinese among themselves, cf. Lattimore, *Manchuria*, 174–5.

118　On the appropriation of Russian words, see also Shi Fang and Gao Ling, *Chuantong yu biange*, 407–9; Ji Fenghui and Duan Guangda, *Lishi huimou*, 117–19.

119　M.N. Levitskii, ed., *V trushchobakh Man'chzhurii*, 374, on *shango*, and more examples of its use in Oglezneva, "Dal'nevostochnyi regiolekt russkogo iazyka." The Chinese transcription of *shang hao* in Mazo and Ivchenko, "Chinese Loanwords in Russian," is doubtful (see the bracketed form in the Glossary); in any case, pidgin words were rarely written in Chinese, remaining in the realm of spoken language. Mazo and Ivchenko consider *khanshin* Chinese, yet they cannot identify its origin. In contrast, Song Xiaolian thought the word *khanshin* Russian and transcribed it as such; see *Song Xiaolian ji*, 19. These and many other pidgin words are also discussed in Bakich, "Did You Speak Harbin Sino-Russian?"

120　See A.I., "Poslednie dni v Man'chzhurii," 163. Bakich, "A Russian City in China," 133, cites a 1923 memoir by Harbin pioneer Vladimir N. Veselovzorov, who claimed that local inhabitants, whom the first party of engineers met on the spot in 1898, "either could not explain the name [Harbin], or interpreted it as a 'merry shore' or a 'merry grave.'"

121　Larisa P. Kravchenko (1929–2003), "Kharbin iznachal'nyi" (Inceptive Harbin), in Taskina and Sel'kina, *Kharbin*, 41.

122　Guan Chenghe, *Ha'erbin kao*, 2–3.

123　Ibid., 3.

124　Compare also with Changling ("prosperous" or "splendid" tomb), a Qing imperial burial site southwest of Beijing. In another context, Jorge Flores, "Distant Wonders: The Strange and the Marvelous between Mughal India and Habsburg Iberia in the Early Eighteenth Century," *Comparative Studies in Society and History* 49, no. 3 (July 2007), 553–81 at 580–1, concludes that "many European views on Asia are less European than we tend to believe," suggesting that "one of the most interesting challenges before future research … is to identify cultural 'hybridities' in western authors, texts, and maps."

125 The theory linking Harbin with the glorious legacy of the Jurchen dynasty and presenting "Harbin" as a corruption of Alejin, a village mentioned in the *History of the Jin*, was first promoted by the above-cited veteran historian Guan Chenghe; see Clausen and Thøgersen, *The Making of a Chinese City*, 4–5.

126 Ji's detective search for Harbin's "roots," initiated as a column in the city paper in 1991, led him to a Manchu document of 1864, which transcribed the place name "Halfiyan" as "Ha'erbin" in its parallel Chinese translation. Ji argued that the written Manchu form would have been pronounced as *ha'erbin* in the dialect then spoken in the area; the word itself meant "flat" and was used as shorthand for an older place name, *halfiyan tun*, or "flat island." Ji Fenghui, *Ha'erbin xungen*, 72–6.

127 The latest presentation is Wang Yulang and Wang Tianzi, "Ha'erbin chengshi jiyuan de zai yanjiu."

128 Stern, "Russische Pidgins," 10, and *passim*, has a useful analysis of the questions involved.

129 I consulted the original editions at the National Library of Latvia: V.K. Arsen'ev, *Po Ussuriiskomu kraiu (Dersu Uzala). Puteshestvie v gornuiu oblast' Sikhote-Alin'* (Vladivostok: Tipografiia 'Ekho', 1921), with acknowledgments to P.V. Shkurkin and note by Shkurkin on the transcription of Chinese place names, dated March 1917 in Harbin; and Arsen'ev, *Dersu Uzala. Iz vospominanii o puteshestvii po Ussuriiskomu Kraiu v 1907 g.* (Vladivostok: Tipo-lit. T-va Izd. 'Svobodnaia Rossiia', 1923).

130 See Arsen'ev, *Dersu Uzala*. The book was widely translated. In 1974 a successful Soviet-Japanese film was made under the same name by director Vladimir Vasil'ev, with scenario by Akira Kurosawa and Iurii Nagibin.

131 "A tiger walks nearby and has eaten a dog. He is a very bad sir. He ought to be killed" (in pidgin). Baikov, *Sobranie*, vol. 2: *V gorakh i lesakh Man'chzhurii*, 245. Stephan, *The Russian Far East*, 96–109, follows the "parallel lives" of Arsen'ev and Baikov between 1900 and 1916.

132 "Kipling was our literature. We Anglo-Indians read him because he wasn't something remote and strange, [and] because he was describing the place in which we lived and the way in which we lived." The longing for England as an idealized home comes up later in the same radio interview of Lawrence Durrell (1912–1985) with Malcolm Muggeridge, broadcast by the BBC on 19 October 1965 (available in *The Spoken Word: Lawrence Durrell*, a British Library CD, 2012).

133 Howard Goldblatt, "Translator's Introduction," in Xiao Hong, *Market Street: A Chinese Woman in Harbin*, 11.

134 "Ouluoba lüguan," in Xiao Hong, *Shangshi jie*, 83. The translation is by Goldblatt, in Xiao Hong, *Market Street*, 15. Cf. the later scene, in which a

flea market hawker asks the author and her companion: " 'Your – what want?' ... He was a Chinese himself, but assumed that all the other Chinese were Japanese or Koreans" (ibid., 44; cf. *Shangshi jie*, 116).

135 Xiao Hong, *Market Street*, 19; cf. *Shangshi jie*, 85.

136 *Market Street*, 90; cf. *Shangshi jie*, 136. Harbin's Market Street of the 1930s is today's Red Glow Street (Hongxia jie).

137 *Market Street*, 82. The 1993 edition of *Shangshi jie* skips over eight of the total forty-two sketches, between no. 29 ("The Book") and no. 38 ("Illness"). For the original text, see *Xiao Hong xuanji*, 110.

138 Cf. Goldblatt, "Life as Art," 352.

139 Chen Wenlong, " 'Wodi' Ouluoba, xunzhao Xiao Hong de Ouluoba."

140 Kradin, *Russkie inzhenery i arkhitektory v Kitae*, 197.

141 Hotel Evropa was owned by Isaak S. Fride (d. December 1927) and Maria K. Fride. *Ves' Kharbin na 1926 god*, ed. Ternavskii, 129, 178, 479; and *Nezabytye mogily*, comp. Chuvakov, vol. 6, bk 2, 699.

4 A Chinese-German Flower

1 On being called "German doctor" and Butaifu (in Budberg's transcription): *Briefe*, 18 December 1907.

2 "Vmesto vstupleniia. Ot izdatelia," in Budberg, *Memuary*, vii.

3 On marrying at nine (ten *sui* by the Chinese count), see a study of the rural banner population in Shuangcheng and Liaoning: Chen et al., "Categorical Inequality and Gender Difference," 413.

4 Budberg's letter to the *St Petersburger Herold* was reprinted in *Rigasche Zeitung* 291 (16 December 1909).

5 Teng, *Eurasian*, 15, 64, 197.

6 Telephone: *Briefe*, 1 August 1906. Dates in the letters follow the Julian calendar, which was still in use in Russia and therefore also in Harbin in the 1900s; to accord them with the standard Gregorian calendar, 13 days should be added. Mindful of this difference, correspondents sometimes indicated the dates in both systems; when Roger Budberg did so, such usage will be reproduced here.

7 Photograph (no. 57) in the Raczynski family album. The address of Budberg's clinic appeared as Samannaia Street 2 in the medical listings of *Kharbinskii vestnik* in September 1907.

8 On most patients coming from New Town, and the pleasures of the Sungari: *Briefe*, 5[18] December 1906. On performing his first operation on a Chinese patient, see 3/18 [*sic*] February 1907.

9 EHA, 402/2/193. See also an entry on Raupach in the database created by Ratmanov, "Rossiiskie vrachi v Kitae."

10 There are several mentions of Dr Göldner in *Briefe*. Dr Kramer corresponded with Roger's father, as cited in ch. 2. See entries on both physicians in Ratmanov, "Rossiiskie vrachi v Kitae."

11 Poletika, *Obshchii meditsinskii otchet*, 10; *Spravochnaia knizhka Kharbina*, 102–3 (my thanks to Pavel Ratmanov for these sources).

12 On work with Dr Raupach at the Central Hospital, *Briefe*, 3/18 February 1907. On the hospital for prostitutes, in a letter to Joseph: 18 December 1907.

13 On his sense of obligation: *Briefe*, 2[15] December 1906. On the impossibility of writing to all siblings: 11[24] July 1908. First publications in Chinese are mentioned in letters to Antoinette and Joseph, 18 December 1907.

14 Budberg's file in the Medical Service of the CER, which he joined in 1907, is in the Russian State Historical Archive of the Far East (RGIA DV), f. 1527 op. 1 d. 7, ll. 144–5. Until 1917, all Russian physicians in the railway zone in Manchuria were subordinate to the CER Chief Physician: see Ratmanov, *Vklad rossiiskikh vrachei v meditsinu Kitaia*, 89.

15 RGIA, f. 688, op. 1, d. 15. There are entries on Richter in BBL, and in Shilov and Kuz'min, *Chleny Gosudarstvennogo soveta Rossiiskoi imperii*. He had been adjutant to Roger Budberg's great-uncle, General Alexander Theodor Budberg. Cf. Plath, "*Heimat*," 68, on the flexible meanings of this term around 1910.

16 As the minister remembered the same scene, it was he who called for a doctor to be brought into the railway car; he mentions an unnamed doctor entering and declaring Itō's condition hopeless. See ch. 4 in Kokovtsov, *Iz moego proshlogo*, vol. 1, 391. For more on An (1879–1910), who was executed by the Japanese in Port Arthur, see Jieun Han and Franklin Rausch, *An Chunggŭn: His Life and Thought in His Own Words* (Leiden: Brill, 2020).

17 An extensive summary of the Berlin article appeared in Riga as "Ein baltischer Augenzeuge über den Tod des Fürsten Ito," *Rigasche Zeitung* 288 (12 December 1909). Cf. *Briefe*, 13[26] October 1909 (wrongly dated 21 October) for a description of the assassination, with a sketch showing his position at the railway station. In a letter of 4[17] December 1909, Budberg complained that the Harbin press had silenced his role in the event.

18 Dr Roger Baron Budberg, "Aus der Mandschurei." This article, as well as "Chinesische Prostitution" and "Zur Charakteristik chinesischen Seelenlebens," were summarized in English in *American Anthropologist*, n.s., 12, no. 4 (October–December 1910), 675–6.

19 Budberg, "Aus der Mandschurei," 172.

20 Ibid., 169.

21 *Briefe*, 11[24] July 1908.

22 Sze, *Reminiscences of His Early Years*, 49. Sze remained in the United States and died in Washington, D.C. The original Chinese is *Shi Zhaoji zaonian huiyi lu* (Taipei: Zhuanji wenxue chubanshe, 1967), here 63.

23 Budberg, "Aus der Mandschurei," 171.

24 See the novella "Atsumi Shibato," titled after the Japanese whom the Russians executed as a spy, in Krieglstein, *Zwischen Weiss und Gelb*, 321, 329–32. A recollection of the incident in Gongzhuling, and of the way the reporter and writer Baron Eugen Binder von Krieglstein (1873–1914) described it, is in Dr. med. Roger Baron Budberg, *Bilder aus der Zeitder Lungenpest-Epidemien*, 121.

25 Dr Roger Baron Budberg,"Chinesische Prostitution." (The Qing edict outlawing the sale of people was issued in early 1910.)

26 This is the argument of Ransmeier, *Sold People*.

27 See the cover image, a photograph by Sidney Gamble showing the entrance to the refuge for prostitutes (*jiliangsuo*) in Peking in the late 1910s, in Remick, *Regulating Prostitution in China*, and her ch. 5, "The *Jiliangsuo*: Prostitute Rescue Institutions."

28 Gamble, *Peking: A Social Survey*, 249, 480–5.

29 Baron Budberg, "Über die Bedingungen des Exporthandels in der Nordmandschurei," 8, 9.

30 Dr. med. Roger Baron Budberg,"Zur Charakteristik chinesischen Seelenlebens," 111–12.

31 Dr R. Baron Budberg, "Bürg- und Haftpflicht im chinesischen Volksleben."

32 Budberg (signed Clemens Goetz), "Die Nationen in der Mandschurei"; and cf. his letter concerning this publication, in *Briefe*, 1 June 1910.

33 Lattimore, *Manchuria*, 176, 296–7.

34 Ibid., 251.

35 *Briefe*, 3[18] February 1907.

36 *Briefe*, 18 March 1907.

37 *Briefe*, 20 September–30 October 1907. For more on the subject, see Gamsa, "Mixed Marriages in Russian-Chinese Manchuria."

38 *Briefe*, 7 August 1907.

39 *Briefe*, 18 December 1907.

40 Budberg, *Memuary*, pt ii, 7, 37–8, 120–1. These mountains are described in Novikov, "Al'chukaskoe fudutunstvo," 18–21.

41 The National Geographic map, "Kirin, Harbin, Vladivostok" (1905), still showed Harbin as the smaller town between "Ashe Ho (Alchuka)" and "Hulan cheng": see Figure I.2.

42 Iastremskii, "Ocherk byta i nravov severnoi Man'chzhurii," 224–5; Novikov, "Al'chukaskoe fudutunstvo," 40–2.

43 See "Girin" (Jilin), entry by the Manchu specialist Aleksei Ivanovskii in *Entsiklopedicheskii slovar' Brokgauz i Efron*, vol. 8a (1893), 753–4; for detailed population data, see Novikov, "Al'chukaskoe fudutunstvo," 30–4, who gives 3,788 Manchu and only 943 Han Chinese households in Ashihe.

44 Budberg, *Bilder aus der Zeit der Lungenpest-Epidemien*, 5–7. "Li-Jui-Dshen" appears in the entry on Roger Budberg in BBL. An autodidact, Budberg improvised his transcription methods. They come closest to, without matching fully, the system of transcribing Chinese into German that he could have found in a textbook published in Germany's leasehold in Shandong: Ferdinand Lessing and Wilhelm Othmer, *Lehrbuch der nordchinesischen Umgangssprache* (Tsingtau, 1912).

45 In the above-cited letter to his sister dated 18 December 1907, Budberg wrote that he had by then been married for two and a half months.

46 See Wang, "Affecting Grandiosity," 168, 173, 179–83.

47 *Briefe*, 16 September 1909. The photographs are in the Popoff and Raczynski family albums.

48 Makaroff had received these photographs, along with photographs of the 1910 plague in Harbin with comments in Roger Budberg's handwriting, from Baron Nikolai Budberg in Germany, who in turn had obtained them from Nikolai Popoff in Belgium (see more on these individuals below). Museum of Russian Culture, miscellaneous materials, folder 26 (microfilm copy at Hoover Institution Archives). I thank Yves Franquien for locating the relevant correspondence at the Museum of Russian Culture.

49 Budberg, *Bilder aus der Zeit der Lungenpest-Epidemien*, 18.

50 Dr Roger Baron Budberg, "Chinesen und Mandschus," extract from article in *St Petersburger Zeitung*, reprinted in *Rigasche Zeitung* 5 (7 January 1912).

51 Budberg, *Memuary*, pt i, 69.

52 Shao, *Remote Homeland*, 35, 75; Chen et al., "Interethnic Marriage in Northeast China, 1866–1913," 948, 953.

53 This would be consistent with bearing a Han surname. See Rhoads, *Manchus & Han*, 54–6; Chen et al., "Interethnic Marriage in Northeast China."

54 *Briefe*, 18 March 1907.

55 Raczynski family album.

56 *Briefe*, 7 August 1907.

57 Popoff and Raczynski family albums.

58 Budberg, "Vom Seelenleben der Chinesen," 59–60. Cf. Budberg, *Memuary*, pt i, 43; *Briefe*, 11[24] September 1908.

59 See Dudbridge, *The Legend of Miaoshan*, for example, 45, on the sword breaking, which thus prevented Miaoshan's execution. I thank Barend ter Haar for additional explanations and the reference to his study, *Practicing Scripture*, 38, 44, 243 n110.

60 *Briefe*, 18 March 1907.

61 *Briefe*, letters to Antoinette and Joseph of 18 December 1907; on his intention to hire a German teacher and his request for German children's

books, 11[24] September 1908; on intensive Chinese studies, see also 17 April 1909.

62 *Briefe*, letter begun on 20 September and completed on 30 October 1907.

63 *Briefe*, 11[24] July 1908. The same letter described his Chinese teacher, his countryside excursions, and his determination to learn spoken Chinese to the highest standard. See also 11[24] September 1908.

64 *Briefe*, 2 November 1922. These people were still there in 1919 and 1920: Budberg, *Memuary*, pt ii, 6, 74.

65 *Briefe*, 7 August 1907.

66 *Briefe*, 16 September 1909.

67 *Briefe*, 1 September 1910.

68 *Briefe*, 11[24] September 1908.

69 Volkov, "Antisemitism as a Cultural Code," 31, 34–5, 45.

70 *Briefe*, 23 July 1906, 31 May[13 June] 1910, 1 June 1910.

71 This article was titled "Russisches Prestige in der Nord-Mandschurei"; cf. *Briefe*, 2 August 1910.

72 He still remembered their names: old Itel'man (probably: Gitel'man) and his daughters, Rosa and Hanna. Budberg, *Memuary*, pt ii, 21. The publisher's introduction went further, claiming that during his youthful studies of the Talmud he corresponded with rabbis. Ibid., ii–iii.

73 See, for example, ibid., pt i, 9, 67; pt ii, 32, 80. Cf. Mark Gamsa, "Letters from Harbin," 33.

74 Esther Kallen, née Komarovskaia (Poltava, 1880–Washington, D.C., 1966), audiotape of interview (in English) with family members, recorded on 17 October 1965 in Washington; and copy of her midwife's diploma, issued by the Medical Faculty of Iur'ev University in 1898, in possession of the Lipkowitz family. Until 1908, the university did not admit women for regular studies in other professions.

75 Cf. Peckham, ed., *Empires of Panic*.

76 See also Gamsa, "The Epidemic of Pneumonic Plague."

77 *Briefe*, 4[17] December 1909. "One of the best China-knowers" was also how the Baltic papers described Budberg when they reported on his decoration; he must have used the same phrase to define himself. The news appeared first in the *Nordlivlandische Zeitung* in Dorpat, was quickly spread by *Rigasche Zeitung* 165 (22 July 1909) and other Baltic German papers, and was then also reported in Estonian, in *Ristirahwa Pühhapäewaleht* 32 (6 August 1909).

78 Shteinfel'd, *Russkoe delo v Man'chzhurii*, 176–8 (the other unnamed person was a Mongol, a former interpreter for the renowned explorer Przhevalsky and presently a commercial agent).

79 Joseph A. Raczynski cited this childhood memory of his elder brother, Sigismund E.A.W. Raczynski, in *Briefe*, 93.

80 "Eguan fu Fujiadian diaocha wenyi" (Russian Officials Come to Fujiadian to Inspect the Plague), in *Yuandong bao*, 20 November 1910, on the arrival and meetings of Dr Bu ("Bu daifu").

81 "Bu yisheng yan Fujiadian zhi fangyi banfa" (Physician Bu on Plague Prevention Methods in Fujiadian), in *Yuandong bao*, 21 November 1910.

82 "E xuetang zhi fangyi" (Plague Prevention at a Russian School), in *Yuandong bao*, 24 November 1910, on these visits; and "Bu daifu bu ganyu Fujiadian fangyi shi" (Dr Bu will not Intervene in Fujiadian Plague Prevention), in *Yuandong bao*, 27 November 1910, on the obstacles he had encountered.

83 Letter printed in the Fujiadian newspaper *Dongchui gongbao* (Eastern Border Gazette) in late November 1910, translated in Martinevskii and Mollaret, *Epidemiia chumy v Man'chzhurii v 1910–1911 gg.*, 169–70.

84 The daily reports on the plague in *Yuandong bao* mentioned Budberg's work at the head of his team on 14, 18, and 21 December 1910.

85 This draws on the detailed exposé in Budberg, *Bilder aus der Zeit der Lungenpest-Epidemien*.

86 *Kharbinskii vestnik*, 1903, no. 9, quoted in Ermachenko, "'V Kharbine vse spokoino,'" 80–1.

87 Budberg, *Bilder aus der Zeit der Lungenpest-Epidemien*, 110–20.

88 Ibid.

89 This pamphlet is mentioned by Budberg in the article cited below and in *Bilder aus der Zeit der Lungenpest-Epidemien*. It was also listed in the bibliographical section of *Vestnik Azii* 8 (1911), 159.

90 Priv.-Doz. Dr. Roger Baron Budberg, "Einige hygienische Prinzipien."

91 Dr. med. Baron Budberg, "Gibt es eine Prädisposition von Geschlecht …?"

92 He told readers of *Zentralblatt für Gynäkologie* in 1901 that treating the navel with alcohol after birth was a method often reported to him by "the simple folk," by which he must have meant Estonian peasants. Roger Freiherr v. Budberg, "Zur Alkoholbehandlung des Nabelschnurrestes" (see n62 to ch. 2 above), 1081.

93 Dr. med. Roger Freiherr von Budberg, "Über die Verwendung des Kampfers in der Gynäkologie."

5 Daily Life in a Mixed City

1 Ermachenko, "Intellektual'naia istoriia i mir veshchei," 322.

2 See ch. 5, "Russian Harbin," in Vassiliev, *Beauty in Exile*.

3 Bickers, "History, Legend and Treaty Port Ideology," 84, makes this observation on parades in expatriate Shanghai.

4 Mao Hong, "Ha'erbin Zhong-E renmin shenghuo zhuangkuang," 119.

5 Liaozuo sanren, *Binjiang chenxiao lu*, 134. The Confucian sage had said: "I have heard of the Chinese converting barbarians to their ways, but not

of their being converted to barbarian ways." *Mencius* (Book 3, part A: 4), trans. D.C. Lau (Harmondsworth: Penguin Books, 1979), 103.

6 Polish sinologist Jerzy Sie-Grabowski (1936–2016), interviewed by Thomas Lahusen in Warsaw in 2012. The interview is included in the documentary film directed by Lahusen, *Manchurian Sleepwalkers* (2017).

7 Mao Hong, "Ha'erbin Zhong-E renmin shenghuo zhuangkuang," 118; Liaozuo sanren, *Binjiang chenxiao lu*, 147–8.

8 See frontispiece in Xiao Hong, *Market Street*.

9 Shi Fang and Gao Ling, *Chuantong yu biange*, 391–2; and on Chinese taking dancing classes, the critical observations in Liaozuo sanren, *Binjiang chenxiao lu*, 129.

10 A good discussion of the connection between hair and national identity in China is Godley, "The End of the Queue"; on the queue and individual identity in the late Qing and early republic, see Chou, *Memory, Violence, Queues*.

11 Smirnov, *Priamurskii krai*, 39; Park, *Sovereignty Experiments*, 81–3, 97, 122, 136.

12 In Peking in the 1870s, one of the most important Western photographers to document life in late imperial China was fascinated by the female Manchu headgear. See Yao, ed., *China: Through the Lens of John Thomson*, photographs on 25–9, 32–43.

13 Christie, *Thirty Years in Moukden*, 14. A local scholar describing Heilongjiang customs in 1891 even claimed that "all city women dress in the Manchu way, while peasants imitate them." Hu Zongliang, *Heilongjiang shuliie*, 83.

14 Philip A. Kuhn, *Soulstealers: The Chinese Sorcery Scare of 1768* (Cambridge, MA: Harvard University Press, 1990), describes a mass panic brought about by a "queue-cutting scare."

15 Golovachev, *Rossiia na Dal'nem Vostoke*, 132, goes so far as to say that dragging Chinese by the queue was commonly done for sport in Vladivostok, as well as at the Harbin railway station.

16 Garin, *Po Koree, Mandzhurii i Liaodunskomu poluostrovu*, 262. Cf. Abrosimov, *Pod chuzhim nebom*, 67, on such scenes in Harbin.

17 Carter, *Creating a Chinese Harbin*, 115, assumes on the basis of "the larger body of colonial and postcolonial studies" that an otherwise straightforward press report on the beating of a white-bearded Russian by a Chinese policeman amounted to an expression of Russian anxiety over the decline of "the white man's prestige." While such anxiety existed, numerous cases of the mistreatment of Russians by Chinese police in Harbin and the CER zone were reported. Many are detailed in the pamphlet *Mémorandum du Comité des Représentants des Institutions Judiciaires à Harbin*, copy Leeds University Library.

18 Vortisch-van Vloten, "Vom gewesenen Zopf," 385; Chou, *Memory, Violence, Queues*, 81, 85. Russians witnessing such scenes were aware of both purposes, as well as of the queue's importance to its wearers; see Runich, "V Man'chzhurii," 629–31.

19 Baikov, "Moi priezd v Man'chzhuriiu," 79–80; cf. Runich, "V Man'chzhurii," 619–20.

20 Tong Yue, *Guandong jiu fengsu*, 110–11.

21 Diabkin and Levchenko, "'Nemets s russkoiu dushoi'."

22 Severnyi, *Farforovyi kitaets kachaet golovoi*; and idem, *Ozero goluboi tsapli*; both books in the collection of Russian émigré literature at Hamilton Library, University of Hawai'i.

23 See entry on him in Sorokina, *Rossiiskoe nauchnoe zarubezh'e*, 124.

24 Magaram, *Zheltyi lik*, copy Fondo Russia Bianca, Università degli Studi di Milano. "Capital of the Yellow Devil" is the opening story in the collection; the two stories on Chinese men's sexual longing for European women are titled "The Wife" and "Dangerous Fun."

25 His stories originally appeared in *Zheltyi lik*, copy National Library of Israel, and in two other Shanghai Russian miscellanies, *The Far East* (1920) and *China* (1923), where he also published his translations from French of Chinese tales and of an essay on Chinese art. See complete contents lists in N.A. Bogomolov, *Materialy k bibliografii russkikh literaturno-khudozhestvennykh al'manakhov i sbornikov, 1900–1937* (Materials for the Bibliography of Russian Literary and Art Miscellanies and Collections) (Moscow: Lanterna-Vita, 1994), vol. 1, nos. 160, 208, 303. Another short introduction to contemporary China, mostly an ethnographic description of Chinese daily life, reflected Magaram's socialist sympathies: see Magaram, *Sovremennyi Kitai*, copy Leeds University Library.

26 Kreid and Bakich, eds., *Russkaia poeziia Kitaia*, 89. Cf. another poem by Baturin on "the strangest love" of a girl from Ningbo, "Luna" (Moon, 1931), in ibid., 91–3. An example from Harbin poetry is "Zhivaia muza" (A Living Muse, 1935) by Nikolai A. Shchegolev (1910–1975), in ibid., 573–4.

27 Ji Xianlin, *Liu De huiyi lu*, 23; Zhu Ziqing, "Xixing tongxun," 368. In pidgin, *babushka* (grandmother, in standard Russian) was applied to Russian women in general.

28 See, for example, Taskina, *Russkie v Man'chzhurii*, 37–46. Ch. 1 of Vengerov, *Reka Kharbinskikh vremen*, is titled "Toska po rodnoi reke Sungari" (Longing for [our] Native Sungari River). The memoirist, who writes, "I had the fortune 'to grow up' on the Sungari, as our whole family spent almost 25 years on this river," left Harbin in 1958. His little book was published by the Harbin and Manchuria Historical Society in Sydney after he revisited Harbin in 1995, and he donated a copy to the State Historical Library in Moscow.

29 Panov, "Zheltyi vopros v Priamur'e," 66, mentions Russians pushing Chinese into the water as a common form of insult. The drowning in Blagoveshchensk in 1900, discussed in ch. 1, may have had similar underpinnings.

30 Liaozuo sanren, *Binjiang chenxiao lu*, 111 (cf. 5). This description is also cited in Ji Fenghui, *Ha'erbin xungen*, 85–6. The Peach Blossom land is the

subject of a celebrated fifth-century poem; the reference to spring employs standard sexual imagery.

31 Catherine Vance Yeh, "Representing the City: Shanghai and its Maps," in David Faure and Tao Tao Liu, eds., *Town and Country in China: Identity and Perception* (New York: Palgrave, 2002), 183.

32 Ch'en, *China and the West*, 388; he does mention conservative opposition to women's liberation.

33 Ianinova, "Zhizn' russkikh v Manchzhurii 1919–1949 gody," 16 February 1956. (Here and below, the instalments of this essay, serialized in the Paris newspaper *Russkaia mysl'*, are cited by date of publication.)

34 Lindt, *Im Sattel durch Mandschukuo*, 195.

35 Ianinova, "Zhizn' russkikh v Manchzhurii," 28 February 1956; cf. Il'in, "Na sluzhbe u iapontsev," no. 80, 201–2.

36 Song Shisheng, "The Brothels of Harbin in the Old Society," available in English translation in Clausen and Thøgersen, *The Making of a Chinese City*, 103–8.

37 Lattimore, *Manchuria*, 271–2.

38 Mart, "Zheltye rabyni." Mart returned to the Soviet Union in 1923 and was executed in Kiev during the Stalinist purges.

39 Another missionary source estimated the total number of prostitutes in Harbin at that time to be as high as 8,000. League of Nations, "Position of Women of Russian Origin in the Far East," 7, 9.

40 Ibid., 1; Il'in, "Na sluzhbe u iapontsev," no. 82, 199–200.

41 Quoted in Shi Fang, Gao Ling, and Liu Shuang, *Ha'erbin Eqiao shi*, 569. The parallel section in the modern edition of Liaozuo sanren, *Binjiang chenxiao lu*, 155–6, is less detailed.

42 Prikashchikov, "K istorii russkogo sadovodstva v Man'chzhurii," 1–2.

43 Ermachenko, "Intellektual'naia istoriia i mir veshchei," 323–4, 327. Cf. an officer's complaint on getting no milk for coffee, in Bekkin, "Pis'ma leitenanta I.I. Isliamova," 32.

44 Novikov, "Al'chukaskoe fudutunstvo," 57, 88.

45 Iashnov, "Pitanie krest'ian v Severnoi Man'chzhurii," 16–17.

46 On Russian farming in Manchuria, see Beloglazov, *Russkaia zemledel'cheskaia kul'tura*.

47 Vitalisov, "Rol' russkikh v razvitii sadovodstva i ovoshchevodstva," 18. However, Khvostov, "Russkii Kitai," pt i, 679, mentions several of the vegetables on this list among Chinese agricultural products in Kwantung, singling out potatoes as a novelty cultivated since the Russians' arrival. Melikhov, *Man'chzhuriia dalekaia i blizkaia*, 270–4, draws heavily on Prikashchikov, "K istorii russkogo sadovodstva v Man'chzhurii," cited above, adding that Russians also introduced horticulture and beekeeping. Cf. Melikhov, *Rossiiskaia emigratsiia v Kitae*, 142–4. Similarly, Kovalevskii, *Zarubezhnaia Rossiia*, 95, quoted his informant V.S. Makarov (Makaroff) on

the introduction of tomatoes into Manchuria by the Russian botanist I.S. Iashkin.

48 The latest list is in Beloglazov, "Kitaiskii vektor tsivilizatsionno-kul'turnogo vzaimodeistviia," 256–7. Shan, *Taming China's Wilderness*, 69, says that "almost all [Chinese settlers in Heilongjiang] grew cabbages, turnips, onions, eggplant, peppers, cucumbers, and potatoes." It is unclear whether any of these vegetables included the botanical species for which Russians claimed credit. In terms of farming technology, Reardon-Anderson, *Reluctant Pioneers*, 182–3, suggests that the Russian plough may have been the only modern innovation that peasants in Jilin and Heilongjiang accepted.

49 Stasiukevich, "Russko-kitaiskoe vzaimodeistvie." While these efforts were largely unsuccessful, the voluntary adoption of some Chinese methods and customs in agriculture, nutrition, and medicine by peasant settlers in the Russian Far East is described in Kaufman, *Po novym mestam*, 167; and Beloglazov, "Kitaiskii vektor," 266–7.

50 Ji Fenghui, *Ha'erbin xungen*, 310–11; Yang Aili, *Sun Yunxuan zhuan*, 8.

51 Hu Zongliang, *Heilongjiang shulüe*, 90. Rice cultivation in Liaoning and southern Jilin began during the Russo-Japanese War and spread more widely by the 1920s, much of it undertaken by Korean settlers. Frizendorf, *Severnaia Man'chzhuriia*, 97–9.

52 Ermachenko, "'V Kharbine vse spokoino,'" 89.

53 Green, "Guobaorou." Chef Zheng's great-grandson still claims to prepare the only authentic *guobaorou* in town. His "Old Chef" restaurant is advertised "since 1907."

54 Cf. Melikhov, *Belyi Kharbin*, 144–9.

55 Ablamskii, who was born in Kiev, lived in Harbin from 1922 (with an interruption for studies in Ghent and Liège, Belgium, between 1930 and 1933) until 1945, when he was deported to the Gulag. A selection of his Harbin photographs was made available by the Irkutsk Municipal History Museum to the "Meeting of Frontiers" project of the Library of Congress and may be seen on the website frontiers.loc.gov.

56 Fujiwara, "Zhenshchiny v Kharbine pri Man'chzhou-Go." Cf. Fialkovskii, "Torgovyi dom I.Ya. Churina v Kharbine." The landmark Matsuura building on Zhongyang dajie also survives, and now houses the Information Department of the adjacent Central Bookstore.

57 Jiang Zhijun and Guo Chonglin, *Songhua jiangpan de minsu yu lüyou*, 16.

58 A frequently reproduced photograph of a peddler selling strings of frozen apples on a Harbin street appears in the unpaginated front matter of Taskina and Sel'kina, *Kharbin*.

59 "'Sblizhenie natsii" ("The Rapprochement of Nations"), *Kharbinskii vestnik*, no. 2247 (14 September 1911).

60 These examples are taken from advertisements placed in an issue of the Harbin daily *Novosti zhizni* (Life News), no. 271 (28 December 1918).

61 Taskina, *Russkie v Man'chzhurii*, 110. The trouble with Lundstrem's oft-repeated memory is that the record, "Dear Old Southland," which he said he had bought "in 1933," was only released in December 1934 (see jazz .ru/2016/08/19/oleg-lundstrem-orchestra-01); his buying it in a Chinese store is more important here.

62 Ermachenko, "'V Kharbine vse spokoino,'" 84–5.

63 Ibid., 88; Starosel'skaia, *Povsednevnaia zhizn' 'russkogo' Kitaia*, 59–60; Rachinskaia, *Pereletnye ptitsy*, 126–30; Grüner, "In the Streets and Bazaars of Harbin."

64 See, for example, Laguta, "Zhiznennyi put'," 144, for a grateful memory. Ushanoff, "Recollections of Life," 9, said that his family "was always in debt to Chinese merchants from one month to the next."

65 Taskina, *Russkie v Man'chzhurii*, 89; on the recipes, see Kapran, *Povsednevnaia zhizn' russkogo naseleniia Kharbina*, 156.

66 See, for example, Nikolaeva, *Iapontsy*, 37, 171.

67 Vinkou, "Vospominaniia o pitanii," 28.

68 Ushanoff, "Recollections of Life," 19.

69 Abrosimov, *Pod chuzhim nebom*, 335. Cf. Reznikova, "V russkom Kharbine," 387–8. Memories of a visit to Fujiadian on the Chinese New Year, with impressions of paper dragons and prostitutes, are in Dvorzhitskaia, "Moi mnogolikii Kharbin," 99–100.

70 The Harbin writer Natal'ia I. Il'ina (1914–1994), who repatriated to the Soviet Union in 1948, left a coded portrait of Eshchin in her memoir, *Vozvrashchenie*, vol. 1, 40–1, 164, 190–4. Eshchin admitted having only poor Chinese in his poem "Iamadzhi" (1928), in Kreid and Bakich, *Russkaia poeziia Kitaia*, 183.

71 As in the opening instalment of Ianinova, "Zhizn' russkikh v Man'chzhurii." Cf. Abrosimov, *Pod chuzhim nebom*, 29, 238.

72 *Song Xiaolian ji*, 101.

73 Norman Smith, *Intoxicating Manchuria*, 25–6, 33–4.

74 Novikov, "Al'chukaskoe fudutunstvo," 50–1, 63–6; Boloban, *Otchet*, 52–7; Li Sui'an, *Ma Zhongjun ji Ha'erbin Dunyuan*, 43.

75 Grüner, "'The Chicago of the East,'" 60–1, 70–3. Il'in, "Na sluzhbe u iapontsev," no. 82, 199, identifies Koreans in Manchuria and Russian employees of the CER as the main opium dealers in the late 1920s, adding that "everybody made a profit in this business." Smith, *Intoxicating Manchuria*, 29, calls Harbin "one of the biggest narcotic markets in East Asia."

76 Sorokina, "Liquor and Opium."

77 Eshchin, "Pro Moskvu" (On Moscow, n.d.), in Kreid and Bakich, *Russkaia poeziia Kitaia*, 180–2. On smoking opium, Nikolai V. Peterets (1907?–1944), "Liubov' – nit'" (Love-Line, n.d.), in ibid., 419–20; on "sitting down with the Chinese in [their] inns," relishing the *khanshin*, see Mikhail Ts. Spurgot

(1901–1993), untitled poem beginning with the lines "Sizhu s kitaitsami v kharchevniakh" (1931), in ibid., 517. Venedikt Mart, an opium addict, also wrote on the subject.

78 Bakich, "Émigré Identity," 53–5. The annual commemoration of Harbin's defence against the Boxers in 1900 was marked as "thrice thirteen" on 13 July 1913 (ibid.).

79 On the "bal poudré": Rachinskaia, *Kaleidoskop zhizni*, 225 (with photograph on 264); for more on these celebrations, see Melikhov, *Belyi Kharbin*, 377–83. The CER anniversary history is Nilus, *Istoricheskii obzor*, vol. 1.

80 Nazemtseva, "Peredacha KVZhD v sobstvennost' SSSR," 168.

81 Qu Qiubai attended Revolution Day in Harbin in 1920: see his *Exiang jicheng*, 271–2.

82 Abrosimov, *Pod chuzhim nebom*, 33–4; Nikolaeva, *Iapontsy*, 35, 148; Ianinova, "Zhizn' russkikh v Manchzhurii," 14 February 1956; E.S. Medvedeva, "Tat'ianin den'," in Taskina, *Russkii Kharbin*, 63.

83 Xiao Hong, *Market Street*, 64–8, 74.

84 Starosel'skaia, *Povsednevnaia zhizn' 'russkogo' Kitaia*, 286.

85 On *tolkai-tolkai* in Russian memory, see, for example, a poem under this title by Harbin poet Vasilii S. Loginov (1891–1945?), quoted in ibid., 61–2; Taskina, *Neizvestnyi Kharbin*, 41.

86 Chen Wenlong, "Yi hao binghua ji ru feng."

87 Zhao Luchen, "Ha'erbin Zhong-E bianyuanyu xiaowang tanyin," 123.

88 Dewar et al., "Harbin, Lanterns of Ice, Sculptures of Snow," 524. Typically, Wang Jingfu, *Ha'erbin bingxue wenhua fazhan shi*, 14, traces the beginnings of the snow festival in 1963 to "the inspiration of ancient ice lanterns."

89 Quoting Taskina, *Neizvestnyi Kharbin*, 41; cf. her *Russkii Kharbin*, 576; Zhernakov, "Reka Sungari v zhizni Kharbina"; Rachinskaia, *Pereletnye ptitsy*, 14–15 (with photograph on 250); Melikhov, *Belyi Kharbin*, 123–8; Mitchell, *Spoils of Opportunity*, 195.

90 Ah Cheng, *Ha'erbin ren*: 124 ff. on beer and kvass; 148 on winter swimming; 152 on the ice festival; 157–8 on the Russian songs; 164 on breakfast habits; 167 on Russian bread. Since 2002, Harbin has also staged an international beer festival every summer, to which young Russian women are flown in as decorations.

91 On Russian Easter in Harbin and paying visits on Easter Sunday, see, for example, V.V. Levitskii, *Pristan' na Sungari*, pt i, 116–18; Melikhov, *Belyi Kharbin*, 319–24. On Chinese New Year, by a Harbin sinologist, I.G. Baranov, "Kitaiskii Novyi god," 42–5 (originally in *Vestnik Man'chzhurii* 1927, no. 1); and idem, *Cherty narodnogo byta v Kitae*, 3–6.

92 Shiliaev, "Obshchestvenno-kul'turnaia, religioznaia i politicheskaia zhizn' Kharbina," 237. On Radonitsa in Harbin, see also Dzemeshkevich, *Kharbintsy*, 97.

93 Ah Cheng, *Ha'erbin ren*, 24. Cf. the comment on this in Ushanoff, "Recollections of Life," 25: "the Chinese people went around and gathered everything which seems to me was a good idea."

94 Laguta, "Zhiznennyi put'," 144 (this recollection may refer either to the speaker's life in Harbin or to his earlier encounters with the Chinese while growing up in a Russian village on the Amur border).

95 Nikitin, "Prazdnik pominoveniia umershikh Chzhun-iuan'-tsze."

96 Shi Laoye (pen name of P.V. Shkurkin), "Den' 'rozhdeniia Buddy,'" *Novaia zhizn'* (Harbin), 27 May 1920. Hoover Institution Archives, Pavel Vasil'evich Shkurkin papers, *Sbornik statei* no. 2.

97 See Il'ina, *Vozvrashchenie*, vol. 1, 182, 202–3; Borodin et al., *Semeinye khroniki*, 44–5.

98 V.P. Ablamskii, "Russkii sport v Kharbine" (1994), in Taskina, *Russkii Kharbin*, 219–20; Kirsanov, "Veitia," on the career of Harbin football player and trainer Viktor Popkov in Shenyang.

99 *Kharbinskii vestnik*, no. 196, (1904), qtd in Ermachenko, "'V Kharbine vse spokoino,'" 92–3, reported that the mixed audience included "generals Du and Zhou Mian with their families, dragomans, secretaries of the diplomatic bureaus," as well as "pupils of the Chinese school" among the public. The comprador official Zhou Mian has been mentioned in ch. 3. Du Xueying was the Binjiang *daotai*.

100 *Kharbinskii vestnik*, 1904, no. 146, quoted ibid., 93.

101 "Feiting renren canguan" (Airplane Exhibition Open to Everyone), *Yuandong bao*, 18 April 1911; and "Feiting jinri you feixing yi" (The Airplane Flew Again Today), *Yuandong bao*, 6 May 1911. Melikhov, *Man'chzhuriia dalekaia i blizkaia*, 230–2, confirms the pull of the aviation show for Chinese spectators.

102 "Laren yuan kaimu zhi sheng" (Successful Opening of Wax Figure Hall), *Yuandong bao*, 30 November 1911.

103 Tikhonov, *Konnozavodstvo Severnoi Man'chzhurii* (copy Russian State Library, Moscow), 16, 20.

104 Advertisements for the Izako circus, with details of the program, as placed in *Yuandong bao* on 16, 23, and 24 December 1916, 11 January 1917, 20 February 1917, 10 February 1918.

105 A report on a charity event at the Tongle Tea Garden (Tongle chayuan), in which Russians participated, appeared in *Yuandong bao* on 9 July 1911.

106 Liu Qun, "Binjiang menghua lu," on the world of traditional Chinese theatre. On that of the operettas, see much in Melikhov, *Belyi Kharbin*.

107 From the memoirs of Jiang Chunfang (1912–1987) on his friendship with painter Jin Jianxiao (1910–1936), qtd in Shi Fang, Gao Ling, and Liu Shuang, *Ha'erbin Eqiao shi*, 420–1. No stranger to the cultural events of Russian Harbin and proficient in Russian, Jin later translated the play

and had it serialized in a newspaper, but he did not manage to stage it in Chinese before being arrested and executed by the Manchukuo regime (Ibid.).

108 Ibid., 284; and cf. Rykunov, "Russkii kinematograf v Kharbine."

109 This may be contrasted with a historian's description of tsarist Georgia: "Literacy, education, and even attendance at the new Tiflis Theater were ... ways in which the peoples of the Caucasus could affirm for Russians their willingness to participate in the civic life of the empire." Jersild, "From Savagery to Citizenship," 108.

110 Data cited in Coulter, "Harbin," 968.

111 Brower, "Islam and Ethnicity," 120; Geraci, "Russian Orientalism at an Impasse," 139.

112 Seide, "Die Russisch-Orthodoxe Kirche in China," 175–6.

113 Elevferii, "Doklad o prebyvanii v Man'chzhurii," 142–7.

114 Wu Baixiang, "Wushi nian zishu," 5, 28, on his arrival in Harbin after the Boxer Uprising, and on being baptized in 1915. Wu was founder of the Tongji department store.

115 Cherkasov-Georgievskii, *Russkii khram na chuzhbine*, 246, 252.

116 Shiliaev, "Obshchestvenno-kul'turnaia, religioznaia i politicheskaia zhizn' Kharbina," 238.

117 However, images of Harbin Russian churches were reproduced not only on Russian postcards but also in a popular Chinese journal like the *Shanghai Pictorial*: see, for example, *Shanghai huabao*, 30 September 1928.

118 In a traditional city such as Mukden, the Scottish Presbyterian missionary and physician Dugald Christie (1855–1936) observed only one-storey houses; he explained this building style by a Chinese belief that towers were for spirits, not humans. See his *Ten Years in Manchuria*, 10. H.E.M. James too saw only one-storey houses when he travelled through Manchuria in 1886: James, *The Long White Mountain*, 135–6.

119 Ji Fenghui, *Ha'erbin xungen*, 288. James, *The Long White Mountain*, 194, cites Rev. Alexander Williamson, *Journeys in North China, Manchuria and Mongolia* (1870) on Chinese fears that "high church-towers, and even telegraph poles and railway signals, will compel good spirits to turn aside in all directions, and so throw everything into confusion."

120 See, for example, Petrov, *Gorod na Sungari*, 35; Melikhov, *Man'chzhuriia dalekaia i blizkaia*, 83; Taskina, *Neizvestnyi Kharbin*, 46.

121 Bakich, "Did You Speak Harbin Sino-Russian?," 30.

122 Pokrovskii et al., *Dukhovnaia literatura staroverov vostoka Rossii*, 132–3. Cf. "Nikola-spasitel' na vodakh" (Nicholas the Saviour on Waters), one of the short stories in Georgievskii, *Tam – na drugom beregu Amura*, 101–3, copy British Library; Nikolaev, *Nikita Ikonnik*, 11–12.

123 Thomas, "History and Anthropology," 14. And cf. 13: "The value of myths or legends to the historian lies in what they tell him about the society in which they were composed, not what he can learn from them about the distant past to which they purport to relate."

124 Cf. Carter, *Creating a Chinese Harbin*, 157–9, for a speculative discussion.

125 Erdberg, *Kitaiskie novelly*, 112.

126 Novikov, "Oskolki russkogo Kharbina," 120. This report on conversations with Harbin's last elderly Russians also restates their belief that a terrible flood and years of drought followed in retribution for the destruction of St Nicholas Cathedral. Cf. Dzemeshkevich, *Kharbintsy*, 11, 227–8.

127 On the popular cult of city gods, see Overmyer, *Local Religion in North China in the Twentieth Century*, 40–1, 56, 158.

128 Obruchev, *Ot Kiakhty do Kul'dzhi*, 5, noticed (in 1892) that Russians had adopted a Buryat superstition regarding the rock called "the shaman's stone" at the source of the Angara River. A report from turn-of-the-century Kiakhta described local Russians honouring a Buddhist temple; see Ular, "Im Brackwasser der Kulturen," 1214. Joseph Baron Budberg, "Zwei Monate im sibirischen Urwalde," 259, observed that Russian hunters had taken up a superstition of the Ostyaks (the Khanty people) about leaving a part of their kill for the forest spirits.

129 Lattimore, "Byroads and Backwoods of Manchuria," 127.

130 Kravkov, *Voina v Man'chzhurii*, 26. More instances of this are described in Runich, "V Man'chzhurii," 627–8. Cf. Novikov, "Al'chukaskoe fudutunstvo," 36.

131 Ushanoff, "Recollections of Life," 29.

132 Bentley, *Old World Encounters*, 8, argues that social conversion and religious syncretism "often took three to five centuries."

133 Quested, *"Matey" Imperialists?*, 90, 124; cf. Matveev, "Kitaitsy na Kariiskikh promyslakh," 30. On hunting "white swans" or "white cranes" (after the traditional clothing of Koreans), "grouse" or "pheasants" (nicknames for the Chinese), see also Legras, *En Sibérie*, 354; Ossendowski, *Man and Mystery in Asia*, 92–3; Shkurkin, *Khunkhuzy*, 7; Stephan, *The Russian Far East*, 69.

134 See Blagoveshchenskii, "Zapiski o Sibiri," 291–300, by an ethnographer vehemently critical of the mores of Siberian villagers. Cf., for example, Keyserling, *Graf Alfred Keyserling erzählt*, 63–6.

135 Garin, *Po Koree, Mandzhurii i Liaodunskomu poluostrovu*, 26, 33. Cf. Hua Meng, "The Chinese Genesis of the Term Foreign Devil," 30–3.

136 Meakin, *A Ribbon of Iron*, 260–1. Vereshchagin, *Po Manchzhurii*, pt ii, 578–9, suggested that this rumour must have been started by hostile Chinese interpreters.

137 Shkurkin, "Kitai i Dal'nevostochnye perspektivy," 46.

138 See Christie, *Thirty Years in Moukden*, 6. Cf. Tian, "Rumor and Secret Space."

139 Cohen, *History in Three Keys*, 160–1; Steve Smith, "Fear and Rumour."

6 Trials and Endings

1 Dr Roger Baron Budberg, "Vom chinesischen Zopf."

2 Martini, "Ueber die Bedeutung der Internationalen Pestkonferenz." There is mention of Martini (1867–1953), and more on German medicine in Shandong, in Eckart, *Medizin und Kolonialimperialismus*.

3 "A Plea for the Pigtail." Uncommented summaries also appeared in the Dutch medical journal *Nederlands Tijdschrift voor Geneeskunde* (Amsterdam), vol. 56 (March 1912), 1507–8, and in the organ of the Theosophical Society in Nuremberg, *Der Theosophische Pfad*, vol. 11, no. 6 (September 1912), 268–9.

4 Dr Roger Baron Budberg, "O kitaiskoi kose," trans. from the *Deutsche medizinische Wochenschrift* by Dr K.A. Liuria, *Kharbinskii vestnik*, no. 2561 (1 September 1912).

5 Idem, "Der chinesische Zopf," *Der Ostasiatische Lloyd*, vol. 26, no. 35 (30 August 1912), 197–8.

6 Vortisch-van Vloten, "Vom gewesenen Zopf." Idem, *Chinesische Patienten und ihre Ärzte*, 73–81, reprinted Budberg's article from the Berlin journal along with Vortisch's response to it. On this author, see *Deutsche Biographische Enzyklopädie*, vol. 10, 312.

7 Dr. med. Baron Budberg, "Europäische Kulturträger und der chinesische Zopf."

8 Cf. Cheng, "Politics of the Queue," 133–8; Harrison, *The Making of the Republican Citizen*, 35–8. The *Draft History of the Qing*, edited by Zhao Erxun, came out in 1927.

9 A summary of this article appeared in *Rigasche Zeitung*, no. 201 (2 September 1913). See also Nilus, *Istoricheskii obzor Kitaiskoi vostochnoi zheleznoi dorogi*, 547–8.

10 National Archives of the United Kingdom, FO 228/1905, includes dispatches on the situation in Harbin following the outbreak of the war, and about the expulsion of German subjects.

11 He died a few weeks later, still to be honoured by an ambassador's burial in the Spanish capital. His tomb was restored in 2015. Mednikov, "Rossiiskii posol v neitral'noi Ispanii"; and "Tribute to the Baron of Budberg, the Last Ambassador of Tsarist Russia to Spain," *The Diplomat*, 12 March 2015.

12 Andreeva, "Pribaltiiskie nemtsy i Pervaia mirovaia voina"; and Deeg, *Kunst & Albers*, ch. 7.

13 Rennikov, *V strane chudes*, 7. See more on Rennikov's publications in Must, *Von Privilegierten zu Geächteten*, 122–39.

14 Lohr, *Nationalizing the Russian Empire*, 21, 77–9, 152–4; Must, *Von Privilegierten zu Geächteten*, 93, 96.

15 Budberg, *Memuary*, pt i, 16, 64.

16 Wilhelm Trautschold (1877–1937) left his post in Harbin, where he had served since 1914, in March 1917. Once he had cleared his name in Petrograd, the Provisional Government reassigned him to Honolulu, Hawai'i. He later immigrated to France. Khisamutdinov, *Rossiiskaia emigratsiia*, 308, referring to his service file in the Archive of Foreign Policy of the Russian Empire.

17 "Harbin Doctor Charged with Treason: Accused of Helping Germans to Escape," *North China Herald*, 13 November 1915. The wire from Harbin is datelined 5 November.

18 RGIA, f. 323, op. 1, d. 824, ll. 35–45 (telegrams to the CER Directorate, 29 and 30 October 1915 O.S.).

19 Budberg, *Memuary*, protocols section following pt i, 3–5. Budberg commented: "I never hid my being a wholeheartedly sinicized German, though not a German-turned-Chink, as von Arnold called me." *Memuary*, pt ii, 19. Budberg often cited this nickname; cf. ibid., 44, 86, 92.

20 Budberg, *Memuary*, pt i, 29, 54–5.

21 Ibid., pt i, 54–6; *Briefe*, 1 April 1924.

22 Sunderland, *The Baron's Cloak*, ch. 7.

23 The first quotation is from an unpublished autobiography by Severnyi, the second from the newspaper *Shankhaiskaia zaria* (The Shanghai Dawn) in 1934. Both are in Diabkin and Levchenko, " 'Nemets s russkoiu dushoi.' "

24 Krusenstern-Peterets, *Vospominaniia* (1975), serialized in *Rossiiane v Azii*, here no. 1 (1994), 93–4, 123.

25 See Happel, "Eine Karte voller Ziele," 69–72. (At 78, Happel mistakes "Chungusen," in an operational order of January 1917, for Tungus natives); Kiselev, " 'Podozritel'nye nemtsy,' " 124, on the Pappenheim mission.

26 There are many references to Stöffler in Budberg's *Memoirs*, his book on the plague in Manchuria, and in the letters to his sister. Cf. Kiselev, " 'Podozritel'nye nemtsy,' " 125, 130.

27 Cf. Schmidt, "Die Beschaffung geheimer Informationen," 116–19. A letter sent by Stöffler from Wujiazhan, his place of service near Bodune, dated 23 October 1912, announcing his decision to leave the mission, yet to stay on in Manchuria ("ma seconde patrie", as he called it), and a biographical sketch, are in the archive of the Société des Missions Étrangères de Paris.

28 Political Archive of the Federal Foreign Office (Berlin), R 18238, Agenten und Nachrichtenwesen in China (January 1915–January 1920), letter by Stöffler from Kassel on 1 August 1919 (also quoted by Schmidt, "Die

Beschaffung geheimer Informationen"). Preparing to return to China, Stöffler described his work during the war while proposing to resume it through his contacts with Baron Budberg in Harbin. German diplomats in Manchuria, such as Otto Hugo Witte, the consul in Mukden, considered Budberg an important promoter of German interests; a letter by Witte in the same file, dated 2 October 1919, mentions a report (now lost) on Budberg's efforts for Germany. See also R 10127, Russland 61: Allgemeine Angelegenheiten Russlands, Bd 180.

29 Budberg testified about meeting two POWs – one of whom he misnamed as Wolff von Tannenfels, or Tannenfeld, or Totenfels – at the apartment of the Shandor brothers in Harbin on 1 April 1915 (OS). *Memuary*, pt i, 41, 44, 50. See Todenwarth, *Eine tolle Flucht*, 148–56, on his sojourn in Harbin. After a night at the "Hotel Belgia" (probably the Bellevue, which belonged to Richard Kegel), he and the Austrian officer Franz Wlad had a secret meeting, at the apartment of two brothers, with "a German, who has lived in Harbin for a long time." This person, coded as "Herr M.," initially suspected they were Russian agents, but he then gave them precious advice on escape routes and contact names in Hulan and Bodune (cf. 163). As the account matches that in *Memuary*, the German resident of Harbin was evidently Budberg; "Herr St.," who assisted the two fugitives in Bodune (188–90), was Stöffler. An early memoir by Todenwarth's companion was even more careful not to identify the individuals who helped them in China: see Wlad, *Meine Flucht durchs mongolische Sandmeer*, 154–6, on Harbin.

30 Kiselev, " 'Podozritel'nye nemtsy,' " 129, 131–2.

31 Mervay, "Austro-Hungarian Refugee Soldiers in China," 50–4.

32 Shkurkin, "Dvoinoe poddanstvo."

33 RGIA DV, f. 1527 op. 1 d. 7, ll. 102–3, 186.

34 State Archive of Irkutsk *oblast* (GAIO), f. 245 op. 4, d. 308. This file, which contains the verdict of the Judicial Chamber, could not be consulted because of its poor state of conservation.

35 Budberg, *Memuary*, pt i, 25, 66–8 (on visits by Riutin, his wife and child, at Budberg's home, and on Riutin's defence of Budberg in a conversation with Khorvat).

36 Riutin then escaped to Irkutsk. He remained active in the Communist Party until he was eliminated for his part in an audacious plot to depose Stalin and the Party leadership. See William A. Clark, "The Ryutin Affair and the 'Terrorism' Narrative of The Purges," *Russian History* 42, no. 4 (November 2015), 377–424.

37 *Zhong-E guanxi shiliao, Dongbei bianfang*, ed. Deng Ruyuan et al., vol. 2, 491 (my thanks to Rachel Lin for noticing this rare mention of Budberg in a Chinese source). Cf. Budberg, *Memuary*, pt i, 69; pt ii, 97.

38 This is the subject of Kuznetsov, *'Gol'd' ukhodit v Kharbin*, who traces the later career of Budberg's steamer in Chinese service until 1932 (see 231). Cf. Melikhov, *Belyi Kharbin*, 360–4.

39 *Briefe*, 15 and 26 April 1921; and more in Budberg, *Memuary*, pt i, 40. Paul Lieven was grandfather of the British historian of imperial Russia, Dominic Lieven.

40 Budberg, *Memuary*, pt ii, 25–8.

41 Ibid., 16, 22, 29, 31, 34, on the Chinese support.

42 Ibid., 61–2. Cf. *Briefe*, 31 March 1920; and 18 November 1924 on accepting a social invitation from "my friend Lopato." See the memoirs of his daughter, a cabaret singer and restaurant owner in Paris, Liudmila Lopato (1914–2004), *Volshebnoe zerkalo vospominanii*. Eliason, who probably came from Tomsk, obtained his medical degree in Paris in 1898. He was chairman of the Society of Harbin Physicians between 1920 and 1922. Cf. entry on him in Ratmanov, "Rossiiskie vrachi v Kitae."

43 Budberg, *Memuary*, pt ii, 126–8. See document 29 in Sisson, *One Hundred Red Days*, 14–15. (Sisson facsimilized the "original" Russian handwriting beside his English translation, in which he misread the reference to Budberg as "Kuzberg"). On the forgery, see Kennan, "The Sisson Documents." The main study is now Startsev, *Nemetskie den'gi i russkaia revoliutsiia*.

44 This letter to Stöffler, dated 11 October 1919, is included in *Briefe*.

45 Zhang Fushan and Zhou Shuzhen, *Ha'erbin geming jiudi shihua*, 381–2.

46 The robbery in February 1920 is described in detail in Budberg, *Memuary*, pt ii, 73–9.

47 A report on the police shooting of the criminal band was reprinted by *Vestnik Kitaiskoi Zheleznoi Dorogi*, vol. 2, no. 10 (March 1921), 18, from Harbin's *Russkii golos*. It identified their ringleader, who had "robbed clean the apartment of Dr Budberg last winter," as Petr Rementov-Gotsulia, nicknamed both Pet'ka-Rumyn (the Romanian) and Pet'ka-shoffer (the chauffeur).

48 See entry in Ratmanov, "Rossiiskie vrachi v Kitae."

49 *North China Hong-List*, pt ii, Harbin Hong-List, 8, 9. On Kirchev, cf. entry in Ratmanov, "Rossiiskie vrachi v Kitae." In 1923 he closed his hospital in Harbin and left for the United States with his family; US immigration and census records show that, after a stay in Hawai'i, they settled in San Diego.

50 *Briefe*, 31 March and 26 April 1920.

51 *Briefe*, 26 April and 9 June 1920; cf. Budberg, *Memuary*, pt ii, 88–9.

52 Ibid., 95–8, 114, 117–18. The last tsarist consul, from 1917 to 1920, was Georgii K. Popov (1879–1929), a graduate of the Faculty of Oriental Languages in Saint Petersburg University, who had served in China since 1903 and was fluent in Chinese. He died as an émigré in Harbin. *Nezabytye mogily*, vol. 5, 596.

53 Cf. Must, *Von Privilegierten zu Geächteten*, 165–6.

54 Li Shuxiao and Li Ting, "Waiguo zhu Ha'erbin lingshiguan yishi."

55 LVVA 2574/2/11/53.

56 *Briefe*, 11 July 1921.

57 *Briefe*, 5 March 1924.

58 A group photograph titled "Public servants of the Estonian colony in Harbin," showing ten unnamed men and one woman, appeared in the illustrated supplement to *Novosti zhizni*, no. 230 (12 October 1924). One of them was an Estonian physician from Tartu, Wilhelm Reni (1882–1941), Honorary Consul of Estonia in Harbin after 1920, who repatriated to Estonia in 1929. *Briefe*, 18 November 1924, mentions Reni as an assistant of Dr Raupach; cf. entry in Ratmanov, "Rossiiskie vrachi v Kitae" (with more information on the website cfe.ee). On Latvians in Harbin in the 1930s, see Katajs, *Zem desmit valstu karogiem*, 63–8.

59 *Baltisches Historisches Ortlexikon*, vol. 2, 93; *Latvijas vēstures atlants*, map on page 40.

60 LVVA 2574/2/11/75.

61 LVVA 2574/2/426; 2574/2/3205/4.

62 The editorial offices and printing shop were on 24 Grosse Neustraße, now Jauniela. LVVA 12/1/29/57, and 12/1/31/452.

63 The confusion began with a lively participant account of the history of the newspaper in David Druck, *Tsu der geshikhte fun der Yudisher prese (in Rusland un Poylen)* (On the History of the Jewish Press in Russia and Poland) (Warsaw: Hacefira, 1920), 65–78. Druck was fascinated with the figure of "the Baron," but he inverted the order of the name and patronymic of Gotgard Aleksandrovich. He reported that the baron's mother had lent essential help to the project by securing permission to publish the newspaper through her personal contacts with the acting Governor General of Livland; he described Budberg's enthusiastic personal involvement and sympathized with the eventual failure of the venture due to poor management. Historians of the Jews in Latvia perpetuated the erroneous reference to the publisher as "Baron Alexander Budberg," while continuing to speculate about his possible motivation.

64 As Roger Budberg testified in his first trial. *Memuary*, pt i, 21.

65 As attested, for example, by Budberg-Magnushof and Höflinger, eds., *Des Jägers Jahrbuch*. No copies of it survive.

66 Joseph (Iosif) Budberg's juridical career is covered by his service files in RGIA, f. 1405, op. 544, d. 1029 (which include petitions for reassignment in 1906) and in the Historical Archive of Omsk *oblast*, f. 25, op. 2, d. 26. It is reflected also in the Tobolsk City Archive, f. И158, op. 1, d. 123, l. 58; and d. 187, l. 35. *Pamiatnaia knizhka Tobol'skoi gubernii na 1914 god* (Memorial Book of the Governorate of Tobolsk for 1914), ed. E.G. Iuferov (Tobolsk: Gubernskaia tipografiia, 1914), 37, 48, 63, attests to his involvement in

Tobolsk public life. He was a regular contributor to a hunters' journal in Riga: both Baron Joseph Budberg, "Eine gefährliche Bärenjagd" (originally a letter to his brother, probably Gotthard), and J. Baron Budberg, "Jagderfolge in Westsibirien," were accompanied by photographs of him with bear trophies on the taiga.

67 Budberg, *Memuary*, pt ii, 24–5. Gotthard's common law wife is unidentified. Berezovka village, mentioned in several of Joseph's hunting reports, is in Uvatskii district of today's Tyumen *oblast*, 122 kilometres from Tobolsk. *Spisok naselennykh mest Tobol'skoi gubernii* (Register of Populated Places in the Governorate of Tobolsk) (Tobolsk: Gubernskaia tipografiia, 1912), 96.

68 *Briefe*, 11 October 1919 and 31 March 1920. The "Tatar village" to which Joseph moved, 16 *versts* (17 km) from Tobolsk according to Roger's memoirs cited above, could refer to the Tatar yurt settlement known as Pushniatskie, located on a road by the Irtysh River. *Spisok naselennykh mest Tobol'skoi gubernii*, 112.

69 Roger then conveyed the news in a letter to Antoinette. *Briefe*, 15 April 1921.

70 V.V. Tsys', *Zapadno-Sibirskoe krest'ianskoe vosstanie 1921 g. na Tobol'skom Severe. Problemy vzaimodeistviia vlasti i obshchestva v usloviiakh politicheskogo krizisa* (The Western Siberian Uprising of 1921 in the Tobolsk North: Problems of Interaction between Power and Society in Conditions of Political Crisis) (Nizhnevartovsk: NVGU, 2018), 125–6.

71 Elfriede Budberg to Roger Budberg, letter copied by him to Antoinette Raczynski. *Briefe*, 9 June 1921.

72 Budberg, *Bilder aus der Zeit der Lungenpest-Epidemien*, 5–8 (the deathbed photograph is also in the Popoff family album), 248–50; and *Briefe*, e.g. 9 June, 1 September and 4 October 1922.

73 Of the four cemeteries extant in Taiping qiao as of 1920, the Quanhe cemetery established in 1917 appears to be her most likely resting place. Cf. Li Xiaoju and Liang Aiying, "Taiping qiao shimo." The photograph of the tomb in the Popoff album shows the date of death as the fifteenth day in the tenth lunar month, ninth year of the Chinese Republic (25 November 1920).

74 *Briefe*, 18 May 1922; and more on such feelings in letters of 25 May (to Marie) and 30 September 1922.

75 In 1909, the siblings' trustee Baron Egon Korff (1861–1930) published a public "warning" regarding the legality of Alexandrine Budberg's management of Magnushof; she responded with a "counter warning," affirming her sole property rights. Another public notice, by Wilhelm, supported his mother and attacked Korff and was met by a joint declaration of the other siblings (apart from Marie, but including Roger) in defence of Korff's actions as the protector of their vital interests.

Dzimtenes Vēstnesis (The Homeland Messenger), no. 115 (23 May 1909), 12; no. 117 (26 May 1909), 1, 3; no. 135 (16 June 1909), 3; no. 153 (8 July 1909), 1 (with front-page critical commentary by the Riga newspaper in that last issue). In 1910, Wilhelm sold his stake in Magnushof to his mother. LVVA 2574/4/3977.

76 *Memuary*, pt i 21, 32.

77 *Briefe*, 9 June 1921 (through the courtesy of Mrs Ute Köhler in Hamburg, granddaughter of Roger Budberg's sister Cecile, I received a typescript copy of this letter, dated 19 June – one of several indications that the letters from Roger were circulated among his siblings). On Bubnik having buried Willy in Ufa, see also *Briefe*, 11 April 1922. In *Memuary*, pt ii, 126, Budberg wrote that Bubnik told him his brother had died of consumption; he gave the cause of death as alcoholism in the letter to Antoinette.

78 *Briefe*, 5 February 1924.

79 *Briefe*, commentary by Joseph A. Raczynski, 180.

80 *Briefe*, 25 April 1922; see also 30 October 1923 and 9 June 1924.

81 *Briefe*, 22 September 1922 and 2 November 1922. As his later letters attest, however, Roger's relations with Marie were never healed.

82 *Briefe*, 26 April 1924.

83 LVVA 2574/4/3977 and 2574/4/5006.

84 *Vestnik Kitaiskoi Zheleznoi Dorogi*, vol. 2, no. 12 (March 1921), 25. The father and daughter could not be traced despite Budberg's efforts. For his criticism of Russian measures against plague, see Budberg, *Bilder aus der Zeit der Lungenpest-Epidemien.*

85 *Briefe*, 9 June and 11 July 1921, described that large hospital, "situated in a splendid garden."

86 Ratmanov, *Vklad rossiiskikh vrachei v meditsinu Kitaia*, 115–16.

87 Cf. *Briefe*, 13 September 1921.

88 "Khronika" (Daily News), *Russkoe slovo* (Harbin), no. 319 (10 August 1921).

89 "Uvol'nenie Budberga" (Budberg's Discharge), *Zaria* (Harbin), no. 243 (3 November 1921).

90 "Istoriia ukhoda Budberga" (The Story of Budberg's Departure), *Zaria*, no. 250 (12 November 1921).

91 "Petitsiia prostitutok" (A Petition by Prostitutes), *Zaria*, no. 221 (7 October 1921); cf. "Lechenie prostitutok" (The Medical Care of Prostitutes), *Russkii golos*, no. 508 (5 April 1922). I am obliged to Pavel Ratmanov for bringing these newspaper articles to my attention.

92 "Sud'ba zheleznodorozhnoi bol'nitsy" (Fate of the Railway Hospital), *Zaria*, no. 275 (7 December 1922); and "Blagodarnye patsienty" (Grateful Patients), *Zaria*, no. 123 (5 June 1923).

93 "Novaia bol'nitsa KhOU" (A New Hospital of the Harbin City Administration), *Novosti zhizni*, no. 176 (8 August 1924).

94 "No study of the Black Death can make sense unless one constantly reminds oneself that this was not primarily a matter of statistics and social trends but of a shock of pain and appalling fear." Philip Ziegler, *The Black Death* (London: Collins, 1969), 143.

95 These photographs, reproduced as illustrations 103, 107, and 115 in Budberg, *Bilder aus der Zeit der Lungenpest-Epidemien*, are also in the Popoff family album.

96 Kegel had lived in the city since its foundation in 1898; after the Russo-Japanese War, he was owner of the restaurant and hotel Bellevue in Old Harbin. Budberg, *Memuary*, protocols section following pt i, 9–10. He died in Budberg's hospital; see *Nezabytye mogily*, vol. 3, 250.

97 Budberg, *Bilder aus der Zeit der Lungenpest-Epidemien*, illust. 62 and 210–13.

98 Oppenheim, review of *[Bilder aus der Zeit der] Lungenpest-Epidemien in der Mandschurei*.

99 "Doktor Budberg i Chernaia Smert'" (Doctor Budberg and the Black Death), *Zaria*, no. 214 (26 December 1923).

100 In order of appearance, this refers to the following reviews: *Mitteilungen zur Geschichte der Medizin und der Naturwissenschaften*, vol. 23, no. 1 (1924), 83, signed by H. Zeiss in Moscow; *Deutsche medizinische Wochenschrift*, vol. 50, no. 18 (2 May 1924), 585, signed Cl. Schilling; *Münchener medizinische Wochenschrift*, vol. 71 (6 June 1924), 756–7, signed Rimpau; and a second review in *Deutsche medizinische Wochenschrift*, vol. 52, no. 17 (23 April 1926), 727, by Geheimrat Kisskalt.

101 Grosberg, "Ein abenteurliches Baltenschicksal." Grosberg would have remembered Budberg's contributions to *St Petersburger Zeitung*. See entry on him in BBL. A memorial plaque marks Grosberg's home in Riga, now the Hotel Gutenberg in the Dom Square.

102 It is unknown who prepared the Russian text, which bears all the hallmarks of Budberg's style, on his behalf. Budberg was not confident enough in his Russian to write directly in that language, but he read and approved the draft and proofs of the *Memoirs*, and was planning to publish a shorter version in German. *Briefe*, 12 May 1922 and 26 April 1924.

103 The term *liang xin* is drawn from the book of Mencius (4th century BC). It was traditionally interpreted within a range of meanings such as the literal "true heart," the philosophical "innate mind" and "true self," and the imperative "moral duty." In modern Chinese, *liangxin* has come to mean "conscience." Gad C. Isay, *The Philosophy of the View of Life in Modern Chinese Thought* (Wiesbaden: Harrassowitz Verlag, 2013), 48, 98–107. Budberg, "Chinesische Prostitution," 319, said that prostitutes lived by the adage *tianli liangxin*, which he explained as "Heaven's law, or providence, and a good conscience."

104 *Briefe*, 10 August 1924.

105 "Mnogoobeshchaiushchie memuary. Kniga doktora Budberga" (Highly
    Promising Memoirs: Doctor Budberg's Book), *Zaria*, no. 460 (29 October
    1924).
106 *Briefe*, 21 December 1924.
107 *Briefe*, 26 October 1923.
108 Copy of the will in Raczynski family archive.
109 Ponosov remained in Harbin until as late as 1961, when he left for
    Brisbane, the city in Australia that took in many Russian émigrés from
    China, including the writer Nikolai Baikov. He was later curator of the
    Anthropology Museum at the University of Queensland. Sorokina,
    Rossiiskoe nauchnoe zarubezh'e, 160; and Alkin, "Arkheologicheskie i
    antropologicheskie issledovaniia."
110 Tolmachev, "Drevnosti Man'chzhurii," 22, 25, and Table 2. Tolmachev
    and Budberg shared another interest. Back in 1913, Budberg identified
    an unusual vertebral column, which the Chinese had found by the
    Sungari, as belonging to a mammoth. A report on this from Harbin's
    Novaia zhizn' was reprinted in *Golos Sibiri* (Irkutsk), no. 4, no. 10
    (19 April 1913). Tolmachev was involved in a similar discovery in
    October 1925: see his "Ostatki mamontov v Man'chzhurii." See also the
    entry on Tolmachev in Sorokina, *Rossiiskoe nauchnoe zarubezh'e*, 195–7, and
    Alkin, "Arkheolog Vladimir Iakovlevich Tolmachev," on this many-sided
    scholar, who moved to Shanghai in the mid-1930s.
111 *Briefe*, 30 September 1922 (on his "rich museum") and 9 June 1924.
112 The illustrations in Tolmachev's essay, including those of the figurines from
    Budberg's collection, are studied along with Jurchen relics from the Soviet
    Far East in Shavkunov, "Antropomorfnye podvesnye figurki iz bronzy."
113 Köhler family album.
114 I. Baranov, "Po kitaiskim khramam Ashikhe." An official Russian
    excursion to Ashihe by members of the Harbin Photographic Society in
    1912 is documented in Gintse, *Russkaia sem'ia doma i v Man'chzhurii*, 183–
    5. A photograph album of Ashihe temples was put together in 1925 by the
    Harbin photographer D. Raninin as *V kitaiskikh kumirniakh gor. Ashikhe*.
    The detailed captions to the images, identifying locally honoured deities,
    suggest collaboration with Ippolit Baranov. The album has been scanned
    by historian Thomas H. Hahn: see hahn.zenfolio.com/p382112314.
115 Hopstock, *Norwegian Members of the Chinese Customs Service*, 14; Huitfeldt,
    The Munthe Collection, 37.
116 See now especially Haakestad, *Porcelain and Revolution*. In 2010 and 2013,
    items from the Munthe collection were stolen from the Bergen museum
    (now called KODE 1); they may have been smuggled back to China.
117 *Briefe*, 9 June 1922.
118 *Briefe*, 13 June 1922.

119 *Briefe*, 9 June 1921 and 7 July 1924. Shkurkin, "Kitai i Dal'nevostochnye
     perspektivy," 46–8, called Yin Chang a notorious Germanophile. Such
     daydreams of marrying into the Qing aristocracy call to mind the novel
     René Leys by Victor Segalen (1878–1919), the French writer and physician,
     who witnessed the fall of the empire in Peking. In Harbin in 1919, Baron
     Roman Ungern-Sternberg married a Manchu Christian convert, who had
     some family connection to the court. Sunderland, *The Baron's Cloak*, 7–8, 152,
     and 280n42. The monarchist Ungern apparently conceived his marriage
     as a political alliance, which the Qing had indeed occasionally practised to
     ensure the loyalty of prominent foreigners: see Teng, *Eurasian*, 46–7.

120 *Briefe*, 2 September, 30 September, and 16 October 1922. Munthe's second
     wife, born in London of noble German extraction (a descendant of the
     eighteenth-century philosopher Johann Gottfried Herder, so Budberg
     believed), was an expatriate writer in English under her name from a
     first marriage, Alexandra E. Grantham. She produced a series of popular
     books on China beginning in 1918. Cf. *Briefe*, 15 April 1921.

121 His opposition to these teachings occupies much space in the
     correspondence – for example, most emphatically, in *Briefe*, 22 and
     23 June 1924, and the last surviving letters from 1925.

122 *Briefe*, 3 October 1925.

123 *Briefe*, 9 October 1925 (the last known letter to Antoinette).

124 *Briefe*, 22 June and 10 August 1924.

125 On his loneliness, see *Briefe*, 15 April 1921, and 16 October 1922.

126 *Briefe*, 1 September and 4 October 1922.

127 *Briefe*, 12 May 1922.

128 *Briefe*, 1 September and 2 September 1922.

129 *Briefe*, 2 November 1922.

130 *Briefe*, 20 January 1925.

131 *Briefe*, 30 September 1922. An introduction to the Rosicrucian Order
     (German: Rosenkreuzertum) is David Katz, *The Occult Tradition*, ch. 2.

132 Burmistrov, "Topography of Russian Esotericism," 81–3. After Japan occupied
     Manchuria, the Russian Rosicrucians moved from Harbin to Shanghai.

133 V. P'iankovich, *Lektsii po okkul'tizmu*, copy Hamilton Library, University
     of Hawai'i. The author died in Tientsin. An obituary by his wife is Sofiia
     P'iankovich, "Svetloi pamiati Viacheslava Nikolaevicha P'iankovicha."

134 Rosov, "Kharbinskie pis'ma P.A. Chistiakova," 77–80, 89. On female
     fortune tellers in Harbin, see also Zolotareva, *Man'chzhurskie byli*, 131–4.

135 Mefodii, *O znamenii obnovleniia sviatykh ikon*, 67–9.

136 Letter to Munthe, in *Briefe*, 23 November 1923. Antonova's address: from
     Ves' Kharbin na 1925 god.

137 Budberg asked his sister to help choose the best school for his nurse's
     daughter; see *Briefe*, 11 July 1921. Cf. the entry in Ratmanov, "Rossiiskie
     vrachi v Kitae."

138 *North China Herald*, 11 May and 16 May 1934.
139 Serafim, *Odigitriia Russkogo Zarubezh'ia*, 125–7; and archive of the Museum of Russian Culture in San Francisco. Nadine Beal was buried in San Francisco in 1978.
140 Budberg, "Zur Charakteristik chinesischen Seelenlebens," 112.
141 *Briefe*, 12 April 1924; young Antoinette's headaches were nonetheless mentioned again in following letters. Budberg quoted at length the words of the "Great Master" (again, a reference to Bubnik), on the unity of all sentient beings in life and death, in a letter of 28 March 1924. In a letter to his sister on 27 October 1922, he had described the uncanny ability of his "friend B." to change the direction of the wind and steer a sailboat by applying his "vital force" (*Lebenskraft*).
142 *Briefe*, 24 May 1923.
143 *Briefe*, 9 June (Bubnik's help), 10 August (living without papers), and 8 November 1924 (properties).
144 *Briefe*, 14 June 1925; cf. 8 April 1924. On physicians' numbers, see Ratmanov, *Vklad rossiiskikh vrachei v meditsinu Kitaia*, 107.
145 Telephone interview with the chess player Efim Krouk (1914–2008) in Sydney, on 24 January 2005.
146 "Ostroumoff Seriously Out of Health: Continued Imprisonment Bringing Him to Point of Death," *North China Herald*, 31 January 1925; "Poslanniki khodataistvuiut za inzh. Ostroumova" (Foreign Envoys Appeal on behalf of Engineer Ostroumov), *Zaria*, no. 32 (13 February 1925). See also Lyandres and Wulff, eds., *A Chronicle of the Civil War*, vol. 2, 260.
147 *Briefe*, 21 December 1924.
148 *Briefe*, 8 October 1925.
149 *Rupor* (Harbin), no. 1307 (5 July 1925). Cf. "V 'mertvom dome'. Kharbinskaia tiur'ma" (In "The House of the Dead": Harbin Prison), *Novosti zhizni*, no. 114 (26 May 1925). Guided by Budberg, the reporter visited the prison hospital and its fifteen patients.
150 "Prikliuchenie doktora Budberga," *Zaria*, no. 167 (4 August 1925).
151 *Rupor*, no. 1345 (13 August 1925). Although the idea that the Sungari water was radioactive was widespread at the time, others thought that this quality made swimming in the river "beneficial, like taking radon baths." Melikhov, *Belyi Kharbin*, 369–70.
152 Mefodii, *O znamenii obnovleniia sviatykh ikon*.
153 Melikhov, *Belyi Kharbin*, 191–7, has a colourful account of Kornilov's criminal career and his final arrest by a Russian-Chinese police force in June 1923; see Budberg, *Memuary*, pt ii, 73, on the arrest of the Kornilov gang in February 1920.
154 "Death Sentence on Foreigner: Korniloff's Execution in Harbin: His Belief That He Would Be Reprieved," *North China Herald*, 8 August 1925.

155 "The N. Manchurian Dynamite Case: Two Soviet Agents Arrested at Pogranitchnaya: Enough to Blow up a Town," *North China Herald*, 10 October 1925 (Harbin report from 28 September). Budberg fully concurred with these suspicions; see *Briefe*, 3 and 8 October 1925.

156 *Rupor*, no. 1421 (1 November 1925). On his passing into Chinese service as of 1 July 1921, see *Briefe*, 9 June 1921. Cf. letter of 11 July, on working for two Chinese ministries, those of Justice and Internal Affairs.

157 "Soviet's [*sic*] Grip on the C.E. Railway: Grandoise [*sic*] Improvements Scheme: Appointees to the Board: Prisons Commissar as Vice-President: Quorum at Last: Brutality of Harbin Police to Russians," *North China Herald*, 21 November 1925.

158 "Uvol'nenie bar. Budberga" (The Discharge of Baron Budberg), *Zaria*, no. 254 (1 November 1925).

159 "Gabid-Ogly umer ot strikhnina" (Gabid-Ogly Died of Strychnine), *Zaria*, no. 270 (18 November 1925).

160 "Zaiavlenie R.A. Budberga" (Statement by R.A. Budberg), *Zaria*, no. 271 (19 November 1925).

161 *Briefe*, 1 April 1924 and 8 October 1925.

162 *Briefe*, 14 June 1925.

163 N. Al'binin, "Na vesakh d-ra barona Budberga" (On the Scales of Dr Baron Budberg), *Molva*, no. 338 (16 January 1926).

164 "Bolezn' d-ra Budberga" (Illness of Dr Budberg), *Zaria*, no. 37 (6 February 1926); "Khronika," *Russkoe slovo*, no. 8 (9 February 1926). The five doctors were Georg von Bergmann (1868–1937), Sergei M. Blumenfeld (1874–1947), Otto Pan (1872–1926), Stepan Migdisov, and Friedrich Raupach. All but Pan were Dorpat graduates. In February 1905, the Kishinev-born Jewish physician Blumenfeld had left Tartu for Manchuria together with Budberg. See entries in Ratmanov, "Rossiiskie vrachi v Kitae"; Blumenfeld's employee files at Tartu University, EHA, 402/3/135 (1901 to 1906); and "Nordlivland. Ärzte auf dem Kriegsschauplatz," *Düna Zeitung*, no. 29 (5 February 1904).

165 Doktor meditsiny R.A. Baron Budberg, *O zhizni*. The cover page of this book again used the adage *tiandi liangxin* as an equivalent of the Budberg heraldic motto in Latin; this time the four Chinese characters were drawn in a circle, and the character *lü*, meaning "law," was added in the middle. Copies of both *Memuary* and *O zhizni* are at the British Library and the National Library of Latvia.

166 "Retsenziia o zhizni" (*sic*; Review on Life) and "Mechenaia shel'ma" (A Marked Scoundrel), both in *Molva*, no. 461 (20 June 1926).

167 The next titles would have been: *O funktsiiakh nashego myshleniia* (On the Functions of Our Thought) and *O zachatii* (On Human Fertilization). The Harbin publisher Vasilii A. Chilikin (1892–after 1969?) moved to Shanghai in September 1926. He eventually repatriated to Soviet Russia. Khisamutdinov, *Rossiiskaia emigratsiia v Aziatsko-Tikhookeanskom regione i Iuzhnoi Amerike*, 335.

168 A description of the route to the resort, its history, the baths treatments, and snakes, is in Kormazov, "Mongol'skii kurort Khalkhin 'Khalun Arshan.'" Cf. Zolotareva, *Man'chzhurskie byli*, 245–9.

169 "Smert' barona Budberg" (Death of Baron Budberg), *Russkoe slovo*, no. 169 (26 August 1926).

170 Letter (n.d.) in Raczynski family archive.

171 *Poslimees*, no. 258 (23 September 1926), 3; *Dorpater Zeitung*, no. 217 (23 September 1926), 4. Notices of Budberg's death also appeared in *Rigasche Rundschau*, no. 218 (29 September 1926), 2; and *Libausche Zeitung* (30 September 1926), 3.

172 Grosberg, "Ein merkwürdiges Leben." This obituary was reprinted in *Revaler Bote* (Tallinn), no. 274 (30 November 1926), 3–4. Grosberg cites a description of the funeral in the daily *Rupor*, no copies of which for August 1926 are known to survive, but the details of his report agree with those in *Molva*, cited below. The biographical article on Budberg in Gottlieb Olpp, *Hervorragende Tropenärzte in Wort und Bild* (Munich: Gmelin, 1932), 57, borrowed the funeral scene from Grosberg.

173 "Pokhorony barona Budberg" (Funeral of Baron Budberg), *Russkoe slovo*, no. 170 (27 August 1926).

174 *Russkoe slovo*, same date. See "Popov, Mikhail Terent'evich" (1884–after 1945), personal file in State Archive of Khabarovsk Region (GAKhK), BREM collection. On the history of the Red Cross Hospital, directed by Friedrich Raupach, see Ratmanov, *Vklad rossiiskikh vrachei v meditsinu Kitaia*, 78, 128–9; on Migdisov's long career in Chinese and ultimately Japanese service, see ibid., 133–4, 167–8, 189.

175 "Smert' d-ra R.A. Budberg" (Death of Dr R.A. Budberg), *Molva*, no. 515 (26 August 1926); "Pokhorony R.A. Budberga" (Funeral of R.A. Budberg), *Molva*, no. 516 (27 August 1926).

176 "Odinokaia dusha. Pamiati R.A. Budberg" (A Lonely Soul: In Memory of R.A. Budberg), *Zaria*, no. 228 (26 August 1926), signed D.D.; this was probably the source of the "love and gratitude" in Grosberg's obituary. On the same page, under the title "Konchina d-ra Budberg" (Decease of Dr Budberg), *Zaria* reported on the circumstances of Budberg's death and summarized his biography. However, neither the popular Harbin daily in Chinese, *Binjiang shibao* (Binjiang Times), nor the important regional paper published in Mukden, *Shengjing shibao* (Shengjing Times), carried a report on the death of "Doctor Bu."

177 Budberg, *Memuary*, pt ii, 16.

178 *Briefe*, 15 April 1921.

179 *Briefe*, 15 June 1922. Cf. Budberg, *Memuary*, pt ii, 6, 24.

180 These thoughts on the contrast between histories based on written sources, on the one hand, and the past as recorded in memory and orally retold, on the other, are inspired by Daniel Woolf, *The Social Circulation of*

the Past: English Historical Culture 1500–1730 (Oxford: Oxford University Press, 2003).

181 Budberg's friend and colleague of Dorpat days, Friedrich Raupach, was council chairman of the Evangelical Lutheran Church in Harbin. *Ves' Kharbin na 1925 god*, 81. On Harbin's Lutherans, see Chernolutskaia, "Religious Communities in Harbin," 90–3.

182 *Russkoe slovo*, no. 185 (15 September 1926).

7 Russians and Chinese under Japanese Rule

1 The available transcription of his given name might refer to Li Yizhen, Yichen, or Yishen. He is not mentioned in the exhaustively documented study by Chi Man Kwong, *War and Geopolitics in Interwar Manchuria*; in personal correspondence, Professor Kwong has suggested Yi Yisan, a senior commander in the Fengtian Army.

2 Mikhail Platonovich Popov, from the gentry of Kharkov governorate, was born in 1869 and died in Liège in 1928 (Popoff family archive).

3 On him, see Melikhov, "Russkie dobrovol'tsy," a useful reading of relevant files in the State Archive of the Russian Federation (GARF), here 274–5. I will refer to this version of the article rather than the partial reproduction in ch. 2 of Melikhov, *Rossiiskaia emigratsiia v mezhdunarodnykh otnosheniiakh*.

4 The entry on Slizhikov in Kuptsov et al., *Belyi generalitet na Vostoke Rossii*, 506–7, adds that he later joined the Japanese-sponsored Russian Fascist Union and died in Dairen.

5 Originally a cavalry officer, Kulebiakin was also trained as a military pilot and served in this capacity with the White Army during the Russian Civil War. Based in Harbin from 1926 to 1934, he served in Chinese aviation. He immigrated again in 1950, this time to the United States from Shanghai. Volkov, *Ofitsery armeiskoi kavalerii*, 293; Museum of Russian Culture, San Francisco.

6 An engineer and architect from the Caucasus, Korganov came to Manchuria in 1921. He built houses in Harbin and spent his last years in Mukden. Kradin, *Russkie inzhenery i arkhitektory v Kitae*, 273.

7 See Bisher, *White Terror*, esp. 68, 81. I owe further information on Kuroki to the kind assistance of Professor Takeshi Nakashima, Tokyo Metropolitan University.

8 Nikolai Baron von Budberg, "Eine europäisch-asiatische Ehe-Allianz." In this article, some of the above names appear in very approximate German transcriptions, obviously converted from Popoff's Russian.

9 See Tat'iana Pang, "The 'Russian Company' in the Manchu Banner Organization," and Giovanni Stary, "A Manchu Document Concerning Russian Teachers in the Manchu Banners' 'Russian Company,' "

Central Asiatic Journal 43, no. 1 (1999), 132–9, 140–6; Andrey V. Ivanov,
  "Conflicting Loyalties: Fugitives and 'Traitors' in the Russo-Manchurian
  Frontier, 1651–1689," *Journal of Early Modern History* 13, no. 5 (2009), 333–58;
  and P.A. Lapin, " 'Russkaia rota' v Pekine. Istoriia albazinskoi diaspory v
  Kitae (XVII – XX vv.)" (The "Russian Company" in Peking: History of the
  Albazinian Diaspora in China, Seventeenth to the Twentieth Centuries),
  in V.P. Nikolaev, ed., *Rossiiskaia diaspora v stranakh Vostoka. Istoriiu i
  sovremennost'* (The Russian Diaspora in Countries of the East: History and
  Present) (Moscow: Russian Academy of Sciences, 2013), 6–11.

10 Borisov, *Dal'nii Vostok*, a pamphlet publicizing Semenov among the
   Russian emigration in Europe.

11 Lin, *Among Ghosts and Tigers*, 69–75, 94, 106–7, 185; Ostrovskii, "Nekotorye
   dannye o kitaiskikh chastiakh."

12 Lin, *Among Ghosts and Tigers*, 101.

13 "Chang Tsung-ch'ang," in *Biographical Dictionary of Republican China*, ed.
   Howard L. Boorman, 5 vols. (New York: Columbia University Press,
   1967–71), vol. 3, 122–7 at 123–4. Cf. Melikhov, "Russkie dobrovol'tsy," 270–1.

14 Ibid., 272. Cf. the Cossack veterans of the Civil War, who entered Zhang
   Zongchang's army having previously been employed in the Fushun coal
   mines. Ibid., 279.

15 Ibid., 284. See photograph of the pilot "General Io," posing in front of an
   airplane with a group of boys identified in the caption as "sons of Zhang
   Zongchang," reproduced in Balmasov, *Beloemigranty*, illustrations between
   224 and 225 (this volume was compiled mostly on the basis of the GARF
   files and the Russian émigré press).

16 See the memoir of one of them, Major-General F. A. Sutton (1884–1944),
   One-Arm Sutton, 276.

17 To quote again from the entry "Chang Tsung-ch'ang," in *Biographical
   Dictionary of Republican China*, ed. Boorman, "[Zhang Zongchang's army]
   included a force of some 4,000 White Russians, aptly labeled 'soldiers
   of misfortune,' who provided a bizarre dimension to the campaigns
   conducted by [Zhang] during that period. Few mercenaries ever fought for
   a cause in which they had less direct concern or faced possible death under
   worse conditions" (124).

18 Melikhov, "Russkie dobrovol'tsy," 274n21.

19 Balmasov, *Beloemigranty*, 25.

20 Karetina, "General U Peifu na politicheskoi stsene Kitaia." By 1925,
   the Soviets had categorized Wu as an agent of British and American
   imperialism.

21 Conversation with Nechaev as reported by General Aleksandr S.
   Lukomskii (1868–1939); quoted in Balmasov, *Beloemigranty*, 39.

22 The same General Lukomskii, an émigré in France rather than in China,
   called this "a fantastic and wild project." Ibid., 24.

23 Mikhail A. Mikhailov, quoted in ibid., 75.

24 Melikhov, "Russkie dobrovol'tsy," 276.

25 Lev Gudkov, *Negativnaia identichnost'. Stat'i 1997–2000 godov* (Negative Identity: Essays, 1997–2000) (Moscow: Novoe literaturnoe obozrenie, 2004), ch. 7, analyses such comparable constructions as *belofinny* (White Finns) and *belopoliaki* (White Poles).

26 This is one of the lesser problems with Balmasov, *Beloemigranty*, which exaggerates the impact of the Russian forces under Nechaev on Chinese and world history.

27 Melikhov, "Russkie dobrovol'tsy," 298.

28 Ibid., 278–9, 283–4, 290, 292.

29 Ibid., 275–7.

30 Balmasov, *Beloemigranty*, 38–9.

31 Melikhov, "Russkie dobrovol'tsy," 289.

32 Ibid., 299–300; Balmasov, *Beloemigranty*, 75.

33 Ibid., 106.

34 Ibid., 69, and see extract from the 1927 diary of Major Stolitsa, 113.

35 Ibid., 48–9, 56, 59–60.

36 For example, ibid., 109–11, part of the diary by Major Stolitsa, combines using the whip on Chinese villagers with caring for his wounded Chinese interpreter. See ibid., 129, on Russians' resistance to having Chinese serve with them.

37 Smirnov, *Rossiiskie emigranty v Severnoi Man'chzhurii*, 42–3.

38 Balmasov, *Beloemigranty*, 80–2, 111–14, 145–7.

39 In Jinan the Russian unit had "a complete cinema crew, which filmed the division's daily life and battle activity." Melikhov, "Russkie dobrovol'tsy," 283. Cf. Balmasov, *Beloemigranty*, 187, for a mention of the "Russian filming detachment," formed by Zhang Zongchang. This was no doubt the team that in 1925 made a documentary in five reels, titled *Modern Warfare in China in 1924–1925*, which was acquired by the Imperial War Museum in London and is now available on the internet. A curiously misinformed article takes this film to be a Soviet production; Arthur Waldron and Nicholas J. Cull, "'Modern Warfare in China in 1924–1925': Soviet Film Propaganda to Support Chinese Militarist Zhang Zuolin," *Historical Journal of Film, Radio, and Television* 15, no. 3 (1995), 407–24.

40 Melikhov, "Russkie dobrovol'tsy," 293–4; Balmasov, *Beloemigranty*, 64–6.

41 Melikhov, "Russkie dobrovol'tsy," 301.

42 Ibid., 302; Balmasov, *Beloemigranty*, 83–6. Images in the collection of the University of Bristol, Historical Photographs of China, reference nos. Ar04–164, Ar04–171, Ar04–175, show the aftermath of this battle and the bodies of fallen Russian soldiers.

43 Melikhov, "Russkie dobrovol'tsy," 304.

44 Ibid., 305–6.

45 Balmasov, *Beloemigranty*, 147–51.

46 Ibid., 136–7.

47 See more in the introduction and commentary in Klerzhe, *Revoliutsiia i grazhdanskaia voina*.

48 Budberg, *Memuary*, pt ii, 120–1.

49 Ibid., pt i, 69 (on the nanny, pt i, 16).

50 *Briefe*, 31 March 1920.

51 *Briefe*, 25 November 1922.

52 *Novosti zhizni*, no. 90, 25 April 1922; *Briefe*, same date.

53 *Briefe*, 23 November 1923 and 1 April 1924.

54 *Briefe*, 22 June and 8 July 1924. "Janja," Anna Eugenie Bubníková (born in Ufa in 1906), began studying medicine at the Czech University in the winter of 1924, graduating in 1928. Archives of Charles University, Faculty of Medicine collection, catalogues of students, medical students (regular), 1924–7, inv. no. 555.

55 *Briefe*, 8 October 1925.

56 Photographs in Popoff family album, and *Briefe*, 26 April 1920 and 12 May 1922, on these trees, which Roger Budberg saw from his window and described in letters to his sister and to General Munthe. On the symbolism of the name Zhong-De-Hua, see Budberg, *Memuary*, pt ii, 27.

57 *Briefe*, 26 March 1924.

58 *Briefe*, 8 November 1924.

59 *Briefe*, 8 July 1924.

60 Commentary by Joseph A. Raczynski in *Briefe*, 153. Bubnik's son Leopold was about to graduate from a Harbin gymnasium in summer 1925; cf. *Briefe*, 8 November 1924.

61 Budberg, *O zhizni*, 43 (the usual number of beads for a Buddhist rosary is 108, corresponding to "the 108 earthly afflictions," although some Buddhist teachings promoted other quantities). Information on the Popoffs' arrival in Belgium and life in Liège comes from my interviews with Victor Popoff, the eldest son, in August 2005.

62 Commentary by Joseph A. Raczynski in *Briefe*, 154.

63 Melikhov, *Belyi Kharbin*, 405. In 1929, Ostroumov moved to Tientsin to work for another Chinese enterprise, the Peking-Mukden Railway. He later lived in Indochina, returning to China shortly before his death in 1944.

64 "Russian Mobs Fight Chinese in Harbin."

65 Cf. Rachinskaia, *Kaleidoskop zhizni*, 233.

66 Grosvenor Coville, "Here in Manchuria," 245, 254. On Pristan' flooded "to a depth of two meters," see Wright, "Legitimacy and Disaster," 208.

67 Grosvenor Coville, "Here in Manchuria," 255; on the cholera, see more in Wright, "Legitimacy and Disaster," 203–5.

68 Ratmanov, *Vklad rossiiskikh vrachei v meditsinu Kitaia*, 123–5.
69 Kapran, *Povsednevnaia zhizn' russkogo naseleniia Kharbina*, 177. Cf. Zolotareva, *Man'chzhurskie byli*, 255.
70 Nestor, *Man'chzhuriia–Kharbin*, 13–15, 20–1, 31–2, 34–5, 38–9. Another Harbin cleric, Bishop Dimitrii (1871–1947), repeated the story of the icon protection in 1924, also telling a colleague in Yugoslavia that in 1935, an old man with a white beard prevented the death of Chinese children playing in a construction site by the Sungari. When one of the children later passed by the icon at the Harbin railway station, he recognized the face of St Nicholas. See St Nikolai Serbskii (Velimirović), *Chudesa bozhii* (The Miracles of God), trans. I.A. Charota (Minsk: Izdatel'stvo Dmitriia Kharchenko, 2013), 179–81.
71 This map was shown to the public as part of the British Library exhibition "Maps and the 20th Century: Drawing the Line." I saw it in London in February 2017. Cf. Bakich, *Harbin Russian Imprints*, no. 3458.
72 Bong, "A 'White Race' without Supremacy," 138, fig. 1. Other estimates suggest that the total population for Manchukuo at the time was even higher – at least 40 million.
73 Argudiaeva, "Istochniki po istoriko-demograficheskim protsessam u russkikh Trekhrech'ia," 69.
74 I.A. D'iakov, "Amaterasu."
75 *"Bushido,"* was written in the United States by a Russian-born Jewish refugee from France, Ossip Alexandre Joseph Pernikoff (1894–1952), who presented it as his revision of a manuscript by a Russian author in Manchuria. The publisher's claim on the jacket flap that "Alexandre Pernikoff has observed the Japanese at close range for over 20 years" was pure invention.
76 Ivanov, "Russkaia koloniia v Man'chzhurii," and his editorial, in the same issue of *Aziia* (copy Cambridge University Library).
77 Ivanov, "Evropa, Aziia, Evraziia."
78 Cf. Smirnov, *Rossiiskie emigranty v Severnoi Man'chzhurii*, 94–6.
79 See "Stroenie" (Construction), in Rerikh, *Sviashchennyi dozor* (copy National Library of Latvia), 80–3.
80 See Rosov, *Nikolai Rerikh*.
81 In Williams, *Russian Art and American Money*, 111–46, Roerich emerges as a swindler exploiting gullible American admirers and as a possible Soviet agent. See more in Andreyev, *The Myth of the Masters Revived*.
82 Summary in DeNio Stephens, "The Occult in Russia Today," 361–5.
83 Stasulane, "Centre of Theosophy in the Baltic Region," 136–7; see also the introduction by Roerich (opening with his praise of Manchukuo) in Kheidok, *Zvezdy Man'chzhurii*.

84 See more on Kheidok's fiction in Gamsa, "On Value Systems of the Russian Émigrés in China."

85 Ivanov's essay on Roerich, "The Painter Thinker" (*Rerikh – khudozhnik myslitel'*, 1937), was included in *Rerikh*, a lavishly illustrated volume, published by the Roerich Museum in Riga in 1939.

86 The opening story in Kheidok, *Zvezdy Man'chzhurii*, "Bezumie zheltykh pustyn'" (The Madness of Yellow Deserts), was about Ungern's soldiers in Mongolia.

87 See also Xiao Hong's later short sketch, "Sleepless Night."

88 Shao, *Remote Homeland*, 289–90; Meyer, *In Manchuria*, 161. Both have translations of the song, on which see also Ah Cheng, *Ha'erbin ren*, 112.

89 An example of this is the fleeting impression of Harbin by a British traveller who passed through on his way to China with the Trans-Siberian in 1936: "My first glimpse of Imperial Japan. Harbin, a dead city already, shops mostly closed, White Russians wandering disconsolate and ill-found." Richard P. Dobson, *China Cycle* (London: Macmillan & Co., 1946), 9–10.

90 On survival strategies in Manchukuo, see Smirnov, *Rossiiskie emigranty v Severnoi Man'chzhurii*, 79–128; Il'in, "Na sluzhbe u iapontsev."

91 Grosvenor Coville, "Here in Manchuria," 238, 235.

92 Ushanoff, "Recollections of Life," 44. In 1974, Ushanoff made his first visit to Russia at the age of seventy. Feeling himself an American, by then he found the Russians strangers (ibid., and 55–6).

93 Clausen and Thøgersen, *The Making of a Chinese City*, 115.

94 Bong, "A 'White Race' without Supremacy"; cf. Teng, *Eurasian*, 200.

95 Ibid., 69.

96 Mao Hong, "Ha'erbin Zhong-E renmin shenghuo zhuangkuang," 119.

97 Liaozuo sanren, *Binjiang chenxiao lu*, 165–6.

98 He added that the same differences in perception held true with regard to learning Chinese, or Russian. Lattimore, *Manchuria*, 247.

99 Dobrynin, "Molodye russkie vrachi."

100 Dement, *Stupeni moei zhizni* (an e-file, privately produced in commemoration of the author after his death in Israel in 2013), 17–18, 21–3, 29–33.

101 See Smirnov and Buiakov, *Otriad Asano*.

102 Price, "Japan Faces Russia in Manchuria," 609, 619, 623, 627. Similarly projecting white racial fear onto the situation in Harbin, a writer for the same journal had in 1929 described it as the city where "the yellow man rules over the white [and] whites work for yellows." Simpich, "Manchuria, Promised Land of Asia," 399–400. Cf. the Harbin scenes of "a Chinese policeman beating a white driver"; "a little ragged Russian girl ... washing windows in a Chinese house"; and mixed children of "the

very low classes," in whose "physiognomy … Chinese blood dominates," all in Gilbreath, "Where Yellow Rules White," 367, 369, 370.

103 An exception in describing Russian beggars and homeless people in Harbin is Zolotareva, *Man'chzhurskie byli*, 104–11.

104 Photographs of these badges are in Danilin, "Nagrady i znaki rossiiskikh vrachei v Kitae," 98.

105 Guins, "Russians in Manchuria," 86–7.

106 Entry on Komarov in *Entsiklopediia literaturnoi zhizni Priamur'ia*, ed. Urmanov, 196–8.

107 Komarov, *Izbrannoe*, 47–82.

108 Smirnov, "Avgust 1945 g. v Severnoi Man'chzhurii"; Moustafine, *Secrets and Spies*, 358–61, 366–7.

109 On Russian looting of Japanese property, and on Japanese suicides in Harbin in 1945, see Il'in, "Na sluzhbe u iapontsev," no. 85, 204; on looting by Russians and Chinese, see Ianinova, "Zhizn' russkikh v Manchzhurii," 15 March 1956.

110 This subject has recently received a great deal of scholarly attention. A pioneering introduction is Tamanoi, *Memory Maps*.

111 See Barshay, *The Gods Left First*.

112 Stolberg, *Stalin und die chinesischen Kommunisten*, 63–5, 72–3.

113 Ibid., 69–71, 111.

114 On the Communist rise to power, beginning from the northeast, see Frank Dikötter, *The Tragedy of Liberation: A History of the Chinese Revolution, 1945–57* (New York: Bloomsbury Press, 2013).

115 Data collected by Bruce Adams, quoted in Wolff, "Returning from Harbin," 99.

116 Galia Katz, "Kharbin (Avgust 1945–1952 gg.)"; and my interview with Mrs Katz (née Volobrinskaia, 1924–2013) in Tel Aviv, 10 January 2005.

117 Testimony about such experiences, which clash with the patriotic celebration of the Red Army victory in the Second World War, is seldom published in Russia. The only mainstream publication to give voice to them is Starosel'skaia, *Povsevdnevnaia zhizn' 'russkogo' Kitaia*, 321–7, which reprints a letter by a rape victim to the Novosibirsk journal *Na sopkakh Man'chzhurii* in the 1990s.

118 Ianinova, "Zhizn' russkikh v Manchzhurii," here 8 and 15 March 1956, also described Red Army soldiers breaking into the author's house and the apparent gang rape of a fifteen-year-old girl. Cf. Il'in, "Sovetskaia armiia v Kharbine," 140; and Zolotareva, *Man'chzhurskie byli*, 196, 200, 204–5, 215, on the robbery and rape of émigrés by Soviet soldiers near Mudanjiang. Other eyewitness accounts of Soviet arrests and terror in Harbin in 1945 are Shapiro, "Kharbin, 1945," and the first two instalments

of her "Zhenskii kontslager'"; Rachinskaia, *Pereletnye ptitsy*, 44–55, 82–5; Stern, *Saitensprünge*, 73–91; and Markizov, *Do i posle 1945*, pt ii.

119　The soldier's name was Ivan Posledov. He was astonished to be told that the mother and son, though native speakers of Russian, were actually Polish. "Vania," in Zdanskii, *Grust'*, 121–30, is a poignant memoir of this encounter by an author who repatriated to Poland in 1952 but spent his entire life between the two cultures.

120　Ianinova, "Zhizn' russkikh v Manchzhurii," 13 and 15 March 1956; Zolotareva, *Man'chzhurskie byli*, 227. The looting and sexual exploitation of Russians in Manchuria by the Soviet Army in 1945 paralleled the situation of displaced Soviet citizens in Europe in the same year. Bernstein, "Ambiguous Homecoming," esp. 208–15.

8 *Kharbintsy* and *Ha'erbin ren*

1　Cf. Sunderland, "Peasant Pioneering," 909–12, which suggests that settlers in the Russian Far East were so lacking in a sense of "imperial mission" as to merit the definition of "un-imperial imperialists."

2　A most unflattering portrait of the greedy *man'chzhurets* is in Torgashev, *Avantiury na Dal'nem Vostoke*, 139–40. The less prejudiced Golovachev, *Rossiia na Dal'nem Vostoke*, 131–40, is no less critical; there are many other descriptions in this vein.

3　Semigorov, "Ocherki Girinskoi provintsii," 391–3, 402–3.

4　Ligin, *Na Dal'nem Vostoke*, 123–32.

5　Shteinfel'd, *Russkoe delo v Man'chzhurii*, 88. This paragraph is also cited by Bakich, "Émigré Identity."

6　Kats, *Dorogami pamiati*, 50–3. I owe this reference to the kind attention of the late Ludmila Rumer.

7　Chuguevskii, "100-letie Kharbina," 118. See Bakich, *Harbin Russian Imprints*, 14; and her "Émigré Identity," 58, for further elaboration.

8　Melikhov, *Rossiiskaia emigratsiia v mezhdunarodnykh otnosheniiakh*, 78, 248–52; Peremilovskii, "Russkaia shkola v Man'chzhurii"; Karasik, "Biulleten' vykhodtsev iz Kitaia," pt ii.

9　See "Kursy kitaiskogo iazyka" (Chinese Language Courses), *Vestnik Azii*, no. 52 (1925), 365–7. Another repercussion of the Mukden agreement was that knowledge of Chinese became useful for Russian lawyers; conversation classes were offered to freshmen at the Faculty of Law in autumn 1924.

10　Bakich, *Harbin Russian Imprints*, 3.

11　A meditation on our connection to place, Alastair Bonnett, *Off the Map: Lost Spaces, Forgotten Islands, Feral Places, and What They Tell Us About the*

World (London: Aurum Press, 2014), never mentions love of country or need for a homeland, to say nothing of a "motherland."

12 Gintse, *Russkaia sem'ia doma i v Man'chzhurii*, 306. On Zheltuga in the collective memory of Russians in Manchuria, see also Gamsa, "California on the Amur," 262–3.

13 Melikhov, *Man'chzhuriia dalekaia i blizkaia*, 8–9, mentions a fort near Qiqihar, which locals supposedly called "Russian Hill," and another, 75 *versts* below Sanxing, discovered in 1909 by A.N. Titov.

14 Shi Fang, Gao Ling, and Liu Shuang, *Ha'erbin Eqiao shi*, 591–2. For good measure, these authors also make sure to denounce Russian imperialism with the help of a quotation from Marx. Ibid., 586–7.

15 Cf. Sunderland, "The 'Colonization Question,'" 221–2; Paine, *Imperial Rivals*, 236.

16 As recalled in Gintse, *Russkaia sem'ia doma i v Man'chzhurii*, 216. Bickers, "History, Legend, and Treaty Port Ideology," 82, offers the neologism "mudflat-ism" for "the common belief that the treaty ports and concessions had been mud flats or marshes before the arrival of Europeans. This, while usually technically true carried the implied and frequently explicit gloss that the Europeans had been solely responsible for constructing the successful ports and industries of modernising China."

17 Dm. D'iakov, "Narodnoe obrazovanie."

18 Shchelkov, "Russko-Kitaiskii Politekhnicheskii Institut," 242–3.

19 "The Young Men's Christian Association / Khristianskii Soiuz Molodykh Liudei v Kharbine," notice published in the first *Annual of the Club of Natural Science and Geography of the YMCA* (Russian text, with titles in Russian and English); Katajs, *Zem desmit valstu karogiem*, 26–7.

20 "Nauchnaia khronika / Scientific Chronicle."

21 *Zapiski Kharbinskogo Obshchestva Estestvoispytatelei i Etnografov*, no. 7 (1947), quoting 33; and *Zapiski Kharbinskogo Obshchestva Estestvoispytatelei i Etnografov*, no. 8 (1950), 75–6 (the name of the Chinese member was Wang Lingxiang).

22 See his memoir: Katajs, *Zem desmit valstu karogiem*.

23 On Svetlana Rimsky-Korsakoff (Vieta Dyer), see William Sima, *China and ANU: Diplomats, Adventurers, Scholars* (Canberra: ANU Press, 2015), 107–8.

24 Introduction by N. Starikova in Starikov, *Po taezhnym tropam*, 3–5.

25 Among persons mentioned in this paragraph, I was fortunate to have known Emmanuel Pratt in Jerusalem and to have corresponded with Edgars Katajs in Riga. My teacher at the Hebrew University of Jerusalem, Professor Irene Eber (1929–2019), discussed Iurii Grause as a translator in her article, "A Critical Survey of Classical Chinese Literary Works in Hebrew," now collected as ch. 4 in Eber, *Jews in China: Cultural*

Conversations, Changing Perceptions (University Park: Pennsylvania State University Press, 2020).

26 Baranov, "Kraevedenie v kartinakh khudozhnika Sungurova" (qting 173; and 175 on his not knowing Chinese); and Rogov, *Antonin Sungurov* (illustrated catalogue, copy British Library). Rogov (1906–1988), at one time the Russian teacher of Xiao Hong in Harbin, was himself a sinologist, translator of modern Chinese literature, and Soviet official.

27 Taskina, "Staryi Kitai na polotnakh russkikh khudozhnikov"; and "A Odisseia de um pintor russo branco," *A Noite Ilustrada* (Rio de Janeiro), 22 June 1954.

28 See information on these exhibitions in the Harbin section of the website artrz.ru (the main portal on Russian artists in emigration).

29 Japanese painters who worked in Harbin were another source of influence. Some Chinese artists from Harbin were trained in France, Japan, and Shanghai. Yu Guanchao, "20 shiji shangbanye Ha'erbin Eqiao," mentions Han Jingsheng (1912–1998), Shi Yi (1921–?) and Gao Mang (1926–2017) as painters taught locally by Japanese and Russian artists. See Gamsa, *The Reading of Russian Literature in China*, 91–2, for more on the Harbin-born painter and prominent translator from Russian, Gao Mang.

30 Alexander Tcherepnine, "Music in Modern China," *The Musical Quarterly* 21, no. 4 (October 1935), 391–400; Ludmila Korabelnikova, *Alexander Tcherepnin: The Saga of a Russian Émigré Composer*, trans. Anna Weinstein (Bloomington: Indiana University Press, 2007), ch. 5. The émigré composer who, more than Tcherepnin, made China central to his creative work, was Aaron A. Avshalomov (1894–1965), a Shanghai resident from 1929 to 1947: see Jacob Avshalomov and Aaron Avshalomov, *Avshalomovs' Winding Way: Composers Out of China – A Chronicle* ([Philadelphia]: Xlibris, 2002).

31 Liu Xinxin and Liu Xueqing, *Ha'erbin xiyang yinyueshi.*

32 See, on Chinese weddings, Stern, *Saitensprünge*; and Katajs, *Zem desmit valstu karogiem*, 70–1; see Nikolaeva, *Iapontsy*, 76, on funerals.

33 Another exception in translating Chinese and Japanese poetry was Nikolai Svetlov (1909–1970), a poet who attended Harbin's Oriental Institute. Kreid and Bakich, *Russkaia poeziia Kitaia*, 693–4.

34 Bakich, *Valerii Pereleshin*, esp. 231. Some specialized translations from the Chinese were made by Harbin sinologists and published in their journal, *Vestnik Azii.*

35 See, for example, Li Xinggeng et al., *Fengyu fuping*, 36–46.

36 The translator was Wen Peiyun (b. 1902), later a victim of the Cultural Revolution. See the biographical note by Wen's children in a revised edition of the anthology in 1984, *Lingluji: Wen Peiyun sanshi niandai yiwen xuan*, 317–26. Xiao Jun, who had known Wen in Harbin and received a copy of *Lingluji* from him (see his introduction to the re-edition, ibid.,

3), evoked poems by "Tolstoy, Pushkin and Lermontov" in his story "Goats" (Yang), published in Shanghai in 1935. In my book, *The Reading of Russian Literature in China*, 85, 177n67, I incorrectly doubted that reference to "Tolstoy's poem." Xiao Jun had in mind "Krai ty moi, rodimyi krai" (1856), by the poet Aleksei K. Tolstoy (1817–1875), which Wen Peiyun had translated as "Zuguo" (The Motherland).

37 Entry on Li Yanling in *Entsiklopediia literaturnoi zhizni Priamur'ia*, ed. Urmanov, 228–30. Cf. the admiring essay by another translator of Russian literature from Harbin (b. 1942), Gan Yuze, "Yi wei Zhongguo de Eluosi shiren." See also Zhelokhovtsev, "Seriia literatury russkikh emigrantov v Kitae."

38 Levoshko, "Pol'sko-russkii arkhitektor Kazimir Skolimovskii," 150. Kravkov, *Voina v Man'chzhurii*, 22, 25–8, was struck by the dragon figures atop CER stations.

39 I.G. Baranov, "Khramy Tszilesy i Konfutsiia v Kharbine" (originally in *Izvestiia Iuridicheskogo Fakul'teta*, vol. 12, 1938), esp. 85–9, 102–5.

40 In 1935, the famous leftist writer Lu Xun (1881–1936) commented on "the perversity of these barely literate characters holding forth on the Thirteen Classics." Lu Xun, "Confucius in Modern China," in David Pollard, ed. and trans., *The Chinese Essay* (New York: Columbia University Press, 2000), 127. Ji Fenghui, *Ha'erbin xungen*, 186–8, explains the political background of the Wenmiao inauguration while poking some fun at the Confucian zeal of warlord Zhang Xueliang.

41 Song Hongyan, *Dongfang xiao Bali*, 127–9, mentions the feng shui. Ch. 5, "A Chinese Place," in Carter, *Creating a Chinese Harbin*, fails to convince that nationalist feeling was more important in the Jilesi and the Wenmiao projects than political calculation and competition between two successive Chinese administrators. The Wenmiao was converted into the Heilongjiang Nationalities Museum in 1985.

42 Ianinova, "Zhizn' russkikh v Manchzhurii," 23 February 1956.

43 Koga, *Inheritance of Loss*, ch. 2.

44 Conversation with editor of the album, historian Li Shuxiao in Harbin, March 2002.

45 Li Shuxiao et al., *Ha'erbin jiuying*, 36.

46 The flood photograph displayed in Hu Hong's café was identical to the top right photograph in *Ha'erbin jiuying*, 128.

47 Chen Jiying, *Sanshi niandai zuojia ji*, 147, 151, on the evacuation of 1932; 168 on returning to the liberated Harbin in 1945; and 171–2 on the immigration to Taiwan.

48 The privately printed booklet *Kharbintsy v Moskve* (copy State Historical Library, Moscow), 34, lists Irina Aleksandrovna Saidakovskaia, née Zhang,

among other members of the Moscow Association "Harbin." Her father had kept a restaurant in Fujiadian and after 1945 managed the restaurant in the Hotel Moderne. He was imprisoned from 1950 to 1956 and died in China in 1960.

49 Sun Yunxuan sent his congratulations on the 80th anniversary of the Polytechnic in 2000. The commemorative exhibition at the Harbin Institute of Technology (the Polytechnic's present name) featured his portrait along with that of Zhang Xueliang (Honorary Chairman of the Board in 1928), which Zhang himself donated in 1995. See introduction in Liu Guixian, *Zoujin Ha gong da*.

50 See, for example, Dzemeshkevich, *Kharbintsy*, 159–60, where the levelling of Russian cemeteries is denounced by an author of chauvinist persuasion. Zylewicz, *V pamiat' ob usopshikh*, documents Harbin Russian graves before their destruction, on the basis of photographs made by the compiler's father in the 1950s.

51 Zhang Tiejiang and Zhao Liantai, "Ha'erbin youtai ren mudi kaocha yanjiu," incorporates results of fieldwork in Huangshan by the Centre for Jewish Research in the Harbin Academy of Social Sciences. See Li Shuxiao et al., eds., *Ha'erbin jiuying*, 106, for *lao maozi fen*. For pride in the preservation of émigré graves at Huangshan, see, for example, Zhang Haiying and Yuan Xiaoguang, "Ha'erbin da mudi" (The Great Harbin Cemetery), *Shenghuo bao* (Harbin), no. 1265 (10 January 1993); and Jiang Xuesong et al., "Shijie yuanju Ha'erbin ren ji houyi canye Huangshan gongmu youtai mudi, dongzhengjiao mudi" (Former Harbinites and Descendants from around the World Pay Homage to the Jewish and Russian Orthodox Cemeteries at Huangshan), *Ha'erbin ribao*, 29 June 2017.

52 Bakich, "Émigré Identity," 67.

53 Kaigorodov, "Man'chzhuriia: avgust 1945," 95. Nonetheless, the Red Army's commanders publicly honoured the dead of 1904 at the largest Russian military cemetery in Port Arthur: see Koval', "Voinskii memorial Rossii v Port-Arture," 162–3.

54 Personal communication with Olga Bakich, January 2018.

55 Evgenii Mar, *My edem v Kitai* (We Travel to China) (Moscow: Detgiz, 1959), 89–93.

56 See, for example, Stolberg, *Stalin und die chinesischen Kommunisten*, 97–8.

57 Gottschang and Lary, *Swallows and Settlers*, 118, has an interview with a former Red Guard who during the Cultural Revolution used his authority to exhume the bones of his father from a grave in a remote Heilongjiang village and then carried them back to Shandong.

58 For an example of such destruction in rural Shandong between 1966 and 1968, cf. Andrew B. Kipnis, *Producing Guanxi: Sentiment, Self, and Subculture in a North China Village* (Durham: Duke University Press, 1997), 141–2.

59 Meng Dongfeng, "Jilin shi faxian Song Xiaolian mu, bei"; and Jing Ai, "Guanyu Ma jia huayuan zhuren Ma Zhongjun de kuang zhiming," on the discovery of Ma's epitaph tablet in Liaoning province in 1985. Rumours that General Shou Shan swallowed gold to commit suicide in 1900 led to the robbery of his tomb near Durbot as early as 1948. Liu Peiran, "Shou Shan jiangjun mukao," 82.

60 Ah Cheng, *Ha'erbin ren*. The book was also published in Taiwan in 1997 as the fourth title in a series on mainland Chinese cities (*Beijing ren*, *Shanghai ren*, and *Chengdu ren* were the first three).

61 Ibid., 13–16.

62 Ibid., 18–19.

63 Ibid., 24–5. The Russian émigré remembered by Ah Cheng wore a common tunic, introduced by Sun Yat-sen and known best as the "Mao suit" – a late-in-the-day adoption of Chinese dress by a foreigner, if the record is exact. Gao Ling et al., *Lishi huimou*, vol. 2, 198–213, has more on the Cultural Revolution in Harbin. For rare visual documentation, see Li Zhensheng, *Red-Color News Soldier*, 72, 94.

Epilogue: The General and the Particular

1 Magris, *Danube*, 194.

2 See Weitz, "From the Vienna to the Paris System."

3 Volkov, *Ofitsery rossiiskoi gvardii*, 82, has entries on Major-General Nikolai Aleksandrovich Budberg (1856–1921) and Major-General Anatolii Aleksandrovich Budberg (1857–1921). The other two brothers were Alexander (1855–1917) and Andreas (1861–1918?). Cf. Budberg-Gemauert-Poniemon, *Beiträge zu einer Geschichte des Geschlechtes*, Table 12, nn 18, 19, 20, 23.

4 *Lebenserinnerung*, 40, and Krebs, *Niederau-Krauthausen und die Herrschaft Burgau*, 129. Condehnen (also Kondehnen) is now called Aistovo.

5 Ibid., 129, 476n317; and ibid.,"Nachfahrentafel der familen von Elmpt and von Keyserlingk."

6 He was assigned to the Eighth Dragoon Regiment of Smolensk. With hindsight, it becomes clear why his father (in 1897) used the past tense when referring to Wilhelm's service in the Dragoon Guards. Budberg-Gemauert-Poniemon, *Beiträge zu einer Geschichte des Geschlechtes*, Table 12, n35.

7 GARF, f. 124, op. 17, d. 1008. On the villages Uspenskoe and Klyshino, located in Il'ino-Zaborskaia *volost'* (lowest administrative unit in tsarist Russia) of Makar'ev County (Makar'evskii *uezd*), see *Spisok naselennykh mest Kostromskoi gubernii* (Register of Populated Places in the Governorate of Kostroma) (Kostroma: Tipografiia T.P. Andronikovoi, 1908), 199–200.

8 LVVA 2574/2/5741 (letter by Wilhelm Budberg, Bogoiavlenie village, to the Minister of Foreign Affairs of Latvia, dated 7 January 1930).

9 LVVA 3234/17/2183 (files related to Wilhelm Budberg's request for a Latvian visa).

10 The paragraph is based on information included by Joseph A. Raczynski in *Lebenserinnerung*, commentary to 12, and in *Briefe*, 169. He dates the beginning of Wilhelm's correspondence with his mother to the second half of the 1920s. The commentary in *Lebenserinnerung* indicates that Wilhelm was living "as a beggar."

11 John Eicher, "A Sort of Homecoming: The German Refugee Crisis of 1929," *German Studies Review* 40, no. 2 (May 2017), 333–52 at 334, 343.

12 *Natsional'nye dvizheniia v period pervoi revoliutsii v Rossii (Sbornik dokumentov iz Arkhiva byv. Departamenta Politsii)* (National Movements during the First Revolution in Russia: A Collection of Documents from the Archive of the Former Police Department), ed. I.D. Kuznetsov (Cheboksary: Chuvashskoe gosudarstvennoe izdatel'stvo, 1935), 139–44.

13 A former factory worker, interviewed in 1967, remembered him as a corpulent German fluent in Russian, who, so he said, was deported to Germany during the First World War after a corruption affair had been discovered, the factory was closed, and Bubnik was suspected of preparing weapons for use by the German army once it reached the Urals. B.G. Akhmetshin, *Gornozavodskoi fol'klor Bashkortostana i Urala* (The Mining and Metallurgical Folklore of Bashkortostan and the Urals) (Ufa: Kitap, 2001), 67, 186. As of 1912, Bubnik was listed as local representative of the Saint Petersburg company that owned the factory. M.I. Rodnov, *Ufimskaia tovarnaia birzha (1905–1917 gody)* (The Ufa Trade Stock Exchange, 1905–17) (Ufa: Al'fa-Reklama, 2016), 178.

14 M.I. Rodnov, *Ufimskii nekropol'* (The Ufa Necropolis) (Saint Petersburg: "Svoe izdatel'stvo," 2015), 28.

15 Announcement by the VATA Partnership in *Zaria*, 16 August 1923.

16 On Bubnik's death: *Russkoe slovo*, no. 1862 (20 May 1932), referenced in *Nezabytye mogily*, vol. 1, 429. Aleksandra Zamesova-Bubnik (1875?–1940) owned a large horse-breeding farm, which her first husband Filipp Ia. Zamesov, an early settler in Manchuria, had established at the Mangou railway station (today's Zhaodong zhan) west of Harbin in the 1910s and managed until his death in 1924. "Zamesova, Aleksandra Georgievna," personal file in BREM collection, GAKhK, includes her obituaries. Cf. Zylewicz, *V pamiat' ob usopshikh*, 137.

17 Labuda et al., eds., *Edward and Atanazy Raczyński*. Another branch was rooted in Russia: see the Harbin poet Elizaveta Rachinskaia (1904–1993), *Kaleidoskop zhizni*, 20–1, 29–30, on the origins of her father, tsarist officer Nikolai Osipovich Rachinskii. Her mother Elizaveta was born to a prominent Baltic German family as Baroness von Maydell; her maternal

aunt Ekaterina married Roman von Arnold, the Harbin Chief of Police. All of these families (other Harbin examples are the Hintze or Krusenstern) intermarried with ethnic Russians and, as memoirs attest, fully identified with imperial Russia and its traditions – an assimilation that Roger Budberg and his siblings largely rejected.

18 In 2013 a copy of Budberg's *Bilder aus der Zeit der Lungenpest-Epidemien*, dedicated by the author to his nephew Andreas and signed in Harbin on 15 October 1923, surfaced in an auction sale in Poland.

19 Douglas, *Orderly and Humane*, quoting 301. Another 900,000 Russian Germans had been deported to the Soviet Asian republics after the German invasion in June 1941. See Naimark, *Fires of Hatred*, 85–107.

20 On receiving the letters in Nakło, northern Poland, in July 1984, see *Briefe*, 1. On transcribing them in Chile, from December 1985 to May 1986, and finishing in Munich in November 1986, see commentary on 273, 276.

21 Kreid and Bakich, *Russkaia poeziia Kitaia*, 679. There are also poems on life in Korea, Manchuria, and Chile, and "the last move" to California in 1961, in Viktoriia Iankovskaia (Victoria Yankovsky, 1909–1996), *Po stranam rasseianiia* (Through the Lands of Exile) (New York: Am-izdat, 1977), 51.

22 As "Lettere dal carcere alla madre M. Budberg," in a special edition of Belloni's journal *L'Idea Repubblicana* in 1957.

23 An obituary by Maria Teresa Gnoli, "Ricordando Maria Belloni," *L'Idea Repubblicana*, nos. 17–18 (1953), mentioned her coming to Italy from the Baltic as an art student. The quotation on Belloni as "romanissimo (ma figlio di madre russa)" comes from "Il Ritorno di Giulio Andrea Belloni," *Il Pensiero Mazziniano*, vol. 30, no. 4 (25 April 1975), 24.

24 Neander and Sakson, eds., *Umgesidelt–Vertrieben*, 54.

25 A vivid example of this is provided by the Yellow Pages and address books of the Baltic region, published under the imprint of Adolf Richter in Riga.

26 Shao, *Remote Homeland*, 71–4, 97–9, 102, 249–51, 259–60; Crossley, *Orphan Warriors*, 185, 201–2 (as he moved to Manchuria from Peking in 1912, one of Crossley's main protagonists wrote: "In three hundred years we had three successive moves. Now after nine generations my youngest son Guandong is once again registered at Changbai").

27 The first mention of Roger Budberg's intention to assist Nikolai financially is in *Briefe*, 16 October 1922.

28 See Volkov, ed., *Belaia bor'ba na Severo-Zapade Rossii*, 89–91, 93–9, 545–50, 653n61. Anatol Lieven was the brother of Roger Budberg's favourite second cousin, Paul Lieven.

29 On the "return home" to Westphalia, see Nicolai Baron von Budberg, "Ein Geschlecht kehrt heim." On him, see Garlinger, "Nikolai Baron von Budberg-Bönninghausen 75 Jahre!"

30 *Baltisches historisches Ortslexikon*, vol. 2, *Lettland*, 92, indicates that this manor, like Gemauert Poniemon (present-day Budberga), passed to the

Barons Budberg from the Barons Grotthuss, who had owned it in the eighteenth century.

31 Documentary film on Nadezhda Āriņš by Dzintra Geka, "… and Igarka, Hope and Butterfly" (Riga, Studija SB, 2008). Conversations with Mrs Āriņš in Riga, on 8–9 October 2011.

32 Cf. Buruma, *Year Zero*.

33 The signed book came to the Riga Town Library, now the Academic Library of the University of Latvia.

34 Entry for Janio Kalatz in Stephen Taylor, ed., *Who's Who in Central and East-Europe 1933/34: A Biographical Dictionary Containing about 10,000 Biographies of Prominent People from Albania, Austria, Bulgaria, Czechoslovakia, Danzig, Estonia, Finland, Greece, Hungary, Latvia, Liechtenstein, Lithuania, Poland, Rumania, Switzerland, Turkey and Yugoslavia* (Zurich: Central European Times Publishing, 1935), 449. Cf. Rasma Zvejniece, ed., *Senatori: Latvijas Senāts 1918–1940* (Riga: Latvijas Republikas Augstākā tiesa, 2008), 26.

35 Budberg, *Memuary*, pt i, 59.

36 "Trimdā miris senators Jānis Kalacs" (Senator Kalacs Dies in Exile), *Tēvzeme* (Hanau, Germany), no. 13 (12 February 1947).

37 *Postimees*, no. 130 (16 June 1897); no. 156 (17 July 1897); and no. 182 (18 August 1897).

38 *Postimees*, no. 26 (2 February 1904), reported on the departure for the battlefield of both Akel and Budberg.

39 Interview with Akel's daughter, in Lauri, ed., *Nenapisannye memuary*, 115–33.

40 See, for example, Dvorzhitskaia, "Moi mnogolikii Kharbin," 94, 96, on being "born in a foreign country" (she was born in Harbin in 1918) and considered an émigré in a city she greatly loved; and the opening pages of her memoir, on the patriotic motivation of repatriates like herself in 1954.

41 See Manchester, "Fusing Russian Nationalism with Soviet Patriotism."

42 Diabkin and Levchenko, " 'Nemets s russkoiu dushoi' "; Severnyi, *Shumit taiga Man'chzhurii*.

43 Saying nothing else about his time in China, Vertinskii, *Chetvert' veka bez rodiny* (first posthumous publication in 1962), 140, identified Shanghai only as the place where the artist finally received the pardon of "our great Mother – the Motherland" (*velikaia Mat' – Rodina*).

44 This is described in detail in Rachinskaia, *Pereletnye ptitsy*, 104–13, 122–6, 131.

45 Archival research by Bruce Adams, quoted in Wolff, "Returning from Harbin," 100; and Katajs, *Zem desmit valstu karogiem*, 230–4.

46 Dvorzhitskaia, "Moi mnogolikii Kharbin," 90–1; Ianinova, "Zhizn' russkikh v Manchzhurii," 15 and 20 March 1956; Rachinskaia, *Pereletnye ptitsy*, 96, 147.

47 Weeks, "Population Politics in Vilnius 1944–1947," 88, on the occasional difficulties of telling Poles apart from Lithuanians.
48 "Splittern des deutschen Volkstums," from Hitler's speech of 6 October 1939. Cf. Łossowski, "The Resettlement of the Germans from the Baltic States," 83.
49 Fitzpatrick, "The Motherland Calls," esp. 323–4, 346–7.
50 See Rachinskaia, *Pereletnye ptitsy*; Moustafine, *Secrets and Spies*, 387–90.
51 Katajs, *Zem desmit valstu karogiem*, 168, 224.
52 The quotation is again from Bakich, *Harbin Russian Imprints*, 3.
53 On "reluctant" cosmopolitanism, cf. the subtitle of Hellmut Stern's memoir *Saitensprünge* in its 3rd edition: *Erinnerungen eines Kosmopoliten wider Willen*.
54 Lattimore, "Wulakai Tales from Manchuria," 272, on the Han banner people, who lived among the Manchus; cf. on this idem, *Manchuria*, 62–3; and see 55–60 on Chinese going native among Mongols (and sometimes going back to being Chinese). On Manchu influence on the Han Chinese, see also Rhoads, *Manchus and Han*, 10, 59–62.
55 The papers of his daughter Anna Eugenie in the Archives of Charles University, Prague, give the father's name as Alois Bubnik and their home community as the village of Homole in the district of České Budějovice (Budweis). Her nationality appears as Czech in some documents and as Russian (referring to her place of birth) in others, but her religion is given consistently as Evangelical Protestant.
56 Archives of the Ministry of Foreign Affairs of the Czech Republic in Prague (AMZV), Fifth Section of the Ministry of Foreign Affairs Nominal Registry 1929–39, "Bubník Ludvík: The Estate of 1935."
57 "Zamesova, Aleksandra Georgievna," personal file in BREM collection, GAKhK.
58 Dolbilov, "Russification and the Bureaucratic Mind."
59 Sunderland, *The Baron's Cloak*, 10, 233. See 72–5 and 120–1 on the groups mentioned.
60 Lieven, "Dilemmas of Empire," 197.
61 Shao, *Remote Homeland*, 168–9, 172, and ch. 6.
62 Budberg, *Memuary*, pt i, 5–6.
63 Tamanoi, "Knowledge, Power, and Racial Classifications."
64 Baker, "Life in the Cities," 470.
65 For these comparisons, cf. my articles "Harbin in Comparative Perspective," and "The Vanishing and Lingering Past in Two Cities: Harbin and Riga."
66 Ristaino, *Port of Last Resort*, 124–5, 282.
67 Keene, "Cities and Cultural Exchange," 24, 26.
68 See, for example, the website myharbin.name and the Harbin section of forum.vgd.ru.
69 Gaiduk, "Vstrecha losianov v Omske."

70 Similarly, after the Second World War, "speaking Estonian or Latvian in Germany, singing their folk songs, using common local recipes, and playing common games were important ways of expressing Baltic German regional belonging." Plath, "*Heimat*," 78.

71 Teddy Kaufman, "Pomnite i znaete li vy proshloe Kharbina?" (The last word should be read with the accent on the final syllable, a declension of the city name that is particular to Harbin Russian speakers.)

72 The Zionist ideal is expressed in the title of a manuscript memoir by Leonfried Heymann, *Meeretz huladeti leeretz moladeti: mitokh dapei ḥayai* (From My Birthland to My Motherland). Born in Harbin, he returned there in 2004 with his daughter and granddaughter on a group tour organized by the Association of Former Residents of China in Israel. At Huangshan cemetery, he prayed at the graves of his parents (both from Courland, they lived in Harbin as Latvian citizens until becoming stateless after the Soviet occupation of Latvia), but the new and unrecognizable Harbin shocked him into realizing that "everything [he] had known existed only in memory." He wondered "how one could have erased it all within only fifty years." Ibid., 40–1, 382–92. I interviewed Mr Heymann (1928–2012) at his home in Haifa on 27 January 2010.

73 Jasanoff, "Cosmopolitan," 407. There are differences in the "unmixing" of cities: while Alexandria and Harbin have lost all, or almost all, of their non-native minorities, Riga or Tallinn have gone through radical change in their ethnic composition without becoming homogeneously Latvian or Estonian.

74 See Briedis, *Vilnius: City of Strangers* (note the title), 229ff., 238; and the conclusion of Kate Brown, *A Biography of No Place: From Ethnic Borderland to Soviet Heartland* (Cambridge, MA: Harvard University Press, 2003). Note also the title of Mark Mazower, *Salonica, City of Ghosts: Christians, Muslims, and Jews, 1430–1950* (New York: Vintage Books, 2006).

75 Mertelsmann, "Tartu–Dorpat–Jur'ev," 220.

76 Rachinskaia, *Pereletnye ptitsy*, 136–37, and the memoirs of Krusenstern-Peterets, among others.

77 My conversation with Mr Zhu in Harbin, winter 1996.

78 Sergei Gribin, *Liubimyi Kharbin*.

79 A main portal of Harbin history fans is the website imharbin.com.

80 Zeng Yizhi, *Cheng yu ren* (a translation of this book into English is being planned); and my conversations with Zeng Yizhi in Harbin, June 2009.

81 See Gamsa, "The Vanishing and Lingering Past in Two Cities."

82 On the "diasporic nationalism" of persons like Wu, who were proud to be Chinese but did not necessarily identify this sense of belonging with living in China, see Frost, "*Emporium in Imperio*," 60–6.

83 Jia Qiuhong, "Yibu shuyuan liangdai qing."

84 Budberg, *Bilder aus der Zeit der Lungenpest-Epidemien*, 75–6, 226–7, 287–8.
85 Jia Qiuhong, "Yibu shuyuan liangdai qing." The same ms, described as "an abridged translation" of the German book, is used in Tang Li, "Tongxiang beican suiyue de 'shijian suidao'. Balun yanzhong de Ha'erbin shuyi (1910–1911)" (A "Time Tunnel" Leading to Tragic Years: The Harbin Plague [1910–11] through Baron's Eyes), *Heilongjiang ribao*, 25 October 2008, a report from the Wu Liande Memorial Hall. A recent historical novel by an American author, which also claims inspiration from Budberg's plague memoir, displays similarly blissful ignorance. Jody Shields, *The Winter Station* (New York: Little, Brown, 2018), turns Budberg into a native of Saint Petersburg and the son of a tsarist diplomat; his Chinese wife "Li Ju" (who is also referred to as a Manchu) is fluent in English thanks to being educated in a Scottish missionary orphanage. Among improbable versions of Chinese and Russian words, names and places, Harbin becomes "Kharbin," and its Russian residents are called, gratingly, "Kharbinskiis."
86 On Petr Chistiakov, see Il'in, "Sovetskaia armiia v Kharbine," 141–4.
87 Shao, *Remote Homeland*, 290–1, 297. On a Chinese family's escape from Manchuria to Taiwan after the Communist takeover and dreams of return to the ancestral home, which have been passed to the second generation, see Yang, *The Odyssey of a Manchurian*.
88 See Tamanoi, *Memory Maps*; and Koga, *Inheritance of Loss*.
89 Kumiko Muraoka, "Mémoires d'une somnambule," 400–1. The film by Thomas Lahusen, "Manchurian Sleepwalkers," focuses on Muraoka's determination not to forget her Harbin while also featuring interviews with Harbinites in Russia, Poland, Germany, and Japan. Cf. Lahusen, "Remembering China, Imagining Israel," 267; for more on the situation of colonists after Japan's defeat, see Watt, *When Empire Comes Home*.
90 *Briefe*, 9 October 1925.
91 Magris, *Danube*, 43.
92 Cf. my article "On Value Systems of the Russian Émigrés in China," and especially the ongoing research by Laurie Manchester on Russians from Manchuria in the Soviet Union from 1954.
93 Leonid Eshchin, "Bezhenets" (1930), in Kreid and Bakich, *Russkaia poeziia Kitaia*, 188. Another poet developed the fantasy of finding a home in China, complete with *fanza* and *kang*, chopsticks and tea, and concluding with the image of a life as clear as Chinese calligraphy on silk: see Boris Beta (1895–1931), "Man'chzhurskie iamby" (Manchurian Iambs, posthumously published in 1935), ibid., 96–8. After moving from Harbin to Shanghai, Beta immigrated again to Serbia in 1924; he died in Marseille (ibid., 670).
94 "Zabludivshiisia argonavt" (Lost Argonaut, 1947). Ibid., 402–3; for the context, see Bakich, *Valerii Pereleshin*, 166.

95 Valerii Pereleshin, "Tri rodiny" (1971; included in a collection by the same title in 1987), original text and English translation in Bakich, *Valerii Pereleshin*, 141.

96 "Izdaleka" (From Afar, 1953), original text and English translation in Bakich, *Valerii Pereleshin*, 137–8; cf. an earlier statement of this vision, in ibid., 71.

97 Khaindrova, *Serdtse poeta*, 275, on *Tri Otchizny*.

98 Ibid., 291–2. For such regrets, cf. Krusenstern-Peterets, *Vospominaniia*, in *Rossiiane v Azii*, no. 5 (1998), 65.

Glossary of Chinese Terms

Acheng 阿城

A'ershan 阿爾山

Ah Cheng: see Wang Acheng

Alchuka 阿勒楚喀

Aihui 愛輝

Ashihc 阿什河

Baoding 保定

Bazhan 八站

Baicheng 白城

bainian 拜年

bangzi 梆子

Bei'an 北安

bingtang hulu 冰糖葫蘆

bilida 壁里搭

Bin County 賓縣

Binjiang 濱江

Boduna 伯都納

Bu *daifu* 卜大夫

budongde 不懂得

Bu men Li shi 卜門李氏

Buteha 布特哈

Butou 埠頭

Changling 昌陵

Chang Shun 長順

Chen Jiying 陳紀瀅

Cheng Dequan 承德全

Cixi 慈禧

da bizi 大鼻子

Dawoer 達斡爾

Daoli 道里

daotai 道太

Daowai 道外

Deng Jiemin 鄧潔民

Dong Dazhi jie 東大直街

Du Xueying 杜學瀛

Dunyuan 遁園

Elunchun 鄂倫春

facai 發財

fangzi 房子

Fenghua 奉化

fengshui 風水

Fengtian 奉天

Feng Yuxiang 馮玉祥

fucuo 浮厝

fudutong 副都統

Fujiadian 傅家甸 (originally 店)

Fujin 富錦

Fularji 富拉爾基

Fuling 福陵

Fuming'a 富明阿

Fushun 撫順

gaoliang 高粱

Gao Mang 高莽

Gaoyijie 高誼街

gewasi 格瓦斯

Gongzhuling 公主嶺

Gucheng 固城

Guan Chenghe 關成和

Guandong 關東

guobaorou 鍋包肉

Guogeli dajie 果戈里

Guo Zongxi 郭宗熙

Ha'erbin 哈爾濱

Haicheng 海城

Hailar 海拉爾

Hailun 海倫

Hanhua 漢化

Han Jingsheng 韓景生

Hanjun 漢軍

Heihe 黑河

Heilongjiang 黑龍江

hong huzi 紅胡子

hong qiang hui 紅槍會

Hongxia jie 紅霞街

Hu'erha 瑚爾哈

Hu Hong 胡泓

Hua-E yuekan 華俄月刊

Huaqiao 華僑

Huang County 黃縣

Huangshan 皇山

Huiningfu 會寧府

Hulunbuir 呼倫貝爾

Hunchun 琿春

hunxue'r 混血儿

huoji 伙計

Ji Fenghui 紀鳳輝

Ji Fengtai 紀鳳台

Jilesi 極樂寺

jiliangsuo 濟良所

Jia Shuhua 賈樹華

Jiandao 間島

Jiang Chunfang 姜椿芳

jiaoshe ju 交涉局

Jiaozhou 膠州

jiefang 解放

Jinan 濟南

Jin Chang 晉昌

Jin Jianxiao 金劍嘯

Jingyu jie 靖宇街

kang 炕

Kuanchengzi 寬城子

Lahasusu 拉哈蘇蘇

Laizhou 萊州

lamatai 喇嘛台

Langhua 郎華

lao maozi 老毛子

laoxiang 老鄉

lidaosi chang 里道斯腸

Li Hongzhang 李鴻章

Li Ruizhen 李瑞珍

Li Shaogeng 李紹庚

Lishu 黎樹

Li Yanling 李延齡

liangbatou 兩把頭

Liaoyang 療陽

Liu Jingyan 劉靜嚴

Liu Zhe 劉哲

Longkou 龍口

Lüshunkou 旅順口

Luxiya 露西亞

luodi shenggen 落地生根

Ma Zhanshan 馬占山

Ma Zhongjun 馬忠駿

magua 馬褂

mashen 馬神

Maimaicheng 買賣城

Maimaigai 買賣街

Majiagou 馬家溝

Mangou zhan 滿溝站

Manzhou 滿洲

Manzhouli 滿州里

Manzi 蠻子

Manzu 滿族

Mao'ershan 帽兒山

maozi 帽子

maozi hua 毛子話

Mudanjiang 牧丹江

Nangang 南岡

neibu 內部

Nenjiang 嫩江

Ni de mingtian banzou, ni de mingtian zou! 你的明天搬走, 你的明天走!

Ning'an 寧安

Ninguta 寧古塔

Ouluoba lüguan 歐羅巴旅館

Penglai 蓬萊

Pikou 皮口

pingju 評劇

Piziwo 貔子窩

Pukou 浦口

Pulandian 普蘭店

Qingdao 青島

Qiqihar 齊齊哈爾

Qiren 旗人

qiong maozi 窮毛子

Qiulin 秋林

Qu Qiubai 瞿秋白

Qu Changliang 曲長亮

Quanhe 圈河

Sanhe qu 三河區

Sanxing 三姓

sao dazi 臊韃子

Shahe 沙河

shang hao 上好 (尚好)

Shangshi jie 商市街

Shangzhi 尚志

Shangzhi dajie 尚志大街

shaojiu 燒酒

shidafu 士大夫

Shi Yi 石揖

Shi Zhaoji 施肇基

Shou Chang 壽長

Shou Shan 壽山

Shuanghesheng 雙合盛

Siping 四平

Songhuajiang 松花江

Song Xiaolian 宋小濂

Songyuan 松原

Suifenhe 綏芬河

Sun Chuanfang 孫傳芳

Sun Yunxuan 孫運璿

Suolun 索倫

Tai'an 泰安

Taiping qiao 太平橋

Tiandi jie 田地街

tiandi liangxin 天地良心

tian'e 天鵝

tianli liangxin 天理良心

Tieling 鐵嶺

Tongfalong 同發隆

Tongji 同記

Tongjiang 同江

Tongjiang jie 通江街

Tongle chayuan 同樂茶園

waiguo gui 外國鬼

Wang Acheng 王阿成

Wang Fengrui 王奉瑞

Wang Yulang 王禹浪

wei 偽

Wenmiao 文廟

Wen Peiyun 溫佩筠

wopeng 窩棚

Wu Baixiang 武百祥

Wujiazhan 五家站

Wu Junsheng 吳俊升

Wu Peifu 吳佩孚

Xi erdao jie 西二道街

Xi sandao jie 西三道街

Xi shidaojie 西十道街

Xiamanjie 霞曼街

Xiangfang 香坊

Xiao Hong 蕭紅

Xiao Jun 蕭軍

Yakeshi 牙克石

Yanbian 延邊

Yantai 煙台

yangqi 洋氣

Ye County 掖縣

Yi Yisan 魏益三

Yilan 依蘭

Yimianpo 一面破

Yin Chang 廕昌

Yingkou 營口

Youyi lu 友誼路

Yuan Chonghuan 袁崇煥

Yuan Erhan 袁爾漢

Yuan Wenbi 袁文弼

yumi bing 玉米餅

Yupi dazi 魚皮韃子

Zaili hui 在理會

Zeng Yizhi 曾一智

Zhabei 閘北

Zhalantun 札蘭屯

Zhang Naiying 張迺瑩

Zhang Tingge 張廷閣

Zhang Xueliang 張學良

Zhang Zongchang 張宗昌

Zhang Zuolin 張作霖

Zhaodong zhan 肇東站

Zhao Erxun 趙爾巽

Zhaolinjie 兆鄰街

Zheng Xingwen 鄭興文

Zhengyang jie 正陽街

Zhifu 芝罘

Zhili 直隸

Zhong-De-Hua 中德花

Zhonghua 中華

Zhongyang dajie 中央大街

Zhou Mian 周冕

Zhu Shipu 朱世樸

Bibliography

Archival and Unpublished Sources

Family Papers in Private Possession

Köhler family albums, Hamburg, Germany.
Popoff family papers and albums, Liège, Belgium. Courtesy of the late Victor
    Popoff.
Raczynski family papers and albums, Santiago, Chile. Courtesy of the
    Raczynski family.
Raczynski, Joseph A., ed. *'Lebenserinnerung' meiner Mutter. Notizen zur*
    Geschichte der Familie Budberg. Unpublished typescript, Munich, 1980–1.
    Courtesy of the Raczynski family. Cited as *Lebenserinnerung.*
– *Roger Budberg: Briefe an seine Schwester Antoinette 1903–1925.* Unpublished
    typescript, Munich, 1986. Courtesy of the Raczynski family. Cited as *Briefe.*

Unpublished Secondary Sources

Lackschewitz, Klas, genealogy of Barons von Bönninghausen gen. Budberg,
    the extinct line Gemauert-Poniemon. Typescript (2002). Courtesy of the
    author.

Interviews

Author's interview with Victor Popoff. Liège, Belgium, August 2005.
Author's interviews in Budberga village, Latvia, October 2008.
Author's interviews with former Harbin residents (identified and dated in the
    text).
Esther Kallen, née Komarovskaia, interview with family members in
    Washington, DC, 17 October 1965. Recording, courtesy of Eugene
    Lipkowitz, Wyckoff, NJ.

Vasily V. Ushanoff, "Recollections of Life in the Russian Community
    in Manchuria and in Emigration," interview by Richard A. Pierce at
    Laguna Beach, CA, July 1981. Typescript, Bancroft Library, University of
    California.

Archives (collections are specified in the text)

Estonian Historical Archives (EHA), Tartu.
Historical Archive of Omsk *oblast*, Omsk.
Hoover Institution Archives, Stanford University.
Latvian State Historical Archives (LVVA), Riga.
Museum of Russian Culture, San Francisco.
National Archives of the United Kingdom, Kew.
Political Archive of the Federal Foreign Office, Berlin.
Russian State Historical Archive (RGIA), St Petersburg.
Russian State Historical Archive of the Far East (RGIA DV), Vladivostok.
Russian State Military History Archive (RGVIA), Moscow.
Société des Missions Étrangères de Paris.
State Archive of Irkutsk *oblast* (GAIO), Irkutsk.
State Archive of Khabarovsk Region (GAKhK), BREM collection.
State Archive of the Russian Federation (GARF), Moscow.
State Archive in Tobolsk City.

Published Sources

A.I. [Anna K. Ivashkevich]. "Poslednie dni v Man'chzhurii (iz lichnykh
    vospominanii)" (Last Days in Manchuria: From Personal Reminiscences).
    Russkoe bogatstvo 10 (October 1900): 143–68.
Abe, Hiroshi. "The Movement to Restore Educational Prerogatives in
    Manchuria during the 1920s: One Aspect of Nationalism in Modern
    Chinese Education." *East Asian Cultural Studies* 21, no. 3 (1981): 1–31.
Ablazhei, Natal'ia N. "Russkie emigranty iz Kitaia. Repatriatsiia, karatel'naia
    politika i trudoispol'zovanie vo vtoroi polovine 1940-kh godov" (Russian
    Émigrés from China: Repatriation, Repressive Measures, and Labour Use
    in the Second Half of the 1940s). *Vestnik Rossiiskogo gumanitarnogo fonda* 4
    (2006): 24–35.
Ablova, Nadezhda E. *KVZhD i rossiiskaia emigratsiia v Kitae. Mezhdunarodnye
    i politicheskie aspekty istorii (pervaia polovina XX veka)* (The CER and the
    Russian Emigration in China: International and Political Aspects of
    History in the First Half of the Twentieth Century). Moscow: Russkaia
    panorama, 2005.
Abrosimov, Igor' A. *Pod chuzhim nebom* (Under an Alien Sky). Moscow:
    Molodaia gvardiia, 1990.

Abrosimov, N.I. "Izuchenie kitaiskogo iazyka i KVZhD" (The Study of the Chinese Language and the CER). *Ekonomicheskii biulleten'* 35 (6 September 1925): 6–8.

Agranovskii, Zalman L. "Evreiskaia obshchina Kharbina 1948–1962" (The Jewish Community of Harbin, 1948–62) [1962]. *Bulletin Igud Yotsei Sin*, nos. 374–381 (2002–4).

Ah Cheng. *Ha'erbin ren* (The Harbin Person). Taipei: Daotian, 1997.

Aleksandrov, V. [Viktor A. Veinshtok]. "Argun' i priargun'e. Putevye zametki i ocherki" (The Argun and Its Adjacent Region: Travel Notes and Sketches). *Vestnik Evropy* 39, no. 5 (September 1904): 281–310.

Alkin, Sergei V. "Arkheolog Vladimir Iakovlevich Tolmachev" (Archaeologist Vladimir Ia. Tolmachev). In *Na pol'zu i razvitie russkoi nauki* (For the Benefit and Development of Russian Science), ed. A.D. Stoliar and Iu.V. Ivanova, 2nd rev. ed., 90–100. Novosibirsk: Sibirskoe Otdelenie RAN, 2005.

– "Arkheologicheskie i antropologicheskie issledovaniia V.V. Ponosova v Man'chzhurii" (The Archaeological and Anthropological Research of V.V. Ponosov in Manchuria). In *Vtorye chteniia im. G.I. Nevel'skogo* (The Second Nevelskoi Readings), 113–17. Khabarovsk: n.p., 1990.

Alpern Engel, Barbara. "In the Name of the Tsar: Competing Legalities and Marital Conflict in Late Imperial Russia." *Journal of Modern History* 77 (March 2005): 70–96.

Altman, Avraham. "Controlling the Jews, Manchukuo Style." In *From Kaifeng ... to Shanghai: Jews in China*, ed. Roman Malek, 279–317. Sankt Augustin: Monumenta Serica Monograph Series, vol. 46, 2000.

Ancelāne, Alma, ed. *Latviešu tautas teikas* (Latvian Folktales). Riga: Latvijas PSR zinātņu akadēmijas izdevniecība, 1961.

Anderson, Benedict. *Imagined Communities: Reflections on the Origin and Spread of Nationalism*, 2nd rev. ed. London and New York: Verso, 2006.

Andreeva, Natal'ia S. "Pribaltiiskie nemtsy i Pervaia mirovaia voina" (Baltic Germans and the First World War). In *Problemy sotsial'no-ekonomicheskoi i politicheskoi istorii Rossii XIX–XX vekov* (Issues of Russian Social-Economic and Political History in the Nineteenth and Twentieth Centuries), ed. A.N. Tsamutali, 461–73. Saint Petersburg: Aleteia, 1999.

Andreyev, Alexandre. *The Myth of the Masters Revived: The Occult Lives of Nikolai and Elena Roerich*. Leiden: Brill, 2014.

Anon. [Aleksei V. Peshekhonov], "Khronika vnutrennei zhizni" (Domestic News), pt 2, *Russkoe bogatstvo* 9 (September 1900): 215–25.

Anrep-Elmpt, Reinhold Graf. *Reise um die Welt. Beschreibung von Land und Meer nebst Sitten- und Kulturschilderungen mit besonderer Berücksichtigung der Tropennatur*, 2 vols. Leipzig: Gressner & Schramm, 1887.

"A Plea for the Pigtail." *British Medical Journal* 2, no. 2710 (7 December 1912), 1633–4.

Argudiaeva, Iulia V. "Istochniki po istoriko-demograficheskim protsessam u russkikh Trekhrech'ia" (Sources on Historical-Demographic Processes among the Russians of Trekhrech'e). *Istoricheskaia demografiia* 1 (2016): 66–70.

Arsen'ev, Vladimir K. *Dersu Uzala*. In *Sobranie sochinenii v shesti tomakh* (Collected Works in Six Vols.), chief ed. P.F. Brovko, vol. 1. Vladivostok: Rubezh, 2007–.

Avenarius, Georgii G. "Shuanchenpu i Shuanchensian'" (Shuangcheng Town and County). *Vestnik Man'chzhurii* 12, no. 8 (August 1934): 114–19.

Baikov, Nikolai A. "Moi priezd v Man'chzhuriiu (1902 god)" (My Arrival in Manchuria in 1902). Reprinted in *Polytechnic* 10 (1979): 76–83.

– *Sobranie* (Collection), in 3 vols. Vladivostok: Rubezh, 2009–12. Vol. 1: *Velikii Van* (The Great Wang). Vol. 2: *V gorakh i lesakh Man'chzhurii* (In the Mountains and Forests of Manchuria). Vol. 3: *Taiga shumit* (The Taiga Rustles).

Baker, Hugh D.R. "Life in the Cities: The Emergence of Hong Kong Man." *China Quarterly* 95 (September 1983): 469–79.

Bakich, Olga. "Did You Speak Harbin Sino-Russian?" *Itinerario* 35, no. 3 (December 2011): 23–36.

– "Émigré Identity: The Case of Harbin." In *Harbin and Manchuria*, ed. Thomas Lahusen, special issue of *South Atlantic Quarterly* 99, no. 1 (2000): 51–73.

– *Harbin Russian Imprints: Bibliography as History, 1898–1961. Materials for a Definitive Bibliography*. New York: Norman Ross, 2002.

– "A Russian City in China: Harbin before 1917." *Canadian Slavonic Papers* 28, no. 2 (June 1986): 129–48.

– "Russian Education in Harbin, 1898–1962." *Transactions of the Association of Russian-American Scholars in the USA* 26 (1994): 269–94.

– "Russian Émigrés in Harbin's Multinational Past: Censuses and Identity." In *Entangled Histories: The Transcultural Past of Northeast China*, ed. Dan Ben-Canaan et al., 83–99. Heidelberg: Springer, 2014.

– *Valerii Pereleshin: Life of a Silkworm*. Toronto: University of Toronto Press, 2015.

Balmasov, Sergei S. *Beloemigranty na voennoi sluzhbe v Kitae* (White Émigrés in Military Service in China). Moscow: Tsentrpoligraf, 2007.

Baranov, Aleksei M. "Doklad Predsedatelia Istoriko-Etnograficheskoi sektsii O.I.M.K." (Report by the Chairman of the Historical-Ethnographic Section). *Izvestiia Obshchestva Izucheniia Man'chzhurskogo Kraia* 2 (January 1923): 4–8.

– "Zadachi sektsii etnografii" (Goals of the Ethnographic Section). *Izvestiia Obshchestva Izucheniia Man'chzhurskogo Kraia* 1 (November 1922): 12–15.

Baranov, Ippolit G. *Cherty narodnogo byta v Kitae (Narodnye prazdniki, obychai i pover'ia)* (Characteristics of Popular Daily Life in China: Folk Festivals, Customs and Beliefs). Harbin: Tipografiia Kit. Vost. zhel. dor., 1928.

– "Khramy Tszilesy i Konfutsiia v Kharbine" (The Jilesi and Confucius Temples in Harbin). In Baranov, Verovaniia i obychai kitaitsev (Beliefs and Customs of the Chinese), ed. K.M. Tertitskii, 85–112. Moscow: Muravei-Gaid, 1999.

– "Kitaiskii Novyi god" (The Chinese New Year). Ibid., 42–67.
– "Kraevedenie v kartinakh khudozhnika Sungurova" (Local Lore Studies in the Works of Painter Sungurov), *Vestnik Man'chzhurii* 3 (1934): 172–5.
– "Po kitaiskim khramam Ashikhe" (Among the Chinese Temples of Ashihe), *Vestnik Man'chzhurii* 1–2 (1926): 120–212.
Barshay, Andrew E. *The Gods Left First: The Captivity and Repatriation of Japanese POWs in Northeast Asia, 1945–1956.* Berkeley: University of California Press, 2013.
Baskhanov, Mikhail K. *Russkie voennye vostokovedy do 1917 goda. Biobibliograficheskii slovar'* (A Bio-bibliographical Dictionary of Russian Military Orientalists before 1917). Moscow: Vostochnaia literatura RAN, 2005.
Bayly, C.A. *The Birth of the Modern World, 1780–1914: Global Connections and Comparisons.* Oxford: Blackwell, 2004.
Becker, Jasper. *The City of Heavenly Tranquillity: Beijing in the History of China.* London: Allen Lane, 2008.
Bekkin, Renat I. "Pis'ma leitenanta I.I. Isliamova k rodnym iz Man'chzhurii. 1904 god" (Letters of Lieutenant Isliamov to Relatives from Manchuria in 1904). *Vostochnyi arkhiv* 1 (2017): 31–5.
Beloglazov, Gennadii P. "Kitaiskii vektor tsivilizatsionno-kul'turnogo vzaimodeistviia" (The Chinese Vector of Civilizational–Cultural Interaction). In *Rossiia i narody Dal'nego Vostoka. Istoricheskii opyt mezhetnicheskogo vzaimodeistviia* (Russia and the Peoples of the Far East: The Historical Experience of Cross-Ethnic Interaction), ed. V.A. Turaev, 250–75. Vladivostok: DVO RAN, 2016.
– *Russkaia zemledel'cheskaia kul'tura v Man'chzhurii (seredina XVII – pervaia tret' XX v.)* (Russian Farming Culture in Manchuria, Mid-Seventeenth Century to the First Third of the Twentieth Century). Vladivostok: Dal'nauka, 2007.
Belov, Evgenii A. "Bor'ba za KVZhD v kontse 1917 – nachale 1918 g." (Struggle for the CER in late 1917–early 1918). *Vostok* 6 (1996): 34–9.
Ben Chi. "Guanyu Songbin yinshe" (On the Songbin Reciting Society). *Ha'erbin yanjiu* 4 (1984): 37–8.
Bentley, Jerry H. *Old World Encounters: Cross-Cultural Contacts and Exchanges in Pre-Modern Times.* New York and Oxford: Oxford University Press, 1993.
Bernstein, Seth. "Ambiguous Homecoming: Retribution, Exploitation, and Social Tensions during Repatriation to the USSR, 1944–1946." *Past and Present* 242 (February 2019): 193–226.
Bickers, Robert A. "History, Legend, and Treaty Port Ideology, 1925–1931." In *Ritual and Diplomacy: The Macartney Mission to China, 1792–1794*, ed. Bickers, 81–92. London: BACS and Wellsweep Press, 1993.
Bisher, Jamie. *White Terror: Cossack Warlords of the Trans-Siberian.* London: Taylor and Francis, 2005.

Bix, Herbert P. "Japanese Imperialism and the Manchurian Economy, 1900–31." *China Quarterly* 51 (July 1972): 425–43.

Blagoveshchenskii [Ivan G. Pryzhov]. "Zapiski o Sibiri. I. Okhota na brodiag. II. Starovery" (Notes on Siberia: 1. Hunting for Rovers. 2. The Old Believers). *Vestnik Evropy* 17, no. 9 (September 1882): 291–325.

Bo Yang. "Lishu diming tanyuan" (An Exploration of the Origins of the Place Name Lishu). *Zhongguo diming* 11 (2014): 67, 71.

Boloban, Andrei P. *Otchet kommercheskogo agenta Kitaiskoi Vostochnoi zheleznoi dorogi A.P. Bolobana po obsledovaniiu v 1911 godu raionov Khei-lun-tszianskoi, Girinskoi i Mukdenskoi provintsii (Severnoi Man'chzhurii), tiagoteiushchikh k Kitaiskoi Vostochnoi zheleznoi doroge, v zemledel'cheskom i khlebopromyshlennom otnosheniiakh* (Report by Commercial Agent of the Chinese Eastern Railway A.P. Boloban on Inspection in 1911 of the Regions of Heilongjiang, Jilin, and Mukden Provinces Adjacent to the CER, with Respect to Agriculture and the Bread Industry). Harbin: Tipografiia Kitaiskoi Vostochnoi zheleznoi dorogi, 1912.

Bong, InYoung. "A 'White Race' without Supremacy: Russians, Racial Hybridity, and Liminality in the Chinese Literature of Manchukuo." *Modern Chinese Literature and Culture* 26, no. 1 (2014): 137–90.

Borisov, B. *Dal'nii Vostok* (The Far East). Vienna: Izdanie Novoi Rossii, 1921.

Böttcher, Bernhard. *Die Kolonne Ihrer Majestät. Briefe eines Arztes aus dem fernen Osten*. Riga: Verlag von Jonck & Poliewsky, 1904.

Borodin, Aleksei, et al. *Semeinye khroniki* (Family Chronicles). Moscow: author's edition, 2000.

Botkin, Evgenii S. "Svet i teni russko-iaponskoi voiny 1904–5 gg." (Light and Shade of the Russo-Japanese War, 1904–5). *Vestnik Evropy* 43, no. 1 (January 1908): 54–82.

Briedis, Laimonas. *Vilnius: City of Strangers*. Budapest: Central European University Press, 2009.

Brower, Daniel. "Islam and Ethnicity: Russian Colonial Policy in Turkestan." In *Russia's Orient: Imperial Borderlands and Peoples, 1700–1917*, ed. Daniel R. Brower and Edward J. Lazzerini, 115–37. Bloomington: Indiana University Press, 1997.

Budberg, Baron Aleksei P. *Dnevnik 1917–1919* (Diary, 1917–19). Moscow: Zakharov, 2016.

Budberg, Baron Joseph. "Eine gefährliche Bärenjagd." *Neue Baltische Waidmannsblätter* 3, no. 19 (1 October 1907), 440–3.

– "Jagderfolge in Westsibirien." *Neue Baltische Waidmannsblätter* 6, no. 10 (15 May 1910), 223.

– "Zwei Monate im sibirischen Urwalde." *Baltische Waidmannsblätter* 4, no. 14 (31 July 1904): 241–4; no. 15 (15 August 1904), 257–9.

Budberg, Baron Nikolai [Nicolai] von. *Budbergiana. Beiträge zur Familiengeschichte*, nos. 1–3. Detmold: author's edition, 1953, 1954, 1955.

– "Ein Geschlecht kehrt heim. Die v. Budberg in Wesfalen, in Livland und wieder in Wesfalen von 13. bis 20. Jahrhundert." *Beiträge zur westfälischen Familienforschung* 11, no. 3 (1952): 1–8.

– "Eine europäisch-asiatische Ehe-Allianz. Dschun-De-Huar = Chinesisch–Deutsche Blume, letzter und jüngster Sproß eines großen Hauses." *Deutsches Adelsarchiv* 9, no. 68 (April 1953): 67–9.

Budberg, Baron Roger. "Aus der Mandschurei: Die Chunchudzen." *Globus* 97, no. 10 (17 March 1910): 149–53; no. 11 (24 March 1910): 168–73.

– *Bilder aus der Zeit der Lungenpest-Epidemien in der Mandschurei 1910/1911 und 1921.* Hamburg: Conrad Behre, 1923.

– "Bürg- und Haftpflicht im chinesischen Volksleben." *Globus* 98, no. 18 (10 November 1910): 285–7.

– "Chinesische Prostitution," *Globus* 97, no. 20 (2 June 1910): 317–19.

– "Die Nationen in der Mandschurei" (signed Clemens Goetz). *Berliner Tageblatt*, 13 May 1910.

– "Einige hygienische Prinzipien im Volksleben der Chinesen." *Deutsche medizinische Wochenschrift* 37, no. 37 (14 September 1911): 1707–8.

– "Europäische Kulturträger und der chinesische Zopf." *Der Ostasiatische Lloyd* 23, no. 3 (17 January 1913): 71–2.

– "Gibt es eine Prädisposition von Geschlecht, Alter und Konstitution bei Infektion durch die Lungenpest?" *Die Therapie der Gegenwart* 52, no. 6 (June 1911): 254–7.

– *Memuary Doktora-Meditsiny R. A. Barona Beningsgauzen-Budberg* (Memoirs of R. A. Baron Boenningshausen-Budberg MD). Harbin: Amerikanskaia tipografiia, 1925.

– *O zhizni. Besedy akushera* (On Life: The Conversations of a Male Midwife). Harbin: Izdatel'stvo V.A. Chilikina, 1926.

– "Über die Bedingungen des Exporthandels in der Nordmandschurei." *Globus* 98, no. 1 (7 July 1910): 7–10.

– "Über die Verwendung des Kampfers in der Gynäkologie." *Zentralblatt für Gynäkologie* 35, no. 37 (16 September 1911): 1313–14.

– "Vom chinesischen Zopf." *Deutsche medizinische Wochenschrift* 38, no. 30 (25 July 1912): 1421–2.

– "Vom Seelenleben der Chinesen." *Deutsche Monatsschrift für Rußland, der baltischen Monatsschrift* 56, no. 1 (January 1914): 57–66.

– "Zur Charakteristik chinesischen Seelenlebens." *Globus* 98, no. 7 (25 August 1910): 111–13.

Budberg-Gemauert-Poniemon, Baron Alexander von. *Beiträge zu einer Geschichte des Geschlechtes der Freiherrn v. Bönninghausen genannt Budberg.* Riga: author's edition, 1897.

Budberg-Magnushof, Baron Gotthard, and Paul Höflinger, eds. *Des Jägers Jahrbuch. Für Russlands Jäger in Nah und Fern.* Riga and Moscow: J. Deubner, 1903.

Buianov, Dmitrii E. "Dukhovnye khristiane v Sibiri i na Dal'nem Vostoke (vtoraia polovina XIX – nachalo XX veka)" (Spiritual Christians in Siberia and the Far East, Second Half of the Nineteenth – Beginning of the Twentieth Centuries). *Vestnik Tomskogo gosudarstvennogo universiteta* 418 (2017): 62–70.

Buianov, Evgenii V. *Dukhovnye khristiane molokane v Amurskoi oblasti vo vtoroi polovine XIX – pervoi treti XX veka* (Molokan Spiritual Christians in the Amur Province, Second Half of the Nineteenth–First Third of the Twentieth Centuries). Blagoveshchensk: Amurskii gosudarstvennyi universitet, 2012.

Burmistrov, Konstantin. "Topography of Russian Esotericism: From Moscow to Harbin and Asunción." In *Capitales de l'ésotérisme européen et dialogue des cultures*, ed. Jean-Pierre Brach et al., 71–84. Paris: Orizons, 2014.

Buruma, Ian. *Year Zero: A History of 1945*. New York: Penguin, 2013.

Carter, James H. *Creating a Chinese Harbin: Nationalism in an International City, 1916–1932*. Ithaca: Cornell University Press, 2002.

Chen, Bijia, et al. "Interethnic Marriage in Northeast China, 1866–1913." *Demographic Research* 38 (March 2018): 929–66.

Ch'en, Jerome. *China and the West: Society and Culture 1815–1937*. London: Hutchinson, 1979.

Chen Jiying. *Sanshi niandai zuojia ji* (Writers of the Thirties: A Memoir). Taibei: Chengwen chubanshe, 1979.

Chen, Shuang. *State-Sponsored Inequality: The Banner System and Social Stratification in Northeast China*. Stanford: Stanford University Press, 2017.

Chen, Shuang, et al. "Categorical Inequality and Gender Difference: Marriage and Remarriage in Northeast China, 1749–1913." In *Similarity in Difference: Marriage in Europe and Asia, 1700–1900*, ed. Christer Lundh and Satomi Kurosu, 393–436. Cambridge, MA: MIT Press, 2014.

Chen Wenlong. " 'Wodi' Ouluoba, xunzhao Xiao Hong de Ouluoba" ("Under Cover" in Europe: Searching for Xiao Hong's Europa). 26 June 2016. imharbin.com/post/20836.

– "Yi hao binghua ji ru feng: xiri Ha'erbin Songhua jiangpan de xueqiao" (A Tangle of Rime Swift Like the Wind: Sleds by the Songhua River in Old-Time Harbin). 23 March 2018. imharbin.com/post/42555.

Chen Yuan, ed. *Wolfgang Seuberlich (1906–1985). Ostasienwissenschaftler und Bibliothekar*. Berlin: Staatsbibliothek zu Berlin, 1998.

Cheng, Weikun. "Politics of the Queue: Agitation and Resistance in the Beginning and End of Qing China." In *Hair: Its Power and Meaning in Asian Cultures*, ed. Alf Hiltebeitel and Barbara D. Miller, 123–42. Albany: SUNY Press, 1998.

Cherkasov-Georgievskii, Vladimir. *Russkii khram na chuzhbine* (The Russian Church Abroad). Moscow: Palomnik, 2003.

Chernolutskaia, Elena N. "Religious Communities in Harbin and Ethnic Identity of Russian Émigrés." In *Harbin and Manchuria*, ed. Lahusen, 79–96.

Chernolutskaia, Elena N., ed. "Ukrainskaia natsional'naia koloniia v Kharbine (pervaia polovina XX v.)" (The Ukrainian National Colony in Harbin in the First Half of the Twentieth Century). In *Slaviane na Dal'nem Vostoke. Problemy istorii i kul'tury* (Slavs in the Far East: Problems of History and Culture), ed. M.S. Vysokov, 87–98. Iuzhno-Sakhalinsk: Sakhalinskii tsentr dokumentatsii noveishei istorii, 1994.

Chernolutskaia, Elena N., et al., eds. *Rossiiane v Aziatsko-Tikhookeanskom Regione, Sotrudnichestvo na rubezhe vekov. Materialy pervoi mezhdunarodnoi nauchno-prakticheskoi konferentsii, Vladivostok, 24–26 sentiabria 1997 g.* (Russians in the Asian-Pacific Region: Proceedings of the First International Conference), pt 2. Vladivostok: DVGU, 1999.

Chernomaz, Viacheslav A. "Obshchestvenno-politicheskaia deiatel'nost' ukrainskoi emigratsii v Kitae (pervaia polovina XX v.)" (The Public and Political Activity of the Ukrainian Emigration in China in the First Half of the Twentieth Century). In Chernolutskaia et al., eds., *Rossiiane v Aziatsko-Tikhookeanskom Regione*, 33–41.

Chiasson, Blaine R. *Administering the Colonizer: Manchuria's Russians under Chinese Rule, 1918–29*. Vancouver: UBC Press, 2010.

Chou, Eva Shan. *Memory, Violence, Queues: Lu Xun Interprets China*. Ann Arbor: Association for Asian Studies Publications, 2012.

Christie, Dugald. *Ten Years in Manchuria: A Story of Medical Mission Work in Moukden, 1883–1893*. Paisley: J. and R. Parlane, 1895.

– *Thirty Years in Moukden, 1883–1913*. London: Constable, 1914.

Chuguevskii, Leonid I. "100-letie Kharbina" (The Hundredth Anniversary of Harbin). *Problemy Dal'nego Vostoka* 3 (1998): 116–22.

Cipko, Serge. "Ukrainians in Manchuria, China: A Concise Historical Survey." *Past Imperfect* 1 (1992): 155–73.

Clausen, Søren, and Stig Thøgersen. *The Making of a Chinese City: History and Historiography in Harbin*. Armonk: M.E. Sharpe, 1995.

Cohen, Paul A. *History in Three Keys: The Boxers as Event, Experience, and Myth*. New York: Columbia University Press, 1997.

Colley, Linda. "Going Native, Telling Tales: Captivity, Collaborations and Empire." *Past and Present* 168 (August 2000): 170–93.

Colquhoun, Archibald R. "Manchuria in Transformation." *Monthly Review* 5, no. 1 (October 1901): 58–72.

Coltman, Robert, Jr, MD. *The Chinese, Their Present and Future: Medical, Political, and Social*. Philadelphia and London: F.A. Davis, 1891.

Coulter, John W. "Harbin: Strategic City on the 'Pioneer Fringe.'" *Pacific Affairs* 5, no. 11 (November 1932): 967–72.

Crossley, Pamela Kyle, *The Manchus*. Oxford: Blackwell, 1997.

– *Orphan Warriors: Three Manchu Generations and the End of the Qing World.*
Princeton: Princeton University Press, 1990.
– *A Translucent Mirror: History and Identity in Qing Imperial Ideology.* Berkeley:
University of California Press, 1999.
Danilin, Iurii. "Nagrady i znaki rossiiskikh vrachei v Kitae" (Awards and
Badges of Russian Physicians in China). *Antikvariat. Predmety iskusstva i
kollektsionirovaniia*, nos. 1–2 (January–February 2015): 94–103.
Datsyshen, Vladimir G. "Inkou. Iz opyta rossiiskoi kolonizatsii" (Yingkou:
From the Russian Colonial Experience). *Vostok* 4 (1995): 78–91.
– "Shou Shan'." *Voprosy istorii* 4 (1998): 152–7.
– *Voina v Priamur'e* (War in the Priamur). In *Voennye sobytiia v Priamur'e.
1900–1902* (The Events of War in the Priamur, 1900–1902), ed. Anatolii
V. Teliuk et al., 160–280. Blagoveshchensk-na-Amure: Amurskaia
iarmarka, 2008.
Deeg, Lothar. *Kunst & Albers. Die Kaufhauskönige von Wladiwostok. Aufstieg und
Untergang eines deutschen Handelshauses jenseits von Sibirien.* Essen: Klartext,
2012.
Deich (Deutsch), Lev G. *16 let v Sibiri. Vospominaniia (1884–1901 gg.)* (16 Years
in Siberia: Memoirs). Geneva: Iskra, 1904.
– *Krovavye dni (epizod iz russko-kitaiskoi voiny)* (Bloody Days: An Episode of the
Russo-Chinese War). Saint Petersburg: Proletariat, 1906.
Dement, Sergei V. *Stupeni moei zhizni* (The Stages of My Life). No place,
publisher or date (privately produced electronic file, 2017).
DeNio Stephens, Holly. "The Occult in Russia Today." In *The Occult in Russian
and Soviet Culture*, ed. Bernice Glatzer Rosenthal, 357–78. Ithaca: Cornell
University Press, 1997.
Derevianko, Il'ia V., ed. *'Belye piatna' Russko-iaponskoi voiny* ("Blind Spots" of
the Russo-Japanese War). Moscow: Iauza and Eksmo, 2005.
Deutsche Biographische Enzyklopädie, ed. Rudolf Vierhaus et al., 2nd ed., 13 vols.
Munich: K.G. Saur, 1995–2003.
Dewar, Keith, et al. "Harbin, Lanterns of Ice, Sculptures of Snow." *Tourism
Management* 22, no. 5 (October 2001): 523–32.
Diabkin, Igor' A., and Anna A. Levchenko. "'Nemets s russkoiu dushoi.'
Russkie pisateli v Kitae (stenogramma besedy s A.P. Severnym)" ("The
German with the Russian Soul": Russian Writers in China [transcript of
a Conversation with A.P. Severnyi]). *Rossiia i Kitai na dal'nevostochnykh
rubezhakh* 11 (2015): 352–62.
D'iakov, Dmitrii A. "Narodnoe obrazovanie v Polose Otchuzhdeniia Kit. Vost.
zhel. dro. [sic]" (Popular Education in the CER Alienation Zone). *Vestnik
Man'chzhurskogo Pedagogicheskogo Obshchestva*, vol. 1, no. 1 (July 1922): 3–7.
D'iakov, Ivan A. "Amaterasu. Pravda o perezhitom v Trekhrech'e za Veru i
Otchiznu" (Amaterasu: The Truth about Experiences in Trekhrech'e for

Faith and Fatherland). In Priest Dionisii Pozdniaev, *Pravoslavie v Kitae (1900–1997)* (The Russian Orthodox Faith in China), 164–243. Moscow: Izdanie Sviato-Vladimirskogo Bratstva, 1998.

Diao Shaohua. *Literatura russkogo zarubezh'ia v Kitae (v g. Kharbine i Shankhae). Bibliografiia (spisok knig i publikatsii v periodicheskikh izdaniiakh)* (Literature of the Russian Emigration in China [Harbin and Shanghai]: A Bibliographical List of Books and Publications in Periodicals). Harbin: Beifang wenyi chubanshe, 2001.

Dobrynin, Petr P. "Molodye russkie vrachi – vypuskniki Kharbinskogo Gosudarstvennogo Meditsinskogo Instituta" (Young Russian Physicians, Graduates of the Harbin State Medical Institute). In *Gody, Liudi, Sud'by. Istoriia rossiiskoi emigratsii v Kitae* (Years, People, Destinies: A History of the Russian Emigration in China), 18–20. Moscow: Institut rossiiskoi istorii RAN, 1998.

Dolbilov, Mikhail. "Russification and the Bureaucratic Mind in the Russian Empire's Northwestern Region in the 1860s." *Kritika: Explorations in Russian and Eurasian History* 5, no. 2 (2004): 245–71.

Domnin, Igor' V., ed. *Voennyi al'bom generala A. P. Budberga. Materialy k biografii. Vospominaniia o voine. 1914–1917* (The War Album of General A.P. Budberg: Materials for a Biography, War Memoirs 1914–17). Moscow: Knizhnitsa, 2014.

Doolittle, Rev. Justus. *Social Life of the Chinese ...*, 2 vols. in one. New York: Harper and Brothers, 1876.

Douglas, R.M. *Orderly and Humane: The Expulsion of the Germans after the Second World War.* New Haven: Yale University Press, 2012.

Drake, F.S. "Religion in a Manchurian City." *The Chinese Register*, February–March 1935, 1–16.

Dubinina, Nina I. *Priamurskii general-gubernator N.I. Grodekov* (The Governor General of the Priamur, N.I. Grodekov). Khabarovsk: Priamurskie vedomosti, 2001.

Dudbridge, Glen. *The Legend of Miaoshan*, rev. ed. Oxford: Oxford University Press, 2004.

Dvorzhitskaia, Alla N. "Moi mnogolikii Kharbin" (My Many-Faced Harbin). *Ural* 12 (1991): 90–112.

Dyatlov, Viktor I. "The Blagoveshchensk Drowning: Story of How Phobias Become a Reality." *Sensus Historiae* 8, no. 3 (2012): 71–90.

– "'The Blagoveshchensk Utopia': Historical Memory and Historical Responsibility." *Sensus Historiae* 8, no. 3 (2012): 115–40.

Dzemeshkevich, Liudmila K. *Kharbintsy* (Harbinites). Omsk: author's edition, 1998.

Eckart, Wolfgang U. *Medizin und Kolonialimperialismus. Deutschland 1884–1945.* Paderborn: F. Schöningh, 1997.

Elevferii, Bishop of Rostov and Taganrog. "Doklad o prebyvanii v Man'chzhurii. Opisanie puteshestviia i prebyvaniia v Kharbine" (Report on Sojourn in Manchuria: Description of Travel and Sojourn in Harbin). Publication by O.V. Kosik, *Vestnik Pravoslavnogo Sviato-Tikhonovskogo gumanitarnogo universiteta*, series 2, no. 2 (2007): 131–53.

Elliott, Mark C. "Ethnicity in the Qing Eight Banners." In *Empire at the Margins: Culture, Ethnicity, and Frontier in Early Modern China*, ed. Pamela Kyle Crossley et al., 27–57. Berkeley: University of California Press, 2006.

Entsiklopedicheskii slovar' Brokgauz i Efron (The Brockhaus and Efron Encyclopedic Dictionary). 82 vols. Saint Petersburg: Brokgauz i Efron, 1890–1907.

Entsiklopediia literaturnoi zhizni Priamur'ia XIX – XXI vekov (Encyclopedia of Literary Life in the Priamur, Nineteenth to Twenty-First Centuries), ed. A.V. Urmanov. Blagoveshchensk: BGPU, 2013.

Erdberg, Oskar S. [O.S. Tarkhanov]. *Kitaiskie novelly* (Chinese Novellas). Moscow: Sovetskii pisatel', 1959.

Erik-Amburger-Datenbank. "Ausländern im vorrevolutionären Russland." dokumente.ios-regensburg.de/amburger.

Ermachenko, Igor' O. "Intellektual'naia istoriia i mir veshchei. Kitaiskaia i iaponskaia predmetnaia sreda v russkikh korrespondentsiiakh iz Man'chzhurii (1904–1905 gg.)" (Intellectual History and the World of Things: The Chinese and Japanese Object Environment in Russian Correspondence from Manchuria, 1904–5). In *Mir Klio* (Clio's World), ed. A. Supriianova, vol. 1, 310–33. Moscow: Institut Vseobshchei istorii RAN, 2007.

– "'V Kharbine vse spokoino.' Povsednevnye mezhkul'turnye kontakty v zerkale gorodskoi gazetnoi khroniki (nachalo XX v.)" ("All is Quiet in Harbin": Daily Cross-Cultural Contacts Mirrored in the City Newspaper Reports at the Beginning of the Twentieth Century). In *Povsednevnost' rossiiskoi provintsii. Istoriia, iazyk i prostranstvo* (The Everyday Life of the Russian Province: History, Language and Space), 75–99. Kazan: Novoe znanie, 2002.

Eropkina, Ol'ga I. "Russkie i kitaiskie shkoly na KVZhD. 20-e gody" (Russian and Chinese Schools on the CER in the 1920s). *Problemy Dal'nego Vostoka* 3 (2001): 132–8.

Esherick, Joseph W. *The Origins of the Boxer Uprising*. Berkeley: University of California Press, 1987.

Feest, David, ed. *Baltisches Biographisches Lexikon digital*. Updated 2012. bbld. de. Cited as BBL.

Feldmann, Hans, and Heinz von zur Mühlen, eds. *Baltisches historisches Ortslexikon*. 2 vols. Cologne and Vienna: Böhlau Verlag, 1990.

Fialkovskii, Petr K. "V ego stenakh my vse byli molody" (Inside Its Walls We All Were Young). *Problemy Dal'nego Vostoka* 3 (1995): 115–18.

– "Torgovyi dom I.Ya. Churina v Kharbine" (The Churin Trade Company in Harbin). *Problemy Dal'nego Vostoka* 3 (1996): 123–5.

Filippovich, K.A. "Sovetskie i kitaiskie shkoly na KVZhD" (CER Soviet and Chinese Schools). *Vestnik Man'chzhurii* 5 (1926): 27–39.

Fitzpatrick, Sheila. "The Motherland Calls: 'Soft' Repatriation of Soviet Citizens from Europe, 1945–1953." *Journal of Modern History* 90, no. 2 (June 2018): 323–50.

Frizendorf (Friesendorff), Maximilian Iu. *Severnaia Man'chzhuriia. Ocherki ekonomicheskoi geografii* (Sketches of the Economic Geography of Northern Manchuria). Khabarovsk: Knizhnoe delo, n.d. [1930].

Fromm, Martin. "Invoking the Ghosts of Blagoveshchensk: Massacre, Memory, and the Post-Mao Search for Historical Identity." In *China's Rise to Power: Conceptions of State Governance*, ed. Joseph Tse-Hei Lee et al., 139–63. New York: Palgrave Macmillan, 2012.

Frost, Mark Ravinder. "*Emporium in Imperio*: Nanyang Networks and the Straits Chinese in Singapore, 1819–1914." *Journal of Southeast Asian Studies* 36, no. 1 (February 2005): 29–66.

Fujiwara, Katsumi. "Zhenshchiny v Kharbine pri Man'chzhou-Go. Vzgliad cherez problemu potrebleniia odezhdy" (Harbin Women in the Manchukuo Period: A View through the Issue of Clothes Consumption). Paper presented at the Ninth World Congress of the International Council for Central and East European Studies, Makuhari, Japan, 5 August 2015.

Gaiduk, Georgii G. "Vstrecha losianov v Omske" (A Reunion of Laoxiang in Omsk). *Na sopkakh Man'chzhurii* 186 (November–December 2014), 1.

Galambos, Imre. "The Blagoveshchensk Massacre of July 1900: Translation from A. Vereshchagin's Account of His Journey down the Amur." *Sinológiai Szemle* 1 (2009): 1–12.

Gamble, Sidney D. *Peking: A Social Survey*. New York: George H. Doran, 1921.

Gamsa, Mark. "Asiatics and Chinamen: Borrowed Idioms of National Self-deprecation in Russia and China (1890s–1930s)." *Monumenta Serica* 65, no. 2 (December 2017): 401–20.

– "California on the Amur, or the 'Zheltuga Republic' in Manchuria (1883–86)," *Slavonic and East European Review* 81, no. 2 (April 2003): 236–66.

– "China as Seen and Imagined by Roger Baron Budberg, a Baltic Physician in Manchuria." In *Eastwards: Western Views on East Asian Culture*, ed. Frank Kraushaar, 23–35. Bern: Peter Lang, 2010.

– "Cross-Cultural Contact in Manchuria: Approaches to Lives in Between, 1900s–1950s." *History and Anthropology* 30, no. 5 (2019): 563–80.

– "The Epidemic of Pneumonic Plague in Manchuria 1910–1911." *Past and Present* 190 (February 2006): 147–83.

– "Harbin in Comparative Perspective." *Urban History* 37, no. 1 (May 2010): 136–49.

– "The Historiography of Harbin and the Imagery of Inter-Ethnic Contact."
    Asiatica Venetiana 10–11 (2009): 63–79.
– "How a Republic of Chinese Red Beards Was Invented in Paris." *Modern
    Asian Studies* 36, no. 4 (October 2002): 993–1010.
– "Letters from Harbin." *Acta Universitatis Latviensis* 779 (*Oriental Studies,*
    2012): 27–38.
– *Manchuria: A Concise History.* London: I.B. Tauris, 2020.
– "The Many Faces of Hotel Moderne in Harbin." *East Asian History* 37
    (December 2011): 27–38.
– "Mixed Marriages in Russian-Chinese Manchuria." In *Entangled Histories:
    The Transcultural Past of Northeast China,* ed. Dan Ben-Canaan et al., 47–58.
    Heidelberg: Springer, 2014.
– *The Reading of Russian Literature in China: A Moral Example and Manual of
    Practice.* New York: Palgrave Macmillan, 2010.
– "On Value Systems of the Russian Émigrés in China," *Archiv Orientální* 86,
    no. 1 (2018): 161–76.
– "The Vanishing and Lingering Past in Two Cities: Harbin and Riga." *Città &
    Storia* 10, no. 2 (July–December 2015): 231–59.
Gan Yuze. "Yi wei Zhongguo de Eluosi shiren. Lun Li Yanling Eyu shige
    chuangzuo" (A Chinese Russian Poet: On Li Yanling's Russian Poetry).
    Eluosi wenyi 1 (2001): 34–6, 67.
Gao Ling, et al. *Lishi huimou – 20 shiji de Ha'erbin. Dongfang zhenzhu, Ha'erbin*
    (Flashback on History: 20th-Century Harbin; Harbin, Pearl of the East),
    vol. 2. Harbin: Ha'erbin chubanshe, 1998.
Garin, Nikolai G. *Po Koree, Mandzhurii i Liaodunskomu poluostrovu (iz
    puteshestviia vokrug sveta)* (Through Korea, Manchuria, and the Liaodong
    Peninsula: From a Voyage around the World). In *Polnoe sobranie sochinenii v
    8 tomakh* (Complete Works in 8 vols.), vol. 5. Petrograd: A.F. Marks, 1916.
Garlinger, H. "Nikolai Baron von Budberg-Bönninghausen 75 Jahre!" *Der
    Märker* 18, no. 2 (1969): 28.
Georgievskii, I. *Tam – na drugom beregu Amura* (There, on the Other Shore of
    the Amur). Harbin: Russko-Man'chzhurskaia knigotorgovlia, 1930.
Geraci, Robert. "Russian Orientalism at an Impasse: Tsarist Education Policy
    and the 1910 Conference on Islam," In *Russia's Orient: Imperial Borderlands
    and Peoples, 1700–1917,* ed. Daniel R. Brower and Edward J. Lazzerini,
    138–61. Bloomington: Indiana University Press, 1997.
Gilbreath, Olive. "Where Yellow Rules White." *Harper's Magazine* 158, no. 945
    (February 1929): 367–74.
Gintse [Hintze], Mikhail A. *Russkaia sem'ia doma i v Man'chzhurii.
    Vospominaniia* (A Russian Family at Home and in Manchuria: Memoirs).
    Sydney: author's typescript edition, 1986.

Glebov, Sergey. *From Empire to Eurasia: Politics, Scholarship, and Ideology in Russian Eurasianism, 1920s–1930s.* DeKalb: Northern Illinois University Press, 2017.

Godley, Michael R. "The End of the Queue: Hair as Symbol in Chinese History." *East Asian History* 8 (December 1994): 53–72.

Goertz, Leon. "Beiträge zur Geschichte der baltischen Internate." In *Arbeiten der Zweiten Baltischen Historikertages zu Reval, 1912*, ed. Ehstländische Litterärische Gesellschaft, 195–216. Reval (Tallinn): Franz Kluge, 1932.

Goldblatt, Howard. "Life as Art: Xiao Hong and Autobiography." In *Woman and Literature in China*, ed. Anna Gerstlacher et al., 345–63. Bochum: Studienverlag Brockmeyer, 1985.

Golovachev, Petr M. *Rossiia na Dal'nem Vostoke* (Russia in the Far East). Saint Petersburg: E.D. Kuskova, 1904.

Gorskii, Aleksandr K., and Nikolai A. Setnitskii. *Sochineniia* (Works), ed. E.N. Berkovskaia (Setnitskaia) and A.G. Gacheva. Moscow: Raritet, 1995.

Gottschang, Thomas R. "Economic Change, Disasters, and Migration: The Historical Case of Manchuria." *Economic Development and Cultural Change* 35, no. 3 (1987): 461–90.

Gottschang, Thomas R., and Diana Lary. *Swallows and Settlers: The Great Migration from North China to Manchuria.* Ann Arbor: Michigan Monographs in Chinese Studies, vol. 87, 2000.

Grauze (Grause), Iurii K. *Kitaiskie fragmenty* (Chinese Fragments). Jerusalem: V. Shkolnikov, 1976.

Green, David. "Guobaorou: Pork Dish of the Gods." *The World of Chinese*, 29 February 2012.

Gribin, Sergei (Sergei Iu. Eremin). *Liubimyi Kharbin. Sbornik rasskazov o samom russkom po svoemu proiskhozhdeniiu i po dukhu iz vsekh kitaiskikh gorodov – Kharbine* (Beloved Harbin: Collected Stories on Harbin, the Most Russian of All Chinese Cities in Origin and Spirit). Vladivostok and Harbin: Izdatel'stvo Morskogo gosudarstvennogo universiteta im. admirala G.I. Nevel'skogo, 2015.

Grigorash, Igor' V. "Budberg Andrei Iakovlevich." In *Ocherki istorii Ministerstva inostrannykh del Rossii* (Sketches on the History of the Russian Foreign Ministry), vol. 3: *Biografii ministrov inostrannykh del. 1802–2002 gg.* (Biographies of Ministers of Foreign Affairs, 1802–2002), ed. Igor' S. Ivanov et al., 48–71. Moscow: Olma-Press, 2002.

Groot, J.J.M. De. *The Religious System of China*, 6 vols. [1892–2010]. Taipei: Ch'eng wen, 1972 (reprint).

Grosberg, Oskar. "Ein abenteurliches Baltenschicksal. Die Memoiren des Dr. med. Roger Baron Budberg." *Rigasche Rundschau* 108 (16 May 1925): 17.

– "Ein merkwürdiges Leben." *Rigasche Rundschau* 251 (6 November 1926): 9.

Grosse, Ernst. *Ostasiatische Erinnerungen eines Kolonial- und Ausland-Deutschen.* Munich: Neuer Filser-Verlag, 1938.

Grosvenor Coville, Lilian. "Here in Manchuria: Many Thousand Lives Were Lost and More Than Half the Crops Destroyed by the Floods of 1932." *National Geographic Magazine* 63, no. 2 (February 1933): 233–56.

Grulev, Mikhail V. "Iz poezdki v Man'chzhuriiu" (From a Trip to Manchuria). *Istoricheskii vestnik* 81, no. 9 (1900): 945–72.

Grüner, Frank. " 'The Chicago of the East': Cross-Border Activities and Transnational Biographies of Adventurers, Shady Characters, and Criminals in the Cosmopolitan City of Harbin." *Comparativ* 23, no. 6 (2013): 52–75.

– "In the Streets and Bazaars of Harbin: Marketers, Small Traders, and Peddlers in a Changing Multicultural City." *Itinerario* 35, no. 3 (2011): 37–72.

– "The Russian Revolution of 1905 at the Periphery: The Case of the Manchurian City of Harbin." In *The Russian Revolution of 1905 in Transcultural Perspective: Identities, Peripheries, and the Flow of Ideas,* ed. Felicitas Fischer von Weikersthal et al., 175–96. Bloomington: Slavica, 2013.

Guan Chenghe. *Ha'erbin kao* (An Investigation of Harbin). Harbin: Ha'erbin shi difangshi yanjiusuo, 1980.

Guins, George C. "Russians in Manchuria." *Russian Review* 2, no. 2 (1943): 81–7.

Guzei, Iana S. *"Zheltaia opasnost'." Predstavleniia ob ugroze s Vostoka v rossiiskoi imperii v kontse XIX – nachale XX v.* ("Yellow Peril": Perceptions of Threat from the East in the Russian Empire, late Nineteenth to early Twentieth Century), PhD diss., European University at Saint Petersburg and Irkutsk State University, 2014.

Haakestad, Jorunn. *Porcelain and Revolution: Johan Munthe and the Chinese Collection in Bergen, Norway,* trans. Peter Cripps. Bergen: Fagbokforlaget, 2018.

Ha'erbin shizhi congkan. Supplement, selections from the *Yuandong bao,* in 12 issues. (1983), no. 4 to (1984), no 8.

Hagemeister, Michael, "Neue Materialien zur Wirkungsgeschichte N.F. Fedorovs. M. Gor'kij und die Anhänger Fedorovs in Moskau und Harbin." In *Studia Slavica,* ed. Hans-Bernd Harder and Bernd E. Scholz, 219–44. Giessen: Wilhelm Schmitz, 1981.

Haltzel, Michael H. "The Russification of the Baltic Germans: A Dysfunctional Aspect of Imperial Modernization." In *Baltic History,* ed. Arvids Ziedonis, Jr, et al., 143–52. Columbus: Association for the Advancement of Baltic Studies, 1974.

Happel, Jörn. "Eine Karte voller Ziele. Deutsche Sabotageträume in Russland während des Ersten Weltkriegs." In *Osteuropa kartiert – Mapping Eastern Europe,* ed. Jörn Happel und Christophe von Werdt, 61–83. Zurich: LIT Verlag, 2010.

Harrison, Henrietta. *The Making of the Republican Citizen: Political Ceremonies and Symbols in China, 1911–1929.* Oxford: Oxford University Press, 2000.

Havard, Colonel Valery, and Colonel John van R. Hoff. *Reports of Military Observers Attached to the Armies in Manchuria during the Russo-Japanese War*, pt 2. Washington, DC: GPO, 1906.

Heretz, Leonid. *Russia on the Eve of Modernity: Popular Religion and Traditional Culture under the Last Tsars*. Cambridge: Cambridge University Press, 2008.

Heymann, Leonfried. *Meeretz huladeti leeretz moladeti. Mitokh dapei ḥayai* (From My Birthland to My Motherland: From the Leaves of My Life). No place, no year [2006?]: author's typescript edition.

Hohlbeck, Dr Otto. "Professor Zoege und die Fliegende Kolonne I.M. der Kaiserin-Mutter Maria." *Beiträge zur Kunde Estlands* 16 (1931): 130–41.

Honey, David B. *Incense at the Altar: Pioneering Sinologists and the Development of Classical Chinese Philology*. New Haven: American Oriental Society, 2001.

Hopstock, Sigfred. *Norwegian Members of the Chinese Customs Service since 1861*. Shanghai: n.p., 1938.

Hosking, Geoffrey. *Russia: People and Empire, 1552–1917*. London: Fontana Press, 1998.

Howgego, Raymond John. *Encyclopedia of Exploration*. 4 vols. Sydney: Hordern House, 2003–8.

Hsu, Chia Yin. "Railroad Technocracy, Extraterritoriality, and Imperial *Lieux de Mémoire* in Russian Émigrés' Manchuria, 1920–1930s." *Ab Imperio* 4 (2011): 59–105.

Hu Zongliang. *Heilongjiang shulüe* (A Brief Account of Heilongjiang), ed. Li Xingsheng and Zhang Jie [1891]. Harbin: Heilongjiang renmin chubanshe, 1985.

Hua Meng. "The Chinese Genesis of the Term Foreign Devil." In *Images of Westerners in Chinese and Japanese Literature*, ed. Hua Meng and Sukehiro Hirakawa, 25–37. Amsterdam: Rodopi, 2000.

Huitfeldt, Johanne. *The Munthe Collection in the West Norway Museum of Applied Art*, trans. E.R. Waaler. Oslo: C. Huitfeldt Forlag, 1996.

Ianinova, O. "Zhizn' russkikh v Manchzhurii 1919–1949 gody" (The Life of Russians in Manchuria, 1919–49). *Russkaia mysl'* (Paris), 1956: 14 February, 16 February, 21 February, 23 February, 28 February, 1 March, 6 March, 8 March, 13 March, 15 March, 20 March.

Iashnov, Evgenii E. "Pitanie krest'ian v Severnoi Man'chzhurii" (The Nutrition of Peasants in Northern Manchuria). *Ekonomicheskii vestnik Man'chzhurii* 45 (9 November 1924): 15–18.

Iastremskii, F.P. "Ocherk byta i nravov severnoi Man'chzhurii" (A Sketch of the Daily Life and Customs of Northern Manchuria). *Istoricheskii vestnik* 95, no. 4 (1904): 223–34.

Il'in, Iosif S. "Na sluzhbe u iapontsev" (In Japanese Service). *Novyi zhurnal* 80 (September 1965): 179–203; no. 82 (March 1966): 193–211; no. 84 (September 1966): 176–99; no. 85 (December 1966): 179–206.

- "Sovetskaia armiia v Kharbine" (The Soviet Army in Harbin). *Novyi zhurnal* 96 (September 1969): 130–52.

Il'ina, Natal'ia I. *Vozvrashchenie* (The Return). 2 vols. Moscow: Sovetskii pisatel', 1969.

Istoricheskii obzor i sovremennoe polozhenie podgotovitel'nykh kursov Kharbinskogo Politekhnicheskogo Instituta (Historical Survey and Current State of the Preparatory Courses at the Harbin Polytechnic). Harbin: Izdanie Pedagogicheskoi Korporatsii Podgotovitel'nykh Kursov, 1932.

Ivanov, Vsevolod N. *Bezhenskaia poema* (A Refugee Poem). Harbin: Bambukovaia roshcha, 1926.

- "Evropa, Aziia, Evraziia. Na poroge novykh kul'tur" (Europe, Asia, Eurasia: At the Doorstep of New Cultures). *Aziia* (Harbin) 3 (1 May 1932): 7–14.

- "Logika Evropy i Kitaia. Kul'turno-filosofskii etiud" (The Logic of Europe and Asia: A Cultural-Philosophical Sketch). *Vestnik Kitaia* 2 (April 1936): 14–19.

- *My na Zapade i na Vostoke. Kul'turno-istoricheskie osnovy russkoi gosudarstvennosti* (We: In the West and in the East: The Cultural-Historical Foundations of Russian Statehood). Saint Petersburg: Tsentr Strategicheskikh Issledovanii, 2005.

- "Ot redaktsii" [Editorial]. *Vestnik Kitaia* 1 (March 1936): 1–2.

- "Poeziia i ieroglif Kitaia" (provided English title: Poesy and the Chinese Character). *Vestnik Kitaia* 1 (March 1936): 9–11.

- "Russkaia koloniia v Man'chzhurii" (The Russian Colony in Manchuria). *Aziia* 1 (10 April 1932): 7–10; no. 2 (20 April 1932): 6–9.

James, Henry E.M. *The Long White Mountain*. London: Longmans, 1888.

Janhunen, Juha. *Manchuria: An Ethnic History*. Helsinki: Finno-Ugrian Society, 1996.

Jasanoff, Maya. "Cosmopolitan: A Tale of Identity from Ottoman Alexandria." *Common Knowledge* 11, no. 3 (2005): 393–409.

Jersild, Austin Lee. "From Savagery to Citizenship: Caucasian Mountaineers and Muslims in the Russian Empire." In *Russia's Orient: Imperial Borderlands and Peoples, 1700–1917*, ed. Daniel R. Brower and Edward J. Lazzerini, 101–14. Bloomington: Indiana University Press, 1997.

Ji Fenghui. *Ha'erbin xungen* (Search for the Roots of Harbin). Harbin: Ha'erbin chubanshe, 1996.

Ji Fenghui and Duan Guangda. *Lishi huimou – 20 shiji de Ha'erbin. Dongfang zhenzhu, Ha'erbin* (Flashback on History: 20th-Century Harbin; Harbin, Pearl of the East), vol. 1. Harbin: Ha'erbin chubanshe, 1998.

Ji Xianlin, *Liu De huiyi lu* (Memoirs of Study in Germany). Hong Kong: Zhonghua shuju, 1993.

Jia Qiuhong, "Yibu shuyuan liangdai qing" (One Book's Destiny, Two Generations' Feelings). 23 April 2018. liandaigou.com/msfc/3058903.htm.

Jiang Zhijun and Guo Chonglin. *Songhua jiangpan de minsu yu lüyou* (Folklore and Travel by the Songhua River). Beijing: Lüyou jiaoyu chubanshe, 1996.

Jing Ai. "Guanyu Ma jia huayuan zhuren Ma Zhongjun de kuang zhiming" (On the Epitaph Tablet of Ma Zhongjun, Master of the Ma Family Garden), *Heilongjiang shizhi* 5 (1985): 18–19.

Jones, Richard. *Harbin as a Russo-Chinese City, 1917–1931*. MPhil thesis in Russian and East European Studies, Oxford University, 2000.

Jordan, J.N. "Notes on a Journey from Vladivostock to Irkutsk." In *British Documents on Foreign Affairs*, pt 1, series A, vol. 2, (Russia, 1881–1905), ed. Dominic Lieven, 322–6. Frederick: University Publications of America, 1983.

Kachanovskii, Iurii V. "Kak zaselialsia Dal'nii Vostok" (How the Far East was Settled). *Problemy Dal'nego Vostoka* 3 (1973): 186–9.

Kaigorodov, Aleksei M. "Man'chzhuriia. Avgust 1945" (Manchuria: August 1945). *Problemy Dal'nego Vostoka* 6 (1991): 94–103.

Kanevskaia, Galina I., and Marina A. Pavlovskaia. "Deiatel'nost' vypusknikov Vostochnogo instituta v Kharbine" (The Activity of Graduates of the Oriental Institute in Harbin). *Izvestiia Vostochnogo instituta* 1 (1994): 72–7.

Kapran, Inessa K. *Povsednevnaia zhizn' russkogo naseleniia Kharbina (konets XIX v. – 50-e gg. XX v.)* (The Everyday Life of the Russian Population of Harbin: Late Nineteenth Century to the 1950s). Vladivostok: Izdatel'stvo Dal'nevostochnogo federal'nogo universiteta, 2011.

Karasik, Vladimir. "Biulleten' vykhodtsev iz Kitaia" (The Bulletin of Former Residents of China). *Vesti-2* (weekly supplement to *Vesti*, Tel-Aviv), pt 1 (11 January 2001): 19; pt 2 (25 January 2001): 19; pt 3 (1 February 2001): 19.

Karetina, Galina S. "General U Peifu na politicheskoi stsene Kitaia" (General Wu Peifu on the Political Arena of China). *Rossiia i ATR* 4 (2010): 116–25.

Karpov, A.B. "Sbornik slov, sinonimov i vyrazhenii, upotrebliaemykh Amurskimi kazakami" (A Lexicon of Words Used by the Amur Cossacks). *Sbornik otdeleniia russkogo iazyka i slovesnosti Imperatorskoi Akademii Nauk 87*, no. 1 (1909).

Karttunen, Frances. *Between Worlds: Interpreters, Guides, and Survivors*. New Brunswick: Rutgers University Press, 1994.

Katajs, Edgars. *Zem desmit valstu karogiem* (Under the Banners of Ten States). Riga: Jumava, 2000.

Katz, David S. *The Occult Tradition: From the Renaissance to the Present Day*. London: Jonathan Cape, 2005.

Katz (Volobrinskaia), Galia M. "Kharbin (Avgust 1945–1952 gg.)" (Harbin from August 1945 to 1952). *Bulletin Igud Yotsei Sin* 382 (November–December 2004): 34–8.

Kats (Katz), Sigizmund A. *Dorogami pamiati: vospominaniia, vstrechi, vpechatleniia (zapiski kompozitora)* (Down Memory Lane: A Composer's Reminiscences, Encounters and Impressions). Moscow: Sovetskii kompozitor, 1978.

Kaufman, Aleksandr A. *Po novym mestam (ocherki i putevye zametki). 1901–1903* (Through New Places: Sketches and Travel Notes, 1901–3). Saint Petersburg: Izdanie t-va "Obshchestvennaia Pol'za," 1905.

Kaufman, Teddy. "Pomnite i znaete li vy proshloe Kharbina?" (Do You Remember and Know the Past of Harbin?). *Bulletin Igud Yotsei Sin* 53, no. 391 (March–April 2007): 30–1.

Keene, Derek. "Cities and Cultural Exchange." In *Cultural Exchange in Early Modern Europe*, vol. 2: *Cities and Cultural Exchange in Europe, 1400–1700*, ed. Donatella Calabi and Stephen Turk Christensen, 3–27. Cambridge and New York: Cambridge University Press and European Science Foundation, 2006–7.

Kennan, George F. "The Sisson Documents." *Journal of Modern History* 28, no. 2 (June 1956): 130–54.

Keyserling, Count Alfred. *Graf Alfred Keyserling erzählt*. Kaunas and Leipzig: Ostverlag der Buchhandlung Pribačis, 1937.

Khaindrova, Lydia Iu. *Serdtse poeta* (A Poet's Heart). Kaluga: Poligraf–Inform, 2003.

Kharbintsy v Moskve. Biograficheskie ocherki v dvukh vypuskakh (Biographical Sketches of Harbinites in Moscow, in 2 issues). Moscow: Assotsiatsiia Kharbin, 1997.

Kheidok [Heidoks], Al'fred P. *Zvezdy Man'chzhurii* (The Stars of Manchuria). Vladivostok: Rubezh, 2011.

Khisamutdinov, Amir A. *Kak russkie izuchali Kitai. Obshchestvo Izucheniia Man'chzhurskogo Kraia* (provided English title: How the Russians Studied China: Society for the Study of the Manchurian Region). Vladivostok: DVGU (electronic file), 2018.

– "Obshchestvo russkikh orientalistov v Kharbine" (The Society of Russian Orientalists in Harbin). *Vostok* 3 (1999): 104–14.

– *Rossiiskaia emigratsiia v Aziatsko-Tikhookeanskom regione i Iuzhnoi Amerike. Biobibliograficheskii slovar'* (A Bio-bibliographical Dictionary of the Russian Emigration in the Asia-Pacific Region and South America). Vladivostok: DVGU, 2001.

– *Rossiiskaia emigratsiia v Kitae. Opyt entsiklopedii* (A Draft Encyclopaedia of the Russian Emigration in China). Vladivostok: DVGU, 2002.

Khvostov, Aleksandr M. "Russkii Kitai. Nasha pervaia koloniia na Dal'nem Vostoke" (A Russian China: Our First Colony in the Far East). *Vestnik Evropy* 37 no. 10 (1902): 653–96; no. 11: 181–208.

Kim, Loretta E. "Saints for Shamans? Culture, Religion and Borderland Politics in Amuria from the Seventeenth to Nineteenth Centuries." *Central Asiatic Journal* 56 (2012–13): 169–202.

Kirkhner, Aleksandr V. *Osada Blagoveshchenska i vziatie Aiguna* (The Siege of Blagoveshchensk and Capture of Aigun). In *Voennye sobytiia v Priamur'e. 1900–1902* (The Events of War in the Priamur, 1900–1902), ed. Anatolii V. Teliuk et al., 6–141. Blagoveshchensk-na-Amure: Amurskaia iarmarka, 2008.

Kirsanov, Igor' V. "Veitia" (Weitiya). *Na sopkakh Man'chzhurii* 182 (April 2014): 2–3.

Kiselev, Dmitrii V. " 'Podozritel'nye nemtsy.' Agenty i voennoplennye Tsentral'nykh derzhav v Man'chzhurii v gody Pervoi mirovoi voiny" ("Suspect Germans": Agents and POWs of the Central Powers in Manchuria during the First World War). *Rossiia i ATR* 2 (2015): 121–38.

Klerzhe, Georgii I. *Revoliutsiia i grazhdanskaia voina. Lichnye vospominaniia* (The Revolution and Civil War: Personal Reminiscences) [Mukden: 1932], ed. A.L. Posadskov. Novosibirsk: GPNTB SO RAN, 2012.

Kobzev, Artem I., and Vladimir V. Serbinenko. "Iz naslediia russkogo filosofa Vl. Solov'eva" (From the Legacy of Russian Philosopher Vladimir Solov'ev). *Problemy Dal'nego Vostoka* 2 (1990): 182–7.

Koga, Yukiko. *Inheritance of Loss: China, Japan, and the Political Economy of Redemption after Empire*. Chicago: University of Chicago Press, 2016.

Kokovtsov, Count Vladimir N. *Iz moego proshlogo. Vospominaniia 1903–1919* (From My Past: Memoirs, 1903–19). 2 vols. Paris: Illiustrirovannaia Rossiia, 1933.

Komarov, Petr S. *Izbrannoe* (Selected Works). Moscow: Gosudarstvennoe izdatel'stvo khudozhestvennoi literatury, 1950.

Koretskii, Aleksei P. "Epopeia russkogo emigranta (bez geroiki)" (The Epic Tale of a Russian Emigrant [without Heroism]). *Rossiiane v Azii* 3 (1996): 111–68.

Kormazov, Vladimir A. "Mongol'skii kurort Khalkhin 'Khalun Arshan'" (The Mongolian Resort Halun-Arshan on Khalkha River). *Ekonomicheskii vestnik Man'chzhurii*, nos. 37–8 (21 September 1924): 11–21.

Korsakov, Vladimir V. "Verovaniia i sueveriia u kitaitsev. Po lichnym nabliudeniiam" (Chinese Beliefs and Superstitions: From Personal Observations). *Vestnik Evropy* 37, no. 12 (December 1902): 655–73.

Kosinova, Oksana A. "Organizatorskaia i pedagogicheskaia deiatel'nost' Nikolaia Viktorovicha Borzova v Kharbine" (The Organizational and Pedagogical Activity of N.V. Borzov in Harbin). *Nauchnye trudy Moskovskogo gumanitarnogo universiteta* 4 (2018): 58–65.

Koval', Aleksandr I. "Voinskii memorial Rossii v Port-Arture" (Russia's Military Memorial in Port Arthur). *Problemy Dal'nego Vostoku* 4 (2003): 158–65.

Kovalevskii, Petr E. *Zarubezhnaia Rossiia. Dopolnitel'nyi vypusk* (Russia Abroad: Additional Issue). Paris: Librairie des Cinq Continents, 1973.

Koz'min, G. *Dal'nii Vostok. Vospominaniia i rasskazy* (Memoirs and Stories of the Far East). Saint Petersburg: V.A. Berezovskii, 1904.

Kradin, Nikolai P. *Russkie inzhenery i arkhitektory v Kitae* (Russian Engineers and Architects in China). Khabarovsk: Khabarovskaia kraevaia tipografiia. 2018.

Kravkov, Vasilii P. *Voina v Man'chzhurii. Zapiski divizionnogo vracha* (War in Manchuria: The Notes of a Divisional Physician), ed. M.A. Rossiiskii. Moscow: Veche, 2016.

Krebs, Helmut. *Niederau-Krauthausen und die Herrschaft Burgau. Die Geschichte einer getrennten Einheit.* Düren: Hahne & Schloemer, 1997.

Kreid, Vadim P., and Ol'ga M. Bakich, eds. *Russkaia poeziia Kitaia* (The Russian Poetry of China). Moscow: Vremia, 2001.

Krieglstein, Eugen von. *Zwischen Weiss und Gelb. Neue Erzählungen aus dem Lande der Verdammnis,* 2nd ed. Berlin-Charlottenburg: Deutsches Verlagshaus Vita, 1909.

Krotova, Maria V. *SSSR i rossiiskaia emigratsiia v Man'chzhurii (1920-e–1950-e gg.)* (The USSR and the Russian Emigration in Manchuria, 1920s–1950s). PhD diss., Saint Petersburg Institute of History, Russian Academy of Sciences, 2014.

Krusenstern-Pererets, Iustina V. *Vospominaniia* (Memoirs) *Rossiiane v Azii* 1 (1994): 17–132; no. 4 (1997): 124–209; no. 5 (1998): 25–83; no. 6 (1999): 29–104; no. 7 (2000): 93–149.

Kuptsov, Ivan V., et al. *Belyi generalitet na Vostoke Rossii v gody Grazhdanskoi voiny. Biograficheskii spravochnik* (Biographical Guide to White Generals in the Russian East during the Civil War). Moscow: Kuchkovo pole, "Voennaia kniga," 2011.

Kuznetsov, Aleksei V. *'Gol'd' ukhodit v Kharbin. Parokhody-emigranty i parokhody-trofei* (The 'Gold' Departs for Harbin: Steamships as Émigrés and as Trophies). Ivanovo: Izdatel'stvo Ivanovo, 2015.

Kuznetsov, Dmitrii V. *"'Arestu podlezhat vse': politicheskie repressii v SSSR i sud'ba tak-nazyvaemykh 'kharbintsev'"* ("All Are to Be Arrested": Political Repressions in the USSR and the Fate of the So-called Harbinites). *Problemy Dal'nego Vostoka* 3 (2015): 136–46.

Kwong, Chi Man. *War and Geopolitics in Interwar Manchuria: Zhang Zuolin and the Fengtian Clique during the Northern Expedition.* Leiden: Brill, 2017.

Kwong, Luke S.K., "The T'i-Yung Dichotomy and the Search for Talent in Late-Ch'ing China." *Modern Asian Studies* 27, no. 2 (May 1993): 253–79.

Labbé, Paul. *Les Russes en Extrême-Orient.* Paris: Hachette, 1904.

Labuda, Adam S., et al., eds. *Edward and Atanazy Raczyński: Works – Personalities – Choices – Era* (trilingual edition in Polish, German, English). Poznań: National Museum, 2010.

Laguta, Nina V. "Zhiznennyi put' amurskogo starozhila v iazykovom voploshchenii (na materiale avtobiograficheskikh rasskazov)" (The Life Path of an Amur Veteran as Expressed in Language, Based on

Autobiographical Narratives). *Slovo. fol'klorno-dialektologicheskii al'manakh* 8 (2010): 137–57.

Lahusen, Thomas. "Remembering China, Imagining Israel: The Memory of Difference." In *Harbin and Manchuria*, ed. Lahusen, special issue of *South Atlantic Quarterly* 99, no. 1 (2000): 253–69.

Lahusen, Thomas, dir. "Manchurian Sleepwalkers." Chemodan Films, 2017.

Lamping, Gerlinde, and Heinrich Lamping. "Die Australienreisen von Reinhold Graf Anrep-Elmpt (1878–1883)." In *Australia: Studies on the History of Discovery and Exploration*, ed. H. Lamping and M. Linke. *Frankfurter Wirtschafts- und Sozialgeographische Schriften* 65 (1994): 183–220.

Lattimore, Owen. "Byroads and Backwoods of Manchuria." *National Geographic Magazine* 61, no. 1 (January 1932): 100–30.

– "The Gold Tribe, 'Fishskin Tatars' of the Lower Sungari." *Memoirs of the American Anthropological Association* 40 (1933): 5–77.

– *Manchuria: Cradle of Conflict*, rev. ed. New York: Macmillan, 1935.

– "Wulakai Tales from Manchuria." *Journal of American Folk-Lore* 46, no. 181 (July–September 1933): 272–86.

Latvijas vēstures atlants (Historical Atlas of Latvia), ed. Jānis Turlajs. Riga: Jāņa sēta, 2011.

Lauri, Lembit, ed. *Nenapisannye memuary* (Unwritten Memoirs), trans. B. Tukh et al. Tallinn: Periodika, 1990.

League of Nations, Traffic in Women and Children Committee. "Position of Women of Russian Origin in the Far East." Official No. A12.1935.IV (Geneva: 1935).

Lee, Robert H.G. *The Manchurian Frontier in Ch'ing History*. Cambridge, MA: Harvard University Press, 1970.

Lee, Sophia. "The Foreign Ministry's Cultural Agenda for China: The Boxer Indemnity." In *The Japanese Informal Empire in China, 1895–1937*, ed. Peter Duus et al., 272–306. Princeton: Princeton University Press, 1989.

Legras, Jules. *En Sibérie*. Paris: A. Colin, 1899.

Lensen, George A. *The Russo-Chinese War*. Tokyo: Sophia University, 1967.

Levitskii, Grigorii V., ed. *Biograficheskii slovar' professorov i prepodavatelei Imperatorskogo Iur'evskogo, byvshego Derptskogo, universiteta za sto let ego sushchestvovaniia (1802–1902)* (Biographical Dictionary of the Professors and Teachers of the Imperial University of Iur'ev, formerly Dorpat, in the Hundred Years of its Existence). 2 vols. Iur'ev: Tipografiia K. Mattisena, 1902–3.

Levitskii, Mitrofan N., ed. *V trushchobakh Man'chzhurii i nashikh vostochnykh okrain* (In the Backwaters of Manchuria and Our Eastern Provinces). Odessa: Tipo-litografiia Shtaba Okruga, 1910.

Levitskii, Vladimir V. *Pristan' na Sungari* (A Wharf on the Sungari), in two parts. Kharkov: author's edition, 1998.

Levoshko, Svetlana S. "Pol'sko-russkii arkhitektor Kazimir Skolimovskii (1862–1923) na fone epokhi" (The Polish-Russian Architect Kazimierz Skolimowski and His Times). *Sztuka Europy Wschodniej/Iskusstvo Vostochnoi Evropy/Art of Eastern Europe* 3 (2015): 145–57.

Li, Lillian M. *Fighting Famine in North China: State, Market, and Environmental Decline, 1690s–1990s.* Stanford: Stanford University Press, 2007.

Li Rong, ed. *Ha'erbin fangyan cidian* (Dictionary of Harbin Dialect). Nanjing: Jiangsu jiaoyu chubanshe, 1997.

Li Shuxiao. "Ha'erbin jieming xiao kao" (A Short Investigation of Harbin Street Names). *Heilongjiang wenwu congkan* 1 (1982): 99–100.

Li Shuxiao. et al., eds. *Ha'erbin jiuying: Old Photos of Harbin.* Beijing: Renmin meishu chubanshe, 2000.

Li Shuxiao and Li Ting. "Waiguo zhu Ha'erbin lingshiguan yishi" (Tales of Foreign Consulates in Harbin). In *Waiguoren zai Ha'erbin* (Foreigners in Harbin), ed. Tong Yueqin et al., 181–8. Harbin: n.p., 2002.

Li Sui'an. *Ma Zhongjun ji Ha'erbin Dunyuan* (Ma Zhongjun and the Harbin Dunyuan Garden). Harbin: Heilongjiang renmin chubanshe, 2000.

Li Xiangchen. "Shou Shan de kenhuang shibian sixiang" (Shou Shan's Ideology of Wasteland Reclamation and Border Defence). *Heilongjiang shizhi* 5 (1994): 33–6.

Li Xiaoju and Liang Aiying. "Taiping qiao shimo" (The Story of Taiping qiao). *Heilongjiang shizhi* 3–4 (1990): 77–8.

Li Xinggeng et al. *Fengyu fuping. Eguo qiaomin zai Zhongguo (1917–1945)* (Rovers through Trial and Hardship: Russian Emigrants in China). Beijing: Zhongyang bianyi chubanshe, 1997.

Li Zhensheng. *Red-Color News Soldier: A Chinese Photographer's Odyssey through the Cultural Revolution*, ed. Robert Pledge. London: Phaidon Press, 2003.

Liaozuo sanren [Liu Jingyan]. *Binjiang chenxiao lu* (A Record of Binjiang Hubbub, 1929), ed. Zhang Yiqing and Yang Lian. Beijing: Zhongguo qingnian chubanshe, 2012.

Lieven, Dominic. "Dilemmas of Empire 1850–1918: Power, Territory, Identity." *Journal of Contemporary History* 34, no. 2 (April 1999): 163–200.

Lieven, Prince Pavel P. "… I teni tekh, kogo uzh net" ("And shadows of those, who are no longer with us"). *Daugava* (Riga), 1991, nos. 5–6: 149–77; nos. 7–8: 178–90.

Ligin, Iur. [Leonid N. Iurovskii]. *Na Dal'nem Vostoke (ocherki)* (In the Far East: Essays). Moscow: Zadruga, 1913.

Lin, Yuexin Rachel. *Among Ghosts and Tigers: The Chinese in the Russian Far East, 1917–1920.* DPhil thesis, St Antony's College, Oxford University, 2015.

Lindgren, Ethel John. "An Example of Culture Contact without Conflict: Reindeer Tungus and Cossacks of Northwestern Manchuria." *American Anthropologist* 40 (October–December 1938): 605–21.

Lindt, August R. *Im Sattel durch Mandschukuo. Als Sonderberichterstatter bei Generälen und Räubern.* Leipzig: F.A. Brockhaus, 1934.

Liu Guixian. *Zoujin Ha gong da* (Approaching the Harbin Institute of Technology). Beijing: Kunlun chubanshe, 2000.

Liu Peiran. "Shou Shan jiangjun mukao" (An Investigation of the Tomb of General Shou Shan). *Heilongjiang wenshi ziliao* 12 (1984): 80–2.

Liu Qun. "Binjiang menghua lu. Lun *Yuandong bao, Binjiang shibao* de xiqu shiliao jiazhi" (Binjiang's Dream of Splendour: On the Value of Historical Materials on Traditional Opera in the *Yuandong bao* and *Binjiang shibao*). *Qiqiha'er daxue xuebao* 2 (2014): 144–7.

Liu Shude. "Wo suo zhidao de Shou Shan jiangjun zhi si" (What I Know about the Death of General Shou Shan). *Heilongjiang wenshi ziliao* 12 (1984): 76–9.

Liu Xinxin and Liu Xueqing. *Ha'erbin xiyang yinyueshi* (The History of Western Music in Harbin). Beijing: Renmin yinyue chubanshe, 2002.

Lobza, Petr F. "Kitaiskie sektanty" (Chinese Sectarians). *Knizhki nedeli* 23, no. 7 (July 1900): 5–23.

– "V Mandzhurii (voennoe ustroistvo i naselenie)" (In Manchuria: The Military Organization and Population). *Mir bozhii* 9, no. 8 (August 1900): 268–83.

Lohr, Eric. *Nationalizing the Russian Empire: The Campaign against Enemy Aliens during World War I.* Cambridge, MA: Harvard University Press, 2003.

Lopato, Liudmila I. *Volshebnoe zerkalo vospominanii* (The Magic Mirror of Memories). Moscow: Zakharov, 2003.

Łossowski, Piotr. "The Resettlement of the Germans from the Baltic States in 1939/1941," trans. Agnieszka Kreczmar. *Acta Poloniae Historica* 92 (2005): 79–98.

Lü Huifen. "Weihu zhuquan cuntu bizheng de Song Xiaolian" (Defender of Sovereign Rights, Fighter for Every Inch of the Land, Song Xiaolian). *Heilongjiang shizhi* (1997): 47–8.

Lyandres, Semion, and Dietmar Wulff, eds. *A Chronicle of the Civil War in Siberia and Exile in China: The Diaries of Petr Vasil'evich Vologodskii, 1918–1925.* 2 vols. Stanford: Hoover Institution Press, 2002.

Magaram, Eliazar E. *Sovremennyi Kitai* (Modern China). Berlin: Izdatel'stvo E.A. Gutnova, 1923.

– *Zheltyi lik. Ocherki kitaiskoi zhizni* (The Yellow Visage: Sketches of Chinese Life). Berlin: O. D'iakova, 1922.

Magris, Claudio. *Danube*, trans. Patrick Creagh. London: Harvill Press, 2001.

Makarov, Vladimir G. "Russkii filosof Nikolai Setnitskii. Ot KVZhD do NKVD" (Russian Philosopher Nikolai Setnitskii from the CER to the NKVD). *Voprosy filosofii* 7 (2004): 136–57.

Manchester, Laurie. "Fusing Russian Nationalism with Soviet Patriotism: Changing Conceptions of Homeland and the Mass Repatriation of Manchurian Russians after Stalin's Death." *Kritika: Explorations in Russian and Eurasian History* 20, no. 3 (2019): 529–58.

– "Repatriation to a Totalitarian Homeland: The Ambiguous Alterity of Russian Repatriates from China to the USSR." *Diaspora: A Journal of Transnational Studies* 16, no. 3 (2007): 353–88.

Mao Hong. "Ha'erbin Zhong-E renmin shenghuo zhuangkuang" (The Life Conditions of Chinese and Russians in Harbin). *Shishi yuebao* 1, no. 2 (1929): 115–22.

Markizov, Leonid P. *Do i posle 1945. Glazami ochevidtsa* (Before and After 1945: An Eyewitness Account). Syktyvkar: "Pokaianie," 2003.

Marks, Steven G. *Road to Power: The Trans-Siberian Railroad and the Colonization of Asian Russia, 1850–1917.* London: I.B. Tauris, 1991.

Mart, Venedikt. "Zheltye rabyni" (The Yellow Slaves, 1923). Excerpts introduced by A.A. Levchenko and A.A. Zabiiako, *Rossiia i Kitai na dal'nevostochnykh rubezhakh* 11 (2015): 339–53.

Martinevskii, Ivan L., and Henri Mollaret. *Epidemiia chumy v Man'chzhurii v 1910–1911 gg. (geroicheskii podvig russkikh i frantsuzskikh vrachei v bor'be s nei)* (The Plague Epidemic in Manchuria, 1910–11: Heroism of Russian and French Physicians in the Fight against It). Moscow: Meditsina, 1971.

Martini [Erich]. "Ueber die Bedeutung der Internationalen Pestkonferenz zu Mukden (Mandschurei) 1911." *Deutsche medizinische Wochenschrift* 38, no. 30 (25 July 1912): 1420–1.

Matignon [Jean-Jacques]. "Moukden, capitale de la Mandchourie." *A Travers le monde*, supplement to *Le Tour du monde* 11 (1905): 241–4, 253–4.

Matveev, Nikolai P. "Kitaitsy na Kariiskikh promyslakh" (Chinese at the Kara Mines). *Russkoe bogatstvo* 12 (December 1911): 29–43.

Mazo, Olga, and Taras Ivchenko. "Chinese Loanwords in Russian." In *Encyclopedia of Chinese Language and Linguistics*, vol. 5, ed. Rint Sybesma, 569–72. Leiden: Brill, 2016.

Meakin, Annette M.B. *A Ribbon of Iron.* Westminster: Archibald Constable, 1901.

Mednikov, Igor' Iu. "Rossiiskii posol v neitral'noi Ispanii baron Fedor Andreevich Budberg (1851–1916)" (The Russian Ambassador in Neutral Spain, Baron Fedor A. Budberg). *Novaia i noveishaia istoriia* 5 (2016): 193–206.

Mefodii, Archbishop. *O znamenii obnovleniia sviatykh ikon* (On the Omen of the Reawakening of Holy Icons) [1925]. Moscow: Palomnik, 1999.

Melikhov, Georgii V. *Belyi Kharbin. Seredina 20-kh* (White Harbin: The Mid-Twenties). Moscow: Russkii put', 2003.

– *Man'chzhuriia dalekaia i blizkaia* (Manchuria Far and Near). Moscow: Nauka, 1991.

– *Rossiiskaia emigratsiia v Kitae (1917–1924 gg.)* (The Russian Emigration in China, 1917–24). Moscow: Institut rossiiskoi istorii RAN, 1997.

– *Rossiiskaia emigratsiia v mezhdunarodnykh otnosheniiakh na Dal'nem Vostoke 1925–1932* (The Russian Emigration in International Relations in the Far East, 1925–32). Moscow: Russkii put', 2007.

– "Russkie dobrovol'tsy v armiiakh kitaiskikh militaristov" (Russian Volunteers in the Armies of Chinese Warlords), *Diaspora. Novye materialy* 6 (2004): 263–308.

Mémorandum du Comité des Représentants des Institutions Judiciaires à Harbin [signed P. Popov and Aleksandr A. Tereikovskii]. Peking: Imp. Na-Che Pao, 1921.

Meng Dongfeng. "Jilin shi faxian Song Xiaolian mu, bei" (The Tomb and Stele of Song Xiaolian Discovered in Jilin City). *Beifang wenwu* 3 (1986): 67.

Merritt, Steven E. "Matushka Rossiia, primi svoikh detei! [Mother Russia, Receive Your Children!]: Archival Materials on the Stalinist Repression of the Soviet Kharbintsy." *Rossiiane v Azii* 5 (1998): 205–29.

Mertelsmann, Olaf. "Tartu–Dorpat–Jur'ev." *Nordost-Archiv*, Neue Folge, vol. 15 (2006): 195–220.

Mervay, Mátyás. "Austro-Hungarian Refugee Soldiers in China." *Journal of Modern Chinese History* 12, no. 1 (2018): 45–62.

Meyer, Kathryn. "Garden of Grand Vision: Economic Life in a Flophouse Complex, Harbin, China 1940." *Crime, Law, and Social Change* 36, no. 3 (2001): 327–52.

Meyer, Michael. *In Manchuria: A Village Called Wasteland and the Transformation of Rural China*. London and New York: Bloomsbury Press, 2015.

Mitchell, Janet. *Spoils of Opportunity: An Autobiography*. London: Methuen, 1939.

Morrison, Alexander. "Russian Settler Colonialism." In *The Routledge Handbook of the History of Settler Colonialism*, ed. Edward Cavanagh and Lorenzo Veracini, 313–26. London and New York: Routledge, 2017.

Moustafine, Mara. *Secrets and Spies: The Harbin Files*. Milsons Point and London: Vintage, 2002.

Muraoka, Kumiko. "Mémoires d'une somnambule." *Revue des études slaves* 73, nos. 2–3 (2001): 387–401.

Must, Aadu. *Von Privilegierten zu Geächteten. Die Repressalien gegenüber deutschbaltischen Honoratioren während des Ersten Weltkrieges*, trans. Marju Mertelsmann and Olaf Mertelsmann. Tartu: University of Tartu Press, 2014.

Nachal'noe obrazovanie na Kitaiskoi Vostochnoi zheleznoi doroge (1898–1907 gg.) (Primary Education on the CER, 1898–1907). Harbin: Tipografiia KVZhD, 1907.

Naimark, Norman M. *Fires of Hatred: Ethnic Cleansing in Twentieth-Century Europe*. Cambridge, MA: Harvard University Press, 2001.

"Nauchnaia khronika/Scientific Chronicle." *Ezhegodnik Kluba Estestvoznaniia i Geografii KhSML/The Annual of the Club of Natural Science and Geography of the YMCA* (Harbin), vol. 1 (1934): 239–45.

Nazemtseva, Elena N. "Peredacha KVZhD v sobstvennost' SSSR. Patrioticheskaia initsiativa russkoi emigratsii ili lovushka sovetskoi diplomatii?" (The Transfer of the CER to Soviet Ownership: A Patriotic

Initiative of the Russian Emigration or a Trap of the Soviet Diplomacy?). In *Nansenovskie chteniia 2016*, ed. M.V. Petrova et al., 164–83. Saint Petersburg: Russkaia emigratsiia, 2018.

Neander, Eckhart, and Andrzej Sakson, eds. *Umgesidelt – Vertrieben. Deutschbalten und Polen 1939–1945 im Warthegau*. Marburg: Herder-Institut, 2010.

Nesterova, Elena I. "Kitaiskii torgovyi dom 'Shuankheshen' (Vladivostok–Kharbin, konets XIX – pervaia polovina XX v.)" (The Chinese Trade Company Shuanghesheng: Vladivostok–Harbin, End of the Nineteenth Century – First Half of the Twentieth Century). *Vestnik DVO RAN* 1 (2011): 36–45.

– "Kitaitsy na rossiiskom Dal'nem Vostoke: liudi i sud'by" (The Chinese in the Russian Far East: People and Destinies). *Diaspory* 2 (2003): 6–28.

Nestor, Bishop. *Man'chzhuriia–Kharbin* (Manchuria–Harbin). Belgrade: Tsarskii Vestnik, 1933.

Nezabytye mogily. Rossiiskoe zarubezh'e, nekrologi 1917–1999 (Unforgotten Tombs: Obituaries of the Russian Emigration), comp. V.N. Chuvakov. 6 vols. Moscow: Rossiiskaia gosudarstvennaia biblioteka, 1999–2007.

Ng, Rudolph. "The *Yuandongbao*: A Chinese or a Russian Newspaper?" In *Entangled Histories: The Transcultural Past of Northeast China*, ed. Dan Ben-Canaan et al., 101–18. Heidelberg: Springer, 2014.

Nikitin, Mstislav I. "Prazdnik pominoveniia umershikh Chzhun-iuan'-tsze" (The Festival of Remembering the Dead, Zhongyuan jie). *Luch Azii* 23 (July 1936): 4–5.

Nikitina, Klavdiia. "Osada Blagoveschenska kitaitsami v 1900 godu (iz vospominanii)" (A Memoir of the Siege of Blagoveschensk by the Chinese in 1900). *Istoricheskii vestnik* 122, no. 10 (October 1910): 207–24.

Nikolaev, Iurii M. *Nikita Ikonnik* (Nikita the Master of Icons). San Francisco: author's edition, 1968.

Nikolaeva, Natalia N. *Iapontsy* (The Japanese). Riga: author's edition, 2016.

Nilus, Evgenii Kh. *Istoricheskii obzor Kitaiskoi vostochnoi zheleznoi dorogi 1896–1923 gg.* (A Historical Survey of the Chinese Eastern Railway, 1896–1923), vol. 1. Harbin: Tipografiia Kit. Vost. zhel. dor. i T-va "Ozo," 1923.

North China Hong-List, with supplements: Harbin, Mukden, Newchwang, and Tsingtao. 1919. Tientsin: The N.C. Advertising Co., 1919.

Novikov, Aleksandr. "Oskolki russkogo Kharbina" (Splinters of Russian Harbin). *Bezhin lug* 4 (1995): 116–30.

Novikov, Nikolai K. "Al'chukaskoe fudutunstvo" (The Brigade-General's District of Alchuka). *Izvestiia Vostochnogo instituta*, vol. 5, bk 10 (1903–4): 1–100.

Oblastnik [Ivan I. Serebrennikov]. "Trekhrechenskaia golgofa" (The Golgotha of Trekhrech'e). *Vol'naia Sibir'* (Prague) 8 (1930): 71–84.

Obruchev, Vladimir A. *Ot Kiakhty do Kul'dzhi. Puteshestvie v Tsentral'nuiu Aziiu i Kitai* (From Kiakhta to Kul'dzha: An Expedition to Central Asia and China). Moscow: AN SSSR, 1940.

Obst, Hermann. "Reinhold Graf Anrep-Elmpts letzte Reise." *Das Ausland* 64, no. 22 (1 June 1891): 421–7; no. 24 (15 June 1891): 477–80; no. 25 (22 June 1891): 491–4.

Oglezneva, Elena A. "Dal'nevostochnyi regiolekt russkogo iazyka. Osobennosti formirovaniia" (The Far Eastern Regiolect of Russian: Particularities of Its Formation). *Russkii iazyk v nauchnom osveshchenii* 2 (2008): 119–36.

Olmert, Mordechai. *Darki bederekh harabim* (provided English title: My Way). Tel Aviv: Or-Am, 1981.

Oppenheim, Franz. Review of *Lungenpest-Epidemien in der Mandschurei*, by Dr Med. Roger Baron Budberg. *The China Medical Journal* 38, no. 11 (November 1924): 952–3.

Ossendowski, Ferdinand. *Man and Mystery in Asia.* London: Edward Arnold, 1924.

Ostrovskii, A.I. "Nekotorye dannye o kitaiskikh chastiakh v Armii Sovetskoi Latvii i Latyshskoi strelkovoi divizii (1919–1920 gg.)" (Some Data on Chinese Units in the Army of Soviet Latvia and the Latvian Riflemen Division, 1919–20). *Obshchestvo i gosudarstvo v Kitae* 16, no. 3 (1985): 207–9.

Ostrovskii, A.V., and M.M. Safonov. "15–17 oktiabria 1905 g. v tsarskoi rezidentsii (iz zapisok A. A. Budberga)" (15–17 October 1905 in the Tsar's Residence: From the Notes of A.A. Budberg). *Ezhegodnik, Sankt-Peterburgskoe nauchnoe obshchestvo istorikov i arkhivistov*, vol. 1 (1997): 391–412.

Overmyer, Daniel L. *Local Religion in North China in the Twentieth Century: The Structure and Organization of Community Rituals and Beliefs.* Leiden: Brill, 2009.

Paine, S.C.M. *Imperial Rivals: China, Russia, and Their Disputed Frontier.* Armonk: M.E. Sharpe, 1996.

Palladii, Archimandrite [signed P.K.]. "O Man'tszakh i koreitsakh" (On *Manzas* and Koreans). *Izvestiia Imperatorskogo Russkogo Geograficheskogo Obshchestva* 6, no. 1 (March 1870): 19–23.

– "Usuriiskie Man'tszy" (*Manzas* of the Ussuri). *Izvestiia Imperatorskogo Russkogo Geograficheskogo Obshchestva* 7, no. 8 (December 1871): 369–77.

Panov, Aleksandr A. "Zheltyi vopros v Priamur'e" (The Yellow Question in the Priamur). *Voprosy kolonizatsii* 7 (1910): 53–116.

Park, Alyssa M. *Sovereignty Experiments: Korean Migrants and the Building of Borders in Northeast Asia, 1860–1945.* Ithaca: Cornell University Press, 2019.

Pavlovskaia, Marina A. "Vostokovedenie na Iuridicheskom Fakul'tete Kharbina (1920–1937 gg.)" (Oriental Studies at the Harbin Faculty of Law, 1920–37). *Izvestiia Vostochnogo instituta* 6 (2001): 11–18.

– "Vostokovedenie v Institute Oriental'nykh i Kommercheskikh Nauk v
    Kharbine (1925–1941 gg.)" (Oriental Studies at the Harbin Institute of
    Oriental and Commercial Studies, 1925–41). In *Rossiiskaia emigratsiia na
    Dal'nem Vostoke* (Russian Emigration in the Far East), ed. Oleg I. Sergeev,
    80–90. Vladivostok: Dal'nauka, 2000.
Peckham, Robert, ed. *Empires of Panic: Epidemics and Colonial Anxieties.* Hong
    Kong: University of Hong Kong Press, 2015.
Peremilovskii, Vladimir V. "Russkaia shkola v Man'chzhurii" (The Russian
    School in Manchuria). *Russkaia shkola za rubezhom* 18 (1926): 601–17.
Pernikoff, Alexandre. *"Bushido": The Anatomy of Terror.* New York: Liveright,
    1943.
Personal der Kaiserlichen Universität zu Dorpat, nebst Beilage. 1889. Semester II.
    Dorpat: Schnakenburg's Buchdruckerei, 1889.
Petrov, Aleksandr I. *Istoriia kitaitsev v Rossii 1856–1917 gody* (A History of the
    Chinese in Russia, 1856–1917). Saint Petersburg: Beresta, 2003.
Petrov, Viktor P. *Gorod na Sungari* (The City on the Sungari). Washington,
    D.C.: Russo-American Historical Institute, 1984.
P'iankovich, Sofiia. "Svetloi pamiati Viacheslava Nikolaevicha P'iankovicha"
    (In Blessed Memory of V.N. P'iankovich). *Okkul'tizm i ioga*, vol. 9 (1937): 130–2.
P'iankovich, Viacheslav N. *Lektsii po okkul'tizmu. Polnyi, podgotovitel'nyi
    k izucheniiu arkanov kurs, chitannyi na mladshei stupeni ezotericheskogo
    kruzhka Kresta rozy v 1923–24 godu* (Lectures in Occultism: A Full Course,
    Preparatory for the Study of Arcana, Read in the Esoteric Circle of the Rose
    Cross, Junior Level, in 1923–24), 2nd rev. and exp. ed. Harbin: Sofiiskaia
    tipografiia, 1928.
Plath, Ulrike. *"Heimat*: Rethinking Baltic German Spaces of Belonging."
    *Kunstiteaduslikke Uurimusi/Studies on Art and Architecture/Studien für
    Kunstwissenschaft* 23, nos. 3–4 (2014): 55–78.
Pokrovskii, Nikolai N., et al., eds. *Dukhovnaia literatura staroverov vostoka
    Rossii XVIII–XX vv.* (Spiritual Literature of Old Believers in East Russia,
    Eighteenth to Twentieth Centuries). Novosibirsk: Sibirskii khronograf,
    1999.
Poletika, Mikhail I. *Obshchii meditsinskii otchet po postroike Kitaiskoi Vostochnoi
    Zheleznoi Dorogi* (A General Medical Report on the Construction of the
    Chinese Eastern Railway). Saint Petersburg: Tipografiia Slovo, 1904.
Polytechnic (Sydney). Jubilee issue 10 (1979).
Ponomareva, Liudmila V., ed. *Evraziia. Istoricheskie vzgliady russkikh emigrantov*
    (Eurasia: The Historical Views of Russian Émigrés). Moscow: Institut
    vseobshchei istorii RAN, 1992.
Pozdneev, Dmitrii M., ed. *Opisanie Man'chzhurii* (A Description of Manchuria).
    2 vols. Saint Petersburg: Izdanie Ministerstva Finansov, 1897.

Price, Willard. "Japan Faces Russia in Manchuria." *National Geographic Magazine* 82, no. 5 (November 1942): 603–34.

Prikashchikov, Nikolai N. "K istorii russkogo sadovodstva v Man'chzhurii" (Towards a History of Russian Gardening in Manchuria). *Zapiski Kharbinskogo Obshchestva Estestvoispytatelei i Etnografov* 6 (1947): 1–4.

Qi Xuejun. "Aihui de bianqian" (The Evolution of Aihui). *Heilongjiang shizhi tongxun* 4 (1984): 18–21.

Qingshi liezhuan (Collected Biographies of Qing History). 20 vols. Beijing: Zhonghua shuju, 1987.

Qu Qiubai. *Exiang jicheng* (A Journey to the Land of Hunger). [1922]. In *Qu Qiubai zuopin jingbian* (The Best of Qu Qiubai), 231–306. Guilin: Lijiang chubanshe, 2004.

Quested, Rosemary K.I. "A Fresh Look at the Sino-Russian Conflict of 1900 in Manchuria." *Journal of the Institute of Chinese Studies of the Chinese University of Hong Kong* 9, no. 2 (1978): 473–501.

– "Further Light on the Expansion of Russia in East Asia: 1792–1860." *Journal of Asian Studies* 29, no. 2 (February 1970): 327–45.

– "An Introduction to the Enigmatic Career of Chou Mien (1843?–1924?)." *Journal of Oriental Studies* 16, nos. 1–2 (1978): 39–48.

– *"Matey" Imperialists? The Tsarist Russians in Manchuria, 1895–1917.* Hong Kong: University of Hong Kong Press, 1982.

R.F. [Raisa Friesse]. "Vospominaniia iz zhizni na Amure" (Memoirs of Life on the Amur). *Russkaia starina* 129, no. 3 (March 1907): 557–68; 130, no. 4 (April 1907): 145–60; no. 5 (May 1907): 353–61; no. 6 (June 1907): 643–50.

Rachinskaia, Elizaveta N. *Kaleidoskop zhizni. Vospominaniia* (The Kaleidoscope of Life: Memoirs). Paris: YMCA-Press, 1990.

– *Pereletnye ptitsy* (Birds of Passage). San Francisco: Globus, 1982.

Räder, T.M.W., and E. Bettac, eds. *Album Curonorum.* Jurjew (Dorpat): n.p., 1903.

Räder, Wilhelm, ed. *Album Curonorum 1808–1932.* Riga: n.p., n.d. [1932].

Raninin, D. *V kitaiskikh kumirniakh gor. Ashikhe. Fotograficheskii al'bom s 32 snimkami* (In the Chinese Temples of Ashihe Town: A Photographic Album with 32 Images). Harbin: n.p., 1925.

Ransmeier, Johanna S. *Sold People: Traffickers and Family Life in North China.* Cambridge, MA: Harvard University Press, 2017.

Ratmanov, Pavel E. "Rossiiskie vrachi v Kitae" (Physicians from Russia in China). Database, sites.google.com/site/russemedecinsenchine.

– *Vklad rossiiskikh vrachei v meditsinu Kitaia (XX vek)* (The Contribution of Russian Physicians to China's Medicine in the Twentieth Century). PhD diss., State Research Institute of Public Health, Russian Academy of Medical Sciences, Moscow, 2010.

Reardon-Anderson, James. *Reluctant Pioneers: China's Expansion Northward, 1644–1937*. Stanford: Stanford University Press, 2005.

Recouly, Raymond. "En Mandchourie. Les populations de Mandchourie au cours de la dernière guerre." *Revue des deux mondes* 30 (November–December 1905): 207–18.

Remick, Elizabeth J. *Regulating Prostitution in China: Gender and Local Statebuilding, 1900–1937*. Stanford: Stanford University Press, 2014.

Remnev, Anatolii V., and Natal'ia Suvorova. "Russians as Colonists at the Empire's Asian Borders: Optimistic Prognoses and Pessimistic Assessments." In *Russia in Motion: Cultures of Human Mobility Since 1850*, ed. John Randolph and Eugene M. Avrutin, 126–49. Urbana: University of Illinois Press, 2012.

– "'Russkoe delo' na aziatskikh okrainakh. 'Russkost" pod ugrozoi ili 'somnitel'nye kul'turtregery'" ("The Russian Cause" in the Asian Periphery: "Russianness" in Danger, or "Dubious Kulturträger"). *Ab Imperio* 2 (2008): 157–220.

Rennenkampff, Lutz von. *Genealogie derer von Rennenkampff*. N.p.: author's edition, 2011.

Rennikov, A. (Andrei M. Selitrennikov). *V strane chudes. Pravda o pribaltiiskikh nemtsakh* (In Wonderland: The Truth about Baltic Germans). Petrograd: Novoe vremia, 1915.

Rerikh [Roerich], Nikolai K. *Sviashchennyi dozor* (The Holy Watch). Harbin: n.p., 1934.

Reznikova, Nataliia S. "V Russkom Kharbine" (In Russian Harbin). *Novyi zhurnal*, nos. 172–3 (September–December 1988): 385–94.

Rhoads, Edward J.M. *Manchus and Han: Ethnic Relations and Political Power in Late Qing and Early Republican China, 1861–1928*. Seattle: University of Washington Press, 2000.

Ristaino, Marcia Reynders. *Port of Last Resort: The Diaspora Communities of Shanghai*. Stanford: Stanford University Press, 2001.

Rogov, Vladimir N. *Antonin Sungurov, khudozhnik-kitaeved* (Antonin Sungurov, a Painter-Sinologist). Harbin: Tipografiia G. Sorokina, 1934.

Rosov, Vladimir A. "Kharbinskie pis'ma P.A. Chistiakova" (The Harbin Letters of Petr Chistiakov). *Vestnik Ariavarty* 1–2 (2005): 72–89.

– *Nikolai Rerikh. Vestnik Zvenigoroda* (Roerich the Herald of Zvenigorod). 2 vols. Moscow: Gosudarstvennyi Muzei Vostoka, 2005.

Ross, Rev. John. *The Boxers in Manchuria*. Shanghai: N.-C. Herald Office, 1901.

Rotshtein, Aleksandr. "Manchzhurskie ocherki. Lichnye nabliudeniia i zametki" (Manchurian Sketches: Personal Observations and Notes). *Vestnik Evropy* 42, no. 1 (1907): 71–93; no. 2: 475–509.

Runich, Sergei. "V Man'chzhurii" (In Manchuria). *Istoricheskii vestnik* 95, no. 2 (1904): 608–32; no. 3, 952–81; no. 4, 235–71.

"Russian Mobs Fight Chinese in Harbin." *New York Times*, 5 January 1932.

Rykunov, Dmitrii E. "Russkii kinematograf v Kharbine (1900–1945 gg.)" (Russian Cinema in Harbin, 1900–1945). *Izvestiia Vostochnogo instituta* 1 (2013): 51–9.

Sablin, Ivan. *Governing Post-Imperial Siberia and Mongolia, 1911–1924: Buddhism, Socialism, and Nationalism in State and Autonomy Building*. London and New York: Routledge, 2016.

Salogub, Iana L. "Stanovlenie smeshannykh sudov v polose otchuzhdeniia KVZhD (1896–1905)" (The Establishment of Mixed Courts in the CER Alienation Zone, 1896–1905). *Obshchestvo i gosudarstvo v Kitae* 46, no. 1 (2016): 647–51.

Salupere, Malle. *Tysiacheletnii Tartu. Gorod molodosti* (Millenary Tartu: The City of Youth), 2nd ed. Tartu: n.p., 2011.

Schlesinger, Jonathan. *A World Trimmed with Fur: Wild Things, Pristine Places, and the Natural Fringes of Qing Rule*. Stanford: Stanford University Press, 2016.

Schmidt, Jürgen W. "Die Beschaffung geheimer Informationen durch amtliche Einrichtungen des Deutschen Reiches in China, 1896–1917." *Berliner China-Hefte* 29 (2006): 102–21.

Seide, Gernot. "Die Russisch-Orthodoxe Kirche in China und in der Mandschurei seit dem Jahre 1918." *Ostkirchliche Studien* 25 (1976): 166–92.

Semigorov. "Ocherki Girinskoi provintsii" (Sketches of Jilin Province). *Russkii vestnik* 6 (1905): 390–440.

Serafim, Bishop. *Odigitriia Russkogo Zarubezh'ia. Povestvovanie o Kurskoi Chudotvornoi Ikone Znameniia Bozhiei Materi i o divnykh chudesakh ee* (Hodegetria of the Russian Emigration: The Story of the Thaumaturgic Icon of Our Lady of the Sign and Her Marvellous Miracles), 2nd rev. ed. Mahopac: Izdanie Novoi Korennoi Pustyni, 1963.

Serebrennikov, Ivan I. *Ocherk ekonomicheskoi geografii Kitaia* (Survey of the Economical Geography of China). *Vestnik Azii* 53 (1925): 1–113.

Setnitskii, Nikolai A. "Russkie mysliteli o Kitae (V. S. Solov'ev i N. F. Fedorov)" (Russian Thinkers on China: V. S. Solov'ev and N.F. Fedorov), *Izvestiia Iuridicheskogo Fakul'teta* (Harbin) 3 (1926): 191–229.

Severnyi, Pavel. *Farforovyi kitaets kachaet golovoi* (A Porcelain Chinaman Nods His Head). Shanghai: Slovo, 1937.

– *Ozero goluboi tsapli* (Blue Heron Lake). Shanghai: Slovo, 1938.

– *Shumit taiga Man'chzhurii* (The Manchurian Taiga Rustles). Moscow: Detgiz, 1960.

Shan, Patrick Fuliang. *Taming China's Wilderness: Immigration, Settlement, and the Shaping of the Heilongjiang Frontier*. Farnham and Burlington: Ashgate, 2014.

Shao Dan. *Remote Homeland, Recovered Borderland: Manchus, Manchoukuo, and Manchuria, 1907–1985*. Honolulu: University of Hawai'i Press, 2011.

Shapiro, Maria L. "Kharbin, 1945" [1956]. *Pamiat'. Istoricheskii sbornik* 1 (1978): 3–92.

– "Zhenskii kontslager'. sud'ba emigrantki" (A Women's Concentration Camp: The Destiny of an Émigré Woman) [1956–58]. *Novyi zhurnal* 150 (March 1983): 225–48; 151 (June 1983): 116–37.

Shavkunov, Ernst V. "Antropomorfnye podvesnye figurki iz bronzy i kul't predkov u chzhurchzhenei" (Anthropomorphic Pendant Figurines of Bronze and the Jurchen Cult of Ancestors). *Sovetskaia etnografiia* 4 (July–August 1975): 110–20.

[Shchelkov, Aleksei A.]. *Kratkii ocherk vozniknoveniia i deiatel'nosti Russko-Kitaiskogo Tekhnikuma v techenie 1920/21 uchebnogo goda i ego zadachi v budushchem* (Brief Sketch of the Foundation and Activity of the Russian-Chinese Technical College in the Academic Year 1920–21 and Its Future Tasks). Harbin: Tipografiia KVZhD, 1921.

Shchelkov, Aleksei A. "Russko-Kitaiskii Politekhnicheskii Institut k nachalu 1925 goda. Gor. Kharbin" (The Russian-Chinese Polytechnic Institute by the Start of 1925, City of Harbin). *Izvestiia Iuridicheskogo Fakul'teta*, no. 1 (1925): 242–8.

Shi Fang and Gao Ling. *Chuantong yu biange. Ha'erbin jindai shehui wenming zhuanxing yanjiu* (Tradition and Change: A Study of the Cultural Evolution of Harbin's Modern Society). Harbin: Heilongjiang renmin chubanshe, 1995.

Shi Fang, Gao Ling, and Liu Shuang. *Ha'erbin Eqiao shi* (The History of Russian Émigrés in Harbin), 2nd ed. Harbin: Heilongjiang renmin chubanshe, 2003.

Shiliaev, Evgenii P. "Obshchestvenno-kul'turnaia, religioznaia i politicheskaia zhizn' Kharbina" (The Social, Cultural, Religious, and Political Life of Harbin). *Transactions of the Association of Russian-American Scholars in the USA* 26 (1994): 211–39.

Shilov, Denis N. *Gosudarstvennye deiateli Rossiiskoi imperii. Glavy vysshikh i tsentral'nykh uchrezhdenii, 1802–1917. Biobibliograficheskii spravochnik* (Statesmen of the Russian Empire, 1802–1917: Heads of Highest and Central Institutions: A Bio-bibliographical Reference Book), 2nd rev. ed. Saint Petersburg: Dmitrii Bulanin, 2002.

Shilov, Denis N., and Iurii A. Kuz'min. *Chleny Gosudarstvennogo soveta Rossiiskoi imperii, 1801–1906. Biobibliograficheskii spravochnik* (Members of the State Council of the Russian Empire, 1801–1906: A Bio-bibliographical Reference Book). Saint Petersburg: Dmitrii Bulanin, 2006.

Shirokogoroff, Sergei M. *Social Organization of the Manchus: A Study of the Manchu Clan Organization*. Shanghai: Royal Asiatic Society, 1924.

Shkurkin, Pavel V. "Dvoinoe poddanstvo" (Double Nationality). *Vestnik Azii* 38–9 (1916): 1–9.

– *Khunkhuzy. Rasskazy iz kitaiskogo byta* (Honghuzi: Stories from Chinese Daily Life). Harbin: Tipo-litografiia t-va "OZO," 1924.

– "Kitai i Dal'nevostochnye perspektivy" (China and Far Eastern Perspectives).
  Russkoe obozrenie (Peking): 1–2 (January–February 1921): 34–50.
Shteinfel'd, Nikolai P. *Russkoe delo v Man'chzhurii s XVII veka do nashikh dnei*
  (The Russian Cause in Manchuria from the Seventeenth Century to Our
  Day). Harbin: Yuandong bao, 1910.
Shul'man, Iakov M. *Goroda i liudi evreiskoi diaspory v Vostochnoi Evrope do
  nachala XX veka. Litva. Panevežys, Kaseiniai, Ukmergė, Švenčionys, Šiauliai
  i Žagarė* (Towns and People of the Jewish Diaspora in Eastern Europe
  before the Beginning of the Twentieth Century: Lithuania). Moscow:
  Paralleli, 2005.
Sibiriakov, N.S. [Nikolai I. Bogomiagkov]. "Konets zabaikal'skogo kazach'ego
  voiska" (The End of the Transbaikal Cossack Host). *Minuvshee. Istoricheskii
  al'manakh* 1 (1990): 193–254.
Silin, Evgenii P. *Kiakhta v XVIII veke. Iz istorii russko-kitaiskoi torgovli* (Kiakhta
  in the Eighteenth Century: From the History of Russian-Chinese Trade).
  Irkutsk: Irkutskoe oblastnoe iz-vo, 1947.
Simpich, Frederick. "Manchuria, Promised Land of Asia." *National Geographic
  Magazine* 56, no. 4 (October 1929): 379–428.
Sisson, Edgar. *One Hundred Red Days: A Personal Chronicle of the Bolshevik
  Revolution.* New Haven: Yale University Press, 1931.
Smirnov, Evgenii T. *Priamurskii krai na Amursko-Primorskoi vystavke 1899 v gor.
  Khabarovske* (The Priamur District at the 1899 Amur-Maritime Exhibition in
  Khabarovsk). Khabarovsk: Tipografiia Kantseliarii Priamurskogo General-
  Gubernatora, 1899.
Smirnov, Sergei V. "Avgust 1945 g. v Severnoi Man'chzhurii. Vooruzhennaia
  bor'ba russkikh emigrantov protiv iapontsev" (August 1945 in Northern
  Manchuria: The Armed Struggle of Russian Émigrés against the Japanese).
  Rossiia i ATR 3 (2015): 82–90.
– *Rossiiskie emigranty v Severnoi Man'chzhurii v 1920–1945 gg. (problema
  sotsial'noi adaptatsii)* (Russian Émigrés in Northern Manchuria in
  1920–45: The Problem of Social Adaptation). Ekaterinburg: Ural'skii gos.
  pedagogicheskii universitet, 2007.
Smirnov, Sergei V., and Aleksei M. Buiakov. *Otriad Asano. Russkie emigranty
  v vooruzhennykh formirovaniiakh Man'chzhou-go (1938–1945)* (The Asano
  Detachment in the Armed Units of Manchukuo, 1938–45). Moscow:
  Algoritm, 2016.
Smith, Norman. *Intoxicating Manchuria: Alcohol, Opium, and Culture in China's
  Northeast.* Vancouver: UBC Press, 2012.
Smith, Steve. "Fear and Rumour in the People's Republic of China in the
  1950s." *Cultural and Social History* 5, no. 3 (September 2008): 269–88.
Sokolova, A. "Vospominaniia o pogrome v Manchzhurii po linii Vostochnoi
  Kitaiskoi Zheleznoi Dorogi v 1898 godu" (Memoirs of a Pogrom in

Manchuria along the Chinese Eastern Railway line in 1898). *Istoricheskii vestnik* 106, no. 10 (1906): 81–106; no. 11: 424–46; no. 12: 810–28.

Sokolovskii, Pavel E. *Russkaia shkola v Vostochnoi Sibiri i Priamurskom Krae* (The Russian School in Eastern Siberia and the Priamur District). Kharkov: Tipografiia i litografiia M. Zil'berberg, 1914.

Song Hongyan. *Dongfang xiao Bali* (provided English title: The Oriental Paris). Harbin: Heilongjiang kexue jishu chubanshe, 2001.

Song Xiaolian. *Song Xiaolian ji* (Collected Works), ed. Meng Bingshu et al. Changchun: Jilin wenshi chubanshe, 1989.

Sonin [Lev G. Deich]. "Bombardirovka Blagoveshchenska kitaitsami. Rasskaz ochevidtsa" (An Eye-witness Account of the Shelling of Blagoveshchensk by the Chinese). Offprint from *Zaria* (Stuttgart): 4 (1902).

Sorokina, M. "Moi KhPI" (My Harbin Polytechnic Institute). *Golos Rodiny* 22 (May 1990), reprinted in *Bulletin Igud Yotsei Sin* 37, no. 314 (November 1990): 28.

Sorokina, Marina Iu. *Rossiiskoe nauchnoe zarubezh'e. Materialy dlia biobibliograficheskogo slovaria* (Russian Science in the Emigration: Materials for a Bio-bibliographical Dictionary), pilot issue 3, *Vostokovedenie. XIX– pervaia polovina XX v.* (Oriental Studies in the Nineteenth–First Half of the Twentieth Century). Moscow: Dom Russkogo Zarubezh'ia im. A. Solzhenitsyna, 2010.

Sorokina, Tat'iana N. "'The Blagoveshchensk Panic' of the Year 1900: The Version of the Authorities." *Sensus Historiae* 8, no. 3 (2012): 91–114.

– "Kitaiskaia immigratsiia na Dal'nii Vostok Rossii v kontse XIX – nachale XX vv." (Chinese Immigration to the Russian Far East in the Late Nineteenth– Early Twentieth Century). *Istoricheskii ezhegodnik* 3 (1998): 13–23.

– "Liquor and Opium: Joint Efforts to Control Contraband Along the Russia– China Border at the Beginning of the Twentieth Century." *Inner Asia* 16, no. 1 (August 2014): 139–51.

Spravochnaia knizhka Kharbina (A Harbin Guidebook). Harbin: Izdanie KVZhD, 1904.

Stackelberg, Reinhold von. "Heinrich Reinhold von Anrep. Ein Lebensbild." *Baltische Monatsschrift* 57 (1904): 19–27.

Starikov, Vladimir S. *Po taezhnym tropam* (Through the Taiga Paths). Leningrad: author's heirs, 1991.

Starosel'skaia, Natal'ia D. *Povsevdnevnaia zhizn' 'russkogo' Kitaia* (The Everyday Life of "Russian" China). Moscow: Molodaia gvardiia, 2006.

Startsev, Vitalii I. *Nemetskie den'gi i russkaia revoliutsiia. Nenapisannyi roman Ferdinanda Ossendovskogo* (German Money and the Russian Revolution: The Unwritten Novel by Ferdynand Ossendowski), 3rd ed. Saint Petersburg: Izdatel'stvo Kriga, 2006.

Stasiukevich, Svetlana M. "Russko-kitaiskoe vzaimodeistvie i agrarnoe razvitie Dal'nego Vostoka v pervoi treti XX veka" (Russian-Chinese Interaction and Agricultural Development of the Far East in the First Third of the Twentieth Century). *Rossiia i Kitai. Istoriia i perspektivy sotrudnichestva* 4 (2014): 116–20.

Stasulane, Anita. "Centre of Theosophy in the Baltic Region – Riga." In *Capitales de l'ésotérisme européen et dialogue des cultures*, ed. Jean-Pierre Brach et al., 133–47. Paris: Orizons, 2014.

Stepanov, Aleksandr N. *Port-Artur.* Moscow: OGIZ, 1944.

Stephan, John J. *The Russian Far East: A History.* Stanford: Stanford University Press, 1994.

Stern, Dieter. "Russische Pidgins." *Die Welt der Slaven* 47, no. 1 (January 2002): 1–30.

Stern, Hellmut. *Saitensprünge. Erinnerungen eines Kosmopoliten wider Willen,* 3rd ed. Berlin: Aufbau Taschenbuch Verlag, 2002.

Stockhorner von Starein, Otto, Freiherrn. *Die Stockhorner von Starein. Versuch der Darstellung.* Vienna: Verlag von Carl Konegen, 1896.

Stolberg, Eva-Maria. *Stalin und die chinesischen Kommunisten 1945–1953. Eine Studie zur Entstehungsgeschichte der sowjetisch-chinesischen Allianz vor dem Hintergrund des Kalten Krieges.* Wiesbaden: Franz Steiner Verlag, 1997.

Sun Rongtu, ed. *Aihui xianzhi* (Gazetteer of Aihui County) [1920]. 2 vols. Taipei: Chengwen chubanshe, 1974.

Sunderland, Willard. *The Baron's Cloak: A History of the Russian Empire in War and Revolution.* Ithaca: Cornell University Press, 2014.

– "The 'Colonization Question': Visions of Colonization in Late Imperial Russia." *Jahrbücher für Geschichte Osteuropas* 48, no. 2 (2000): 210–32.

– "Peasant Pioneering: Russian Peasant Settlers Describe Colonization and the Eastern Frontier, 1880s–1910s." *Journal of Social History* 34, no. 4 (2001): 895–922.

Sutton, Major-General F. A. *One-Arm Sutton.* New York: The Viking Press, 1933.

Swope, Kenneth M. *The Military Collapse of China's Ming Dynasty, 1618–44.* London and New York: Routledge, 2014.

Sze, Sao-ke Alfred. *Reminiscences of His Early Years, as Told to Anming Fu,* trans. Amy C. Wu. Washington, D.C.: n.p., 1962.

Tamanoi, Mariko Asano. "Knowledge, Power, and Racial Classifications: The 'Japanese' in 'Manchuria.'" *Journal of Asian Studies* 59, no. 2 (May 2000): 248–76.

– *Memory Maps: The State and Manchuria in Postwar Japan.* Honolulu: University of Hawai'i Press, 2008.

Taskina, Elena P. *Neizvestnyi Kharbin* (Unknown Harbin). Moscow: Prometei, 1994.

– *Russkie v Man'chzhurii* (Russians in Manchuria). Moscow: MBA, 2012.

– , ed. *Russkii Kharbin* (Russian Harbin), 2nd rev. and enlarged ed. Moscow: MGU, 2005.

– "Sinologi i kraevedy Kharbina" (Harbin's Sinologists and Researchers of Local Lore). *Problemy Dal'nego Vostoka* 2 (1997): 124–9.

– "Staryi Kitai na polotnakh russkikh khudozhnikov (1920–40-e gody)" (Old Harbin on the Canvasses of Russian Painters, 1920s to 1940s). *Problemy Dal'nego Vostoka* 2 (1996): 93–9.

Taskina, Elena P., and D.G. Sel'kina, eds. *Kharbin. Vetka russkogo dereva* (Harbin: A Branch of the Russian Tree). Novosibirsk: Novosibirskoe knizhnoe iz-vo, 1991.

Teng, Emma Jinhua, *Eurasian: Mixed Identities in the United States, China, and Hong Kong, 1842–1943*. Berkeley: University of California Press, 2013.

Ter Haar, Barend. *Practicing Scripture: A Lay Buddhist Movement in Late Imperial China*. Honolulu: University of Hawai'i Press, 2014.

Thomas, Keith. "History and Anthropology." *Past and Present* 24 (April 1963): 3–24.

Thompson, Laurence G. *Chinese Religion: An Introduction*, 4th ed. Belmont: Wadsworth, 1989.

Tian, Xiaoli. "Rumor and Secret Space: Organ-Snatching Tales and Medical Missions in Nineteenth-Century China." *Modern China* 41, no. 2 (2015): 197–236.

Tikhonov, A.N. *Konnozavodstvo Severnoi Man'chzhurii i ego rol' v voprose uluchsheniia mestnogo konevodstva* (The Horse Breeding of North Manchuria and Its Role in the Issue of Improving Local Horse Raising). Harbin: Tipografiia KVZhD, 1928.

Todenwarth, Frieherr [Paul] von. *Eine tolle Flucht*. Leipzig: K.F. Koehler Verlag, 1935.

Tolmachev, Vladimir Ia. "Drevnosti Man'chzhurii. Razvaliny Bei-chena" (Antiquities of Manchuria: The Ruins of Baicheng). Offprint from *Vestnik Man'chzhurii* 1–2 (1925).

– "Ostatki [sic] mamontov v Man'chzhurii" (The Remains of Mammoths in Manchuria). *Izvestiia Obshchestva Izucheniia Man'chzhurskogo Kraia* 6 (March 1926): 51–5.

Tong Yue. *Guandong jiu fengsu* (Old Customs East of the Pass). Shenyang: Liaoning daxue chubanshe, 2001.

Torgashev, Pavel I. *Avantiury na Dal'nem Vostoke. Iz-za chego my voevali s Iaponiei* (Shady Ventures in the Far East: Why We Fought against Japan). Moscow: Tip. F. Ia. Burche, 1907.

Tytgat, Charles. *Un reportage en Chine. Le tour du monde par le Transsibérien*. Brussels: Imprimerie Polleunis & Ceuterick, 1901.

Ular, Alexander. "Im Brackwasser der Kulturen." *Die Neue Rundschau* 15, no. 2 (October 1904): 1212–35.

V. [Nikolai P. Vishniakov]. "Blagoveshchenskaia 'utopiia'" (The Noyade in Blagoveshchensk). *Vestnik Evropy* 45, no. 7 (July 1910): 231–41.

Vasilenko, Nadezhda A. "Shkol'noe obrazovanie v polose otchuzhdeniia KVZhD (konets XIX v.–nachalo 30-kh godov XX v.)" (School Education in the CER Alienation Zone, Late Nineteenth Century–Early 1930s). In *Rossiiskaia emigratsiia na Dal'nem Vostoke* (Russian Emigration in the Far East), ed. Oleg I. Sergeev, 90–9. Vladivostok: Dal'nauka, 2000.

Vasil'chikov, Prince Boris A. *Vospominaniia* (Memoirs). Moscow and Pskov: Nashe nasledie, 2003.

Vassiliev, Alexandre. *Beauty in Exile: The Artists, Models, and Nobility Who Fled the Russian Revolution and Influenced the World of Fashion*, trans. Antonina W. Bouis and Anya Kucharev. New York: Harry N. Abrams, 2000.

Vengerov, Vladimir. *Reka Kharbinskikh vremen* (The River of Harbin Times). Sydney: Kharbinskoe i Man'chzhurskoe Istoricheskoe Obshchestvo, 1998.

Veresaev, Vikentii V. *Zapiski vracha. Na iaponskoi voine* (A Doctor's Notes, and In the Japanese War). Moscow: Pravda, 1986.

Vereshchagin, Aleksandr V. *Po Manchzhurii 1900–1901 gg. Vospominaniia i rasskazy* (Through Manchuria: Memoirs and Stories). *Vestnik Evropy* 37, no. 1 (1902): 103–48; no. 2: 573–627; no. 3: 130–73.

Vertinskii, Aleksandr N. *Chetvert' veka bez rodiny. Stranitsy minuvshego* (Quarter of a Century without the Motherland: Leaves of Years Past). Kiev: Muzychna Ukraina, 1989.

Ves' Kharbin na 1925 god. Adresnaia i spravochnaia kniga Gor. Kharbina (A Harbin City Phonebook and Yellow Pages for 1925), ed. S.T. Ternavskii. Harbin: Tipografiia KVZhD, 1925.

Ves' Kharbin na 1926 god. Adresnaia i spravochnaia kniga, ed. S.T. Ternavskii. Harbin: Tipografiia KVZhD, 1926.

Vespa, Amleto. *Secret Agent of Japan: A Handbook to Japanese Imperialism*. London: Victor Gollancz, 1938.

Vinkou (Likhomanova), Dina. "Vospominaniia o pitanii v period moego kharbinskogo detstva" (Memories about Nutrition during my Harbin Childhood). *Bulletin Igud Yotsei Sin* 57, no. 401 (April–May 2010): 28–32.

Vitalisov, V.M. "Rol' russkikh v razvitii sadovodstva i ovoshchevodstva v Man'chzhurii" (The Role of Russians in the Development of Horticulture and Vegetable Cultivation in Manchuria). *Zapiski Kharbinskogo Obshchestva Estestvoispytatelei i Etnografov* 6 (1947): 17–18.

Volkov, Sergei V. *Ofitsery armeiskoi kavalerii. Opyt martirologa* (Draft Martyrology of Officers of the Military Cavalry). Moscow: Russkii put', 2004.

– *Ofitsery rossiiskoi gvardii. Opyt martirologa* (Draft Martyrology of Officers of the Russian Imperial Guard). Moscow: Russkii put', 2002.

Volkov, Sergei V., ed. *Belaia bor'ba na Severo-Zapade Rossii* (The White Struggle in the Russian Northwest). Moscow: Tsentrpoligraf, 2003.

Volkov, Shulamit. "Antisemitism as a Cultural Code: Reflections on the History and Historiography of Antisemitism in Imperial Germany." *The Leo Baeck Institute Year Book* 23, no. 1 (January 1978): 25–46.

Vortisch-van Vloten, Hermann. *Chinesische Patienten und ihre Ärzte. Erlebnisse eines deutschen Arztes.* Gütersloh: Druck und Verlag von C. Bertelsmann, 1914.

– "Vom gewesenen Zopf." *Der Ostasiatische Lloyd* 22, no. 43 (25 October 1912): 385–6.

Waley-Cohen, Joanna. *Exile in Mid-Qing China: Banishment to Xinjiang, 1758–1820.* New Haven: Yale University Press, 1991.

Wang Fengrui. *Wang Fengrui xiansheng fangwen jilu* (Interview with Wang Fengrui; recorded by Shen Yunlong in 1965). Taipei: Institute of Modern History, 1985.

Wang, Gary. "Affecting Grandiosity: Manchuness and the *Liangbatou* Hairdo-Turned-Headpiece circa 1870s–1930s." In *Fashion, Identity, and Power in Modern Asia*, ed. Kyunghee Pyun and Aida Yuen Wong, 169–92. New York: Palgrave Macmillan, 2018.

Wang Jingfu. *Ha'erbin bingxue wenhua fazhan shi* (The Development History of Harbin's Ice and Snow Culture). Harbin: Heilongjiang renmin chubanshe, 2005.

Wang Peiyue. "Kuayue liang ge lishi shiqi de Heilongjiang sheng xingzheng zhangguan – Song Xiaolian" (Song Xiaolian: Senior Official of Heilongjiang Who Transcended Two Historical Periods). *Heilongjiang shizhi* 5 (1986): 23.

Wang Yulang and Wang Tianzi. "Ha'erbin chengshi jiyuan de zai yanjiu" (A Reconsideration of the Beginnings of Harbin History). *Ha'erbin xueyuan xuebao* 37, no. 1 (January 2016): 1–14; no. 2 (February 2016): 1–13.

Watt, Lori. *When Empire Comes Home: Repatriation and Reintegration in Postwar Japan.* Cambridge, MA: Harvard University Press, 2010.

Weeks, Theodore R. "Population Politics in Vilnius 1944–1947: A Case Study of Socialist-Sponsored Ethnic Cleansing." *Post-Soviet Affairs* 23, no. 1 (2007): 76–95.

Weitz, Eric D. "From the Vienna to the Paris System: International Politics and the Entangled Histories of Human Rights, Forced Deportations, and Civilizing Missions." *American Historical Review* 113, no. 5 (December 2008): 1313–43.

Wen Peiyun. *Lingluji. Wen Peiyun sanshi niandai yiwen xuan* (Scattered Dew: A Selection from Wen Peiyun's Translations of the 1930s). Changchun: Jilin renmin chubanshe, 1984.

Weulersse, Georges. "Au Petchili et sur les frontières de Mandchourie." *Le Tour du monde* 7, no. 9 (2 March 1901): 97–108; no. 10 (9 September 1901): 109–20; no. 11 (16 March 1901): 121–32.

Williams, Robert C. *Russian Art and American Money, 1900–1940.* Cambridge, MA: Harvard University Press, 1980.

Winning, Alexa von. "The Empire as Family Affair: The Mansurovs
and Noble Participation in Imperial Russia, 1850–1917." *Geschichte und
Gesellschaft* 40, no. 1 (2014): 94–116.

Wlad, Franz. *Meine Flucht durchs mongolische Sandmeer.* Berlin and Vienna:
Verlag Ullstein & Co, 1918.

Wolf, Arthur P. "Gods, Ghosts, and Ancestors." In *Religion and Ritual in
Chinese Society,* ed. Wolf, 131–82. Stanford: Stanford University Press, 1974.

Wolff, David. "Returning from Harbin: Northeast Asia, 1945." In *Voices from
the Shifting Russo-Japanese Border: Karafuto/Sakhalin,* ed. Svetlana Paichadze
and Philip A. Seaton, 92–102. Abingdon and New York: Routledge, Taylor &
Francis, 2015.

– *To the Harbin Station: The Liberal Alternative in Russian Manchuria, 1898–1914.*
Stanford: Stanford University Press, 1999.

Wrangel (Vrangel'), Baron Petr. "Manchzhurskie pis'ma. Iz epokhi voiny s
Iaponieiu" (Manchurian Letters: From the Period of the War with Japan).
Vestnik Evropy 43, no. 6 (1908): 377–94.

Wright, Tim. "Legitimacy and Disaster: Responses to the 1932 Floods in
Northern Manchuria." *Modern China* 43, no. 2 (2017): 186–216.

Wu Baixiang. "Wushi nian zishu" (Autobiography at Fifty [1929]). In *Wu
Baixiang yu Tongji* (Wu Baixiang and Tongji), collectively edited, 1–60.
Harbin: Heilongjiang renmin chubanshe, 1989.

Xia Chongwei. "Aihui xuehuo" (The Blood and Fire of Aihui). *Heihe xuekan* 6
(1999): 70–5; 1 (2000): 62–7.

Xiao Hong. *The Field of Life and Death and Tales of Hulan River,* trans. Howard
Goldblatt. Boston: Cheng and Tsui, 2002.

– *Market Street: A Chinese Woman in Harbin,* trans. Howard Goldblatt, 2nd ed.
Seattle: University of Washington Press, 2015.

– *Shangshi jie* (Market Street). Beijing: Beijing guangbo xueyuan chubanshe,
1993.

– "Sleepless Night," trans. Amy D. Dooling and Kristina M. Torgeson. In
*Writing Women in Modern China: An Anthology of Women's Literature from
the Early Twentieth Century,* ed. Dooling and Torgeson, 363–6. New York:
Columbia University Press, 1998.

– *Xiao Hong xuanji* (Selected Works). Beijing: Renmin wenxue chubanshe, 1981.

Xin Peilin. "Ma Zhongjun xiansheng shilüe" (Short Biographical Account of
Ma Zhongjun). *Ha'erbin wenshi ziliao* 6 (1985): 1–22.

Xue Lianju. *Ha'erbin renkou bianqian* (Harbin Population Changes). Harbin:
Heilongjiang renmin chubanshe, 1998.

Yakobson, Helen. *Crossing Borders: From Revolutionary Russia to China to
America.* Tenafly: Hermitage, 1994.

Yang Aili. *Sun Yunxuan zhuan* (Biography of Sun Yunxuan). Taipei: Tianxia
zazhi, 1989.

Yang, Belle. *The Odyssey of a Manchurian*. New York: Harcourt Brace, 1996.

Yao, Betty, ed. *China: Through the Lens of John Thomson 1868–1872*, rev. ed. Bangkok: River Books, 2015.

Young, Walter C. "Chinese Immigration and Colonization in Manchuria." In *Pioneer Settlement: Coöperative Studies by Twenty-Six Authors*, ed. W.L.G. Joerg, 330–59. New York: American Geographical Society special publication No. 14, 1932.

"The Young Men's Christian Association/Khristianskii Soiuz Molodykh Liudei v Kharbine." *Ezhegodnik Kluba Estestvoznaniia i Geografii KhSML/The Annual of the Club of Natural Science and Geography of the YMCA* 1 (1934): 253–4.

Yu Guanchao. "20 shiji shangbanye Ha'erbin Eqiao de Xihua chuanbo yu yingxiang" (The Dissemination and Influence of Western Art by Russian Émigrés in Harbin in the First Half of the 20th Century). *Meishu* 8 (2014): 107–10.

Zatsepine, Victor. *Beyond the Amur: Frontier Encounters between China and Russia, 1850–1930*. Vancouver: UBC Press, 2017.

– "The Blagoveshchensk Massacre of 1900: The Sino-Russian War and Global Imperialism." In *Beyond Suffering: Recounting War in Modern China*, ed. James Flath and Norman Smith, 107–29. Vancouver: UBC Press, 2011.

Zdanskii, Konstantin [Konstanty Zdański]. *Grust'* (Sadness). Privately produced e-file, after 2007.

Zeng Yizhi. *Cheng yu ren. Ha'erbin gushi* (provided English title: The City and the People: The Stories of Harbin). Harbin: Heilongjiang renmin chubanshe, 2003.

Zhang Fushan and Zhou Shuzhen. *Ha'erbin geming jiudi shihua* (provided English title: History of the Sites of Harbin Revolution). Harbin: Heilongjiang renmin chubanshe, 2001.

Zhang Jiangcai. *Dongguan Yuan dushi houyi kao* (A Study of the Descendants of Supervisor Yuan from Dongguan). In *Jing-Jin fengtu congshu* (Conditions and Customs of Beijing and Tianjin; 1938), ed. Zhang Jiangcai, 215–74. Taipei: Jinxue shuju, 1969.

Zhang Tiejiang and Zhao Liantai. "Ha'erbin youtai ren mudi kaocha yanjiu" (Investigation of the Jewish Cemetery in Harbin). *Heilongjiang shehui kexue* 1 (2002): 54–7.

Zhao Luchen. "Ha'erbin Zhong-E bianyuanyu xiaowang tanyin" (An Exploration of Causes for the Dying Out of the Sino-Russian Border Language in Harbin). *Ha'erbin Shangye daxue xuebao (shehui kexue ban)* 4 (2004): 123–4.

Zhao Zhongfu [Chao Chung-fu]."Qingdai dongsansheng beibu de kaifa yu Hanhua" (The Opening and Sinicization of Northern Manchuria in the Qing). *Zhongyang yanjiu yuan jindai shi yanjiusuo jikan* 15, no. 2 (1986): 1–16.

– *Qingji Zhong-E dongsansheng jiewu jiaoshe* (Late Qing Chinese-Russian Negotiations over the Manchurian Border Issue), 2nd ed. Taipei: Institute of Modern History, Academic Sinica, 1998.

– "The Role of the Government in Inter-Regional Migration and Agricultural Development: A Case Study of Manchuria, 1668–1911." *Zhongyang yanjiuyuan jindai shi yanjiusuo jikan* 8 (1979): 217–33.

Zhelokhovtsev, Aleksei N. "Seriia literatury russkikh emigrantov v Kitae. V 5 tomakh" (A Series of Russian Émigré Literature in China in 5 Volumes). *Problemy Dal'nego Vostoka* 6 (2003): 172–5.

Zhernakov, Vladimir N. "Reka Sungari v zhizni Kharbina" (The River Sungari in Harbin Life). *Kharbinskie kommercheskie uchilishcha Kit. vost. zhel. dor.* (San Francisco) 12 (1974): 50–5.

Zhong-E guanxi shiliao, Dongbei bianfang. Zhonghua minguo 6 nian zhi 8 nian (Historical Materials on Chinese-Russian Relations: Northeast Border Defence, 1917–19), ed. Deng Ruyuan et al. 2 vols. Taipei: Zhongyang yanjiuyuan jindaishi yanjiusuo, 1960.

Zhu Ziqing. "Xixing tongxun" (Letters from a Travel to the West). In *Zhu Ziqing quanji* (Complete Works), vol. 1, 365–73. Nanjing: Jiangsu jiaoyu chubanshe, 1988–97.

Zolotareva, Tat'iana I. *Man'chzhurskie byli* (Manchurian Tales), ed. Nikolai Zaika. Sydney: Kharbinskoe i Man'chzhurskoe Istoricheskoe Obshchestvo, 2000.

Zylewicz, Tat'iana V. *V pamiat' ob usopshikh v zemle man'chzhurskoi i kharbintsakh* (provided English title: In Memory of Deceased in Harbin, Manchuria). Melbourne: author's edition, 2000.

Index